Community Mental Health and Well-Being in the New Normal

Remya Lathabhavan
Indian Institute of Management, Bodh Gaya, India

Prabir Chandra Padhy
VIT Business School, Vellore Institute of Technology, Vellore, India

A volume in the Advances in Psychology, Mental Health, and Behavioral Studies (APMHBS) Book Series

IGI Global
PUBLISHER of TIMELY KNOWLEDGE

Published in the United States of America by
IGI Global
Information Science Reference (an imprint of IGI Global)
701 E. Chocolate Avenue
Hershey PA, USA 17033
Tel: 717-533-8845
Fax: 717-533-8661
E-mail: cust@igi-global.com
Web site: http://www.igi-global.com

Library of Congress Cataloging-in-Publication Data

Names: Lathabhavan, Remya, 1984- editor. | Padhy, Prabir Chandra, 1985- editor.
Title: Community mental health and well-being in the new normal / edited by Remya Lathabhavan, Prabir Chandra Padhy.
Description: Hershey, PA : Information Science Reference, [2023] | Includes bibliographical references and index. | Summary: "The novel Coronavirus (COVID-19) affected the mental health of people globally(Lathabhavan, 2021). The reasons for the mental health concerns include the fear of infection, concern about loved one's health, high death tools, non-socialization and so on (Tandon, 2021). The indirect impacts such as economic distress, social isolation etc. also led to impact the mental health of people (Lathabhavan & Padhy, 2022). After around two years of pandemic, though it still raises the concerns of different variants, the countries start relaxing the restrictions and coming back to normalcy. The opening of public places, offices and educational institutions raises another concern such as fear of infection, difficulty in socialization etc. This book discusses the mental health concerns of individuals during the pandemic, new normal and in the transition stage"-- Provided by publisher.
Identifiers: LCCN 2022054943 (print) | LCCN 2022054944 (ebook) | ISBN 9781668472217 (hardcover) | ISBN 9781668472224 (paperback) | ISBN 9781668472231 (ebook)
Subjects: LCSH: Mental health. | COVID-19 Pandemic, 2020- | Community mental health services. | Public health.
Classification: LCC RA790.5 .C625 2023 (print) | LCC RA790.5 (ebook) | DDC 362.2--dc23/eng/20221223
LC record available at https://lccn.loc.gov/2022054943
LC ebook record available at https://lccn.loc.gov/2022054944

This book is published in the IGI Global book series Advances in Psychology, Mental Health, and Behavioral Studies (APMHBS) (ISSN: 2475-6660; eISSN: 2475-6679)

British Cataloguing in Publication Data
A Cataloguing in Publication record for this book is available from the British Library.
All work contributed to this book is new, previously-unpublished material.

For electronic access to this publication, please contact: eresources@igi-global.com.

Advances in Psychology, Mental Health, and Behavioral Studies (APMHBS) Book Series

ISSN:2475-6660
EISSN:2475-6679

MISSION

The complexity of the human mind has puzzled researchers and physicians for centuries. While widely studied, the brain still remains largely misunderstood.

The **Advances in Psychology, Mental Health, and Behavioral Studies (APMHBS)** book series presents comprehensive research publications focusing on topics relating to the human psyche, cognition, psychiatric care, mental and developmental disorders, as well as human behavior and interaction. Featuring diverse and innovative research, publications within APMHBS are ideally designed for use by mental health professionals, academicians, researchers, and upper-level students.

COVERAGE

- Counseling & Therapy
- Trauma & Stress
- Mental Health & Disorders
- Psychiatry
- Cognition
- Developmental Disorders
- Personality Disorders
- Treatment & Care
- Neurological Disorders
- Socialization

The Advances in Psychology, Mental Health, and Behavioral Studies (APMHBS) Book Series (ISSN 2475-6660) is published by IGI Global, 701 E. Chocolate Avenue, Hershey, PA 17033-1240, USA, www.igi-global.com. This series is composed of titles available for purchase individually; each title is edited to be contextually exclusive from any other title within the series. For pricing and ordering information please visit http://www.igi-global.com/book-series/advances-psychology-mental-health-behavioral/110200. Postmaster: Send all address changes to above address.

Titles in this Series

For a list of additional titles in this series, please visit:
http://www.igi-global.com/book-series/advances-psychology-mental-health-behavioral/110200

Perspectives on Stress and Wellness Management in Timesof Crisis
Rohit Bansal (Vaish College of Engineering, India)
Information Science Reference • © 2023 • 381pp • H/C (ISBN: 9781668485651) • US $245.00

Facilitating Social Justice, Service Delivery, and Advocacy Through Multicultural Counseling Competencies
Keith B. Wilson (University of Kentucky, USA) and Si-Yi Chao (University of Kentucky, USA)
Information Science Reference • © 2023 • 315pp • H/C (ISBN: 9781668461556) • US $215.00

Perspectives and Considerations on Navigating the Mental Healthcare System
Susan Van Alstyne (Centenary University, USA)
Medical Information Science Reference • © 2023 • 300pp • H/C (ISBN: 9781668450499) • US $305.00

Managing Pandemic Isolation With Literature as Therapy
Antonio Cortijo Ocaña (University of California, Santa Barbara, USA) Vicent Martines (ISIC-IVITRA, University of Alicante, Spain) and Veronica Orazi (Università degli Studi di Torino, Italy)
Information Science Reference • © 2023 • 281pp • H/C (ISBN: 9781668447352) • US $240.00

Latinx Mental Health From Surviving to Thriving
Edward A. Delgado-Romero (University of Georgia, USA)
Medical Information Science Reference • © 2023 • 353pp • H/C (ISBN: 9781668449011) • US $305.00

For an entire list of titles in this series, please visit:
http://www.igi-global.com/book-series/advances-psychology-mental-health-behavioral/110200

IGI Global
PUBLISHER of TIMELY KNOWLEDGE

701 East Chocolate Avenue, Hershey, PA 17033, USA
Tel: 717-533-8845 x100 • Fax: 717-533-8661
E-Mail: cust@igi-global.com • www.igi-global.com

Table of Contents

Detailed Table of Contents

The spread of the Covid pandemic has impacted every aspect of life including the educational system throughout the world. It has transformed the way of learning as well as teaching activities to online studies, and the use of different digital platforms which were supposed to be conducted in face-to-face classes. This remarkable shift to online learning has brought up issues for the students including psychological and health problems, lack of social integration, problems with the platforms and devices they use, and so forth. It also had a negative influence on the activities of professors such as technical problems, teaching from home, lack of interaction, etc. Therefore, this study attempts to explain the challenges and satisfactions during the online classes due to the pandemic and how they have impacted students' and teachers' well-being.

The COVID-19 epidemic has made social isolation the norm. Isolation from society and routines such as hand-washing and wearing masks are examples of necessary lifestyle adjustments. In addition to suffering from pandemic stress, the individual is housebound and able to work remotely. This chapter analyses the effects of behavioural changes, social isolation, a lack of community support, and working

The pandemic has brought about hitherto unimaginable transformations. Anxiety, loss, and sadness have taken their toll resulting in various frightening results, such as disruptive conduct in younger children and aggression and bullying tendencies in older people. Thus, mental health education is essential. However, mental health education not only helps combat the different challenges in our society but also contributes to many sectors that are not always evident to the human eye and are sometimes overlooked. This chapter addresses how mental health education might help students create their businesses. Through an appended assessment of existing research, this chapter covers the components of mental health education and the various linked dimensions of entrepreneurial readiness/competencies. A thorough examination of present and possible ways for providing adequate mental health education has allowed this chapter to offer explicit content. The chapter concludes with a review of the relationships and alignments shared by the areas of mental health education and entrepreneurship.

Higher education is affected by the COVID-19 outbreak, which forced thousands of schools and educational institutions to close in a short amount of time in order to enact social segregation measures. Educational institutions, particularly in India, face considerable challenges in their system of planning, implementing, and assessing. The main purpose of the study was to gather qualitative data about the pandemic-related worries of college students from various part of the country. Education, personal and public safety, mental health, job security and financial instability, future uncertainty, pandemic's effects on social relationships, misleading news and information, politics, the economy, and travel were among the main topics of concern. Universities must seize the potential to enhance their evidence-based practices, provide readily accessible mental health therapies, and modify their courses to meet the needs of the contemporary world.

Infertility has been one of the most pressing challenges in recent years. Infertility services have been postponed and rescheduled globally due to the start of this deadly pandemic. The current study investigated the psychological distress and social consequences of infertile couples during the COVID-19 pandemic. This review study examined articles on infertility, psychosocial effects, and infertility-related stress and pandemic. From the reviewed data, it can be concluded that the pandemic has affected the mental health of childless couples. Increased anxiety, stress, feelings of hopelessness, and fear of uncertainty were common psychological distress experienced by infertile patients during the pandemic. The results of the investigations aid in identifying the psychological concerns of the COVID-19 pandemic on childless couples, knowledge gaps, contemporary patterns, and cutting-edge psychotherapeutic approaches to handling distress.

Ultimately, every individual will find themselves in a caregiving or care-receiving situation at some point in life. As a family caregiver, an individual's effort to support their loved one during difficult times leaves them in a laborious situation. A remarkable number of caregivers caring for a loved one suffering from an acute illness experience a sense of meaning, fulfillment, and profound emotional and psychological rewards. However, lifelong caregiving for a significant one diagnosed with a chronic illness or disability could be onerous. The current book chapter elucidates to the readers the lived experiences of family caregivers of children with neurodevelopmental disorders. The caregivers of children with neurodevelopmental disorders go through a life-long caregiving process. Thus, this book chapter will attempt to illustrate narratives of primary caregivers of children with neurodevelopmental disorders and the paradigm shift they experienced during COVID-19. This research is a determined effort to ensure that the stories of these unsung heroes reach a wider audience.

Over recent times, multitudinous internal health apps (MHapps) have been developed and made available to smartphone druggies. The pandemic, of course, has put employees under a kind of mental strain few have likely experienced before, so it's no wonder more businesses are looking for ways to help workers who are struggling with anxiety, depression, and sleeplessness. In recent years, apps aiming to address all of those issues have proliferated. The boon of mental health application downloads during Covid-19 soared, and while interest will remain, there are bound to be some digital health apps that disappear. During those strange times, people couldn't go and see a doctor face to face about their mental ill-health or go to therapy appointments. Just as with most areas of healthcare impacted by the pandemic, mental health had to go digital. Digital mental health products and digital and virtual therapy have been shown to be comparable to real-life therapy for many patients.

The chapter will give a broad overview of the changes in the well-being of individuals in the workplace during and post-pandemic. The chapter focuses on the problems faced by the people in the pandemic era, which has affected their physical and mental well-being, and some recommendations to be taken by them post-pandemic. The well-being term is complicated as the authors define it in many other ways. In simple words, well-being means dealing with how well a person's mind works and how happy a person is. The whole chapter consists of two major parts: First, based on the role, and second based on demographic factors. Based on role, there are two categories: employees, and employers and business owners. There are three demographic factors: Age, gender and sexuality, race and religion. In the end, two case studies of reputed organizations are given, which came up with innovative measures to improve employees' well-being.

Preface

The novel Coronavirus (COVID-19) affected the mental health of people globally. The reasons for the mental health concerns include the fear of infection, concern about loved one's health, high death tools, non-socialization and so on. The indirect impacts such as economic distress, social isolation etc. also led to impact the mental health of people. After around two years of pandemic, though it still raises the concerns of different variants, the countries start relaxing the restrictions and coming back to normalcy. The opening of public places, offices and educational institutions raises another concern such as fear of infection, difficulty in socialization etc. This book discusses the mental health concerns of individuals during the pandemic, new normal and in the transition stage.

ORGANIZATION OF THE BOOK

Chapter 1: Online Student and Professor Satisfactions and Challenges During the Pandemic Period of 2020-2021

The spread of the Covid pandemic has impacted every aspect of life including the educational system throughout the world. It has transformed the way of learning as well as teaching activities to online studies and using of different digital platforms which were supposed to be conducted in face-to-face classes. This remarkable shift to online learning has brought up issues for the students including psychological and health problems, lack of social integration, problems with the platforms and devices they use, and so forth. It also had a negative influence on the activities of professors such as technical problems, teaching from home, lack of interaction, etc. Therefore, this study attempts to explain the challenges and satisfactions during the online classes due to the pandemic and how they have impacted students' and teachers' well-being.

Chapter 2: Mental Health Post Pandemic – A Socio-Behavioural Perspective of Change in the Working Class

The COVID-19 epidemic has made social isolation the norm. Isolation from society and routines such as hand-washing and wearing masks are examples of necessary lifestyle adjustments. In addition to suffering from pandemic stress, the individual is housebound and able to work remotely. This chapter analyses the effects of behavioural changes, social isolation, a lack of community support, and working from home on mental health in social and professional settings during the pandemic. The financial impact of the pandemic on different kinds of workmen. The chapter concludes by discussing how the pandemic's impact affected mental health and how people overcame it.

Chapter 3: Women and Mental Health Concerns in the New Normal

Women have been hit harder than men by the Covid-19 pandemic, both on the job and at home. Women's transition to a new normal is influenced by biological, social, psychological, and economic factors. One of the main concerns when it comes to psychological elements is mental health. This had an impact on sadness, anxiety, posttraumatic stress, losing a loved one, and having inadequate coping mechanisms. As a result, it is critical to examine the impact of COVID-19 on the mental health of working women in terms of challenges and concerns as the pandemic transitions to the new normal. The primary goal of this research is to identify factors influencing women's mental health as they move from the COVID-19 pandemic to the new normal. Hence, we consolidated the research with the aid of secondary data and to examine the effects of COVID 19 on working women's mental health in terms of difficulties and worries during the transition from the COVID-19 paradigm to the new normal. Stress, anxiety, depression, insomnia, denial, anger, and fear were the most commonly reported mental health issues.

Chapter 4: Well-Being of Organizational Leaders in the New Normal

This chapter discusses that well-being is a skill that has to be mastered by every professional by practicing meditation, sleep, exercise, nutrition, belonging to a community, a spiritual connection, and other factors such as mindfulness training, maintaining the positive psychological capital, and psychological contract in our day-to-day life. This chapter focuses on the impact of mindfulness, psychological capital, and psychological contract on the well-being of organisational leaders. It concludes with the impact of mindfulness, psychological capital, and psychological contract on the well-being of organisational leaders in the new normal.

Chapter 5: Mental Health Education – A Pathway for Entrepreneurial Readiness

The pandemic has brought about hitherto unimaginable transformations. Anxiety, loss, and sadness have taken their toll resulting in various frightening results, such as disruptive conduct in younger children and aggression and bullying tendencies in older people. Thus, mental health education is essential. However, mental health education not only helps combat the different challenges in our society but also contributes to many sectors that are not always evident to the human eye and are sometimes overlooked. This chapter addresses how mental health education might help students create their businesses. Through an appended assessment of existing research, this chapter covers the components of mental health education and the various linked dimensions of entrepreneurial readiness/competencies. A thorough examination of present and possible ways for providing adequate mental health education has allowed this chapter to offer explicit content. The chapter concludes with a review of the relationships and alignments shared by the areas of mental health education and entrepreneurship.

Chapter 6: Mental Health Challenges of Higher Education Students During the COVID-19 Pandemic – Concerns and Considerations in the New Normal

Higher education is affected by the COVID-19 outbreak, which forced thousands of schools and educational institutions to close in a short amount of time in order to enact social segregation measures. Educational institutions, particularly in India, face considerable challenges in their system of planning, implementing, and assessing. The main purpose of the study was to gather qualitative data about the pandemic-related worries of college students from various part of the country. Education, personal and public safety, mental health, job security and financial instability, future uncertainty, pandemic's effects on social relationships, misleading news& information, politics, the economy, and travel were among the main topics of concern. Universities must seize the potential to enhance their evidence-based practices, provide readily accessible mental health therapies, and modify their courses to meet the needs of the contemporary world.

Chapter 7: Psychological Impact of the COVID-19 Pandemic on Childless Couples – A Review

Infertility has been one of the most pressing challenges in recent years. Infertility services have been postponed and rescheduled globally due to the start of this deadly pandemic.The current study investigated the psychological distress and social consequences of infertile couples during the COVID-19 Pandemic. This review study examined articles on infertility, psychosocial effects, and infertility-related stress and pandemic. From the reviewed data, it can be concluded that the pandemic has affected the mental health of childless couples. Increased anxiety, stress, sense of hopelessness, and fear of uncertainty were common psychological distress experienced by infertile patients during the pandemic. The results of the investigations aid in identifying the psychological concerns of the COVID-19 pandemic on childless couples, knowledge gaps, contemporary patterns, and cutting-edge psychotherapeutic approaches to handling distress.

Chapter 8: Family Carers During the COVID-19 Pandemic – A Paradigm Shift in Caregiving

Ultimately, every individual will find themselves in a caregiving or care-receiving situation at some point in life. As a family caregiver, an individual's effort to support their loved one during difficult times leaves them in a laborious situation. A remarkable number of caregivers caring for a loved one suffering from an acute illness experience a sense of meaning, fulfillment, and profound emotional and psychological rewards. However, lifelong caregiving for a significant one diagnosed with a chronic illness or disability could be onerous. The current book chapter elucidates to the readers the lived experiences of family caregivers of children with neurodevelopmental disorders. The caregivers of children with neurodevelopmental disorders go through a life-long caregiving process. Thus, this book chapter will attempt to illustrate narratives of primary caregivers of children with neurodevelopmental disorders and the paradigm shift they experienced during COVID-19. This research is a determined effort to ensure that the stories of these unsung heroes reach a wider audience.

Chapter 9: Mental Health and Well-Being Products/Apps and Their Challenges

Over recent times, multitudinous internal health apps (MHapps) have been developed and made available to smartphone druggies. The pandemic, of course, has put employees under a kind of mental strain few have likely experienced before, so it's no wonder more businesses are looking for ways to help workers who are struggling with anxiety, depression, and sleeplessness. In recent years, apps aiming to address all of those issues have proliferated. The boon of mental health application downloads during COVID-19 soared, and while interest will remain, there are bound to be some digital health apps that disappear. During those strange times, we couldn't go and see a doctor face to face about our mental ill-health or go to therapy appointments. Just as with most areas of healthcare impacted by the pandemic, mental health had to go digital. Digital mental health products and digital and virtual therapy have been shown to be comparable to real-life therapy for many patients.

Chapter 10: Workplace Well-Being During and Post Pandemic

The chapter will give a broad overview of the changes in the well-being of individuals at the workplace during and post-pandemic. The chapter focuses on the problems faced by the people in the pandemic era, which has affected their physical and mental well-being, and some recommendations to be taken by them post-pandemic. The well-being term is complicated as the authors define it in many other ways. In simple words, well-being means dealing with how well a person's mind works and how happy a person is. The whole chapter consists of two major parts: First, based on the role, and second based on demographic factors. Based on role, there are two categories: Employees and Employers and Business Owners. There are three demographic factors: Age, Gender & LGBTQ+, Race & Religion. In the end, two case studies of reputed organizations are given, which came up with innovative measures to improve employees' well-being.

Chapter 11: A Detailed Post-Pandemic Perspective of Indian Families

Indian households have prioritised health and hygiene since the pandemic. Due to increased awareness of social distancing, handwashing, and mask use, families can protect themselves and their loved ones from infectious diseases. Because of this, people are making healthier choices and appreciating preventative healthcare more. Indian families and households have benefited from the pandemic, despite its many negative effects. Digital technology, family ties, gender equality, and health and hygiene will all benefit Indian society in the long run.

Remya Lathabhavan
Indian Institute of Management, Bodh Gaya, India

Prabir Chandra Padhy
VIT Business School, Vellore Institute of Technology, Vellore, India

Chapter 1
Online Student and Professor Satisfactions and Challenges During the Pandemic Period of 2020-2021

Fatma Guneri
Université Catholique de Lille, France

Gulrenk Hayircil
University of Duisburg-Essen, Germany

Abdul Halim Hasanzada
Université Catholique de Lille, France

ABSTRACT

The spread of the Covid pandemic has impacted every aspect of life including the educational system throughout the world. It has transformed the way of learning as well as teaching activities to online studies, and the use of different digital platforms which were supposed to be conducted in face-to-face classes. This remarkable shift to online learning has brought up issues for the students including psychological and health problems, lack of social integration, problems with the platforms and devices they use, and so forth. It also had a negative influence on the activities of professors such as technical problems, teaching from home, lack of interaction, etc. Therefore, this study attempts to explain the challenges and satisfactions during the online classes due to the pandemic and how they have impacted students' and teachers' well-being.

DOI: 10.4018/978-1-6684-7221-7.ch001

INTRODUCTION

Since its outbreak in December 2019, the Covid-19 crisis has affected every crucial sector in the world including but not limited to education. The main negative impact of this pandemic was the closure of educational buildings and the transition from face-to-face classes to online classes. This affected all the parties involved in the education chain from the students to colleges, professors, and even vocational institutions.

As a result, the learning and teaching process encountered a revolution. The schools had to change their educational systems to a more digitalized system by using online platforms such as Zoom and Microsoft Teams, their planning and schedule for the year ought to be changed. On the other hand, the teachers who used to come to class every day had to bring a significant change in their routine and start online classes from home which of course causes numerous issues. They had to change their pedagogical approach and teaching methodology in addition to the struggles of working from home. Likewise, students which are the core of this circle confronted many challenges and shortcomings in their student life. They suddenly stopped going to school, seeing their classmates and friends and dedicated their study time to a screen in front of them.

Furthermore, in the following periods of Covid-19 where face-to-face teaching has restarted, telepresence robots replacing absent students and allowing them to be present via the robots transform the classes into a new form via human-machine interactions. Guneri, Deligny and Faye (2022) realized a focus group study to collect students' view about the telepresence. Therefore, most of the participants rejected the existence of the machine rather than humans. One of the important reasons for this objection was the need for students to develop empathy and engage in spontaneous dialogue with their teachers. These difficulties were common among students and teachers.

Teachers faced their own problems when preparing lessons at home, interacting online with students, and communicating with them outside of class. For this reason, this chapter presents the impact of online learning in the context of Covid-19 from two main perspectives: Challenges for professors and challenges for students.

DIGITALIZATION AND ONLINE CLASSES

Online education is a popular choice for many because of its convenience and accessibility. However, this form of education has also been criticised for its declining quality, lack of student support and inflexibility.

The digitization of education is not a new phenomenon, but an important issue, and relevant stakeholders have a responsibility and need to develop practical academic and pedagogical solutions to provide better solutions (Bond et al., 2018). This shift and development of digital use in the education sector demonstrates the combined use of technologies such as remote presence in classrooms to address unsafe Covid-19 conditions (Abad-Segura, 2020; Güneri, Deligny, and Faye 2022). However, research has shown that this dramatic shift to online learning brings many challenges and problems. This is because online education removes the human element of learning that exists in face-to-face courses. As a result, both academic performance and interpersonal relationships are negatively impacted by this shift.

One of the main problems with online education is that it removes the personal element from learning in face-to-face courses. This means that online students have limited ability to interact with teachers. You cannot do this through text or email communications. Instead, they must meet with the professors in person. This limits the time students have to complete assignments and reduces their chances of academic success. It also makes it difficult for students to develop relationships with the people who grade their assignments. As a result, academic performance dropped significantly when online learning became the only learning option.

To take online classes, students must use a computer or other digital device with a good internet connection to attend the class. A study (Adedoyin & Soykan, 2020) showed that students experienced technical issues while taking online courses, which greatly reduced the efficiency of the learning process. In this study, students reported that their digital devices suddenly turned off. Of course, it will take some time to restart the device and resume classes. Students have already lost some of their classes during this period; imagine how students would be affected when classes were suddenly suspended during exams. In addition, WiFi and Internet connectivity issues are also among the barriers identified in this study. Some students had slow internet connections and experienced delays in their video conferences. Some others don't have WiFi and have to buy internet data packages. This makes it difficult for students to catch up with their peers, pass exams without pressure, and generally have a consistent curriculum.

Despite these negative effects, online education has some advantages over traditional learning methods. It is possible to set up special housing or programs for people with disabilities or other situations where face-to-face teaching is inappropriate or unhelpful. This makes the learning activity available for people who would otherwise not be able to attend the class.

PROFESSORS' CHALLENGES WITH ONLINE TEACHING

Today, professors should use whatever technology is available to communicate with students. This includes the use of email, blackboard, web chat, message boards and video conferencing. The rise of online courses has increased the need for teachers to update their courses regularly. It is also important that students with disabilities still have access to courses. All of these factors require frequent interaction with students via email and other communication channels.

A study (Rosalina & Nasrullah & Eka Puteri, 2020) shows that most teachers and professors born after the 19th century are tech novices or "digital immigrants". However, younger students are native digital learners, which creates a significant gap between teachers and students in terms of digital proficiency. Today, students know more about their teachers when it comes to technology and digital devices. This makes it difficult for the two parties to form a synergistic effect. In order to have an efficient class, all parties should be in harmony with each other. "We had an older but experienced professor who wasted about 15-20 minutes in each meeting sharing his screen via Microsoft Teams and was barely able to do it," one student described.

There's also noise and distractions that affect the quality of online courses. When teaching at home, distractions from people and even pets play a challenging role in the teaching process as well as student attention in online classrooms (Manfuso, 2020). This can happen, for example, when a family member suddenly enters the room and asks for something, or the children make strange noises, or the baby starts crying for no reason. In addition, teachers with pets at home experience situations such as dogs barking or cats running over desks, disrupting videoconferencing.

PROFESSORS' SATISFACTION WITH ONLINE TEACHING

Many colleges and universities now offer courses over the Internet to meet the growing demand for online courses. These lessons are also a great way for teachers to supplement their regular curriculum. These courses are especially beneficial for teachers teaching subjects that are difficult to demonstrate in the field, such as: Science and Math courses. Teachers teaching online have found that their students tend to be more professional and engaged than their students in the classroom. They also found that the quality of their teaching was better when they could interact directly with students. By addressing some of the challenges of online teaching, university administrators can help increase the number of online courses offered by their institutions.

One of the main benefits of teaching online is that it allows professors to teach their students in ways that wouldn't be possible on campus. Most instructors opt for online classes where both students and instructors interact via chat rooms or email chains. This allows for much greater engagement between teacher and students while reducing the cost of class operation.

Online courses are also useful for courses that are often seminar courses or require intense interaction between teachers and students. For example, an astronomy teacher could host regular webinars where answers to student questions are broadcast live and teachers answer questions via webcam. Alternatively, Geography and Environment courses can be discussed on a Google+ page, where both students and teachers can participate directly on the web. This allows both parties to interact more efficiently while saving time running the virtual classroom.

STUDENTS' CHALLENGES WITH ONLINE LEARNING

Due to the Covid-19 outbreak and the eventual closure of schools and educational institutions, students have reported various mental health issues during this period. (Wen Jun, 2020). A study conducted in Changzhi Province, China, surveyed more than 7,100 college students. Results of the study showed that about 1% of these students experienced severe anxiety, 2.7% experienced moderate anxiety, and more than 21% of respondents experienced mild anxiety while studying during the pandemic and lockdown. Furthermore, in this study, researchers tried to find out the correlation between external factors and students' anxiety. These factors were the student's economic and financial situation, infected relatives, and living in an urban or rural area. The results showed that all of these external factors were associated with the type of anxiety students experienced.

According to data collected from 30 students in India, the majority of students have physical, emotional and mental health problems. The survey results show that most students are at a loss and stressed about their academic progress due to delayed exams, a lack of university-related activities, the ambiguity of pursuing higher education at foreign universities and the uncertainty of university reopenings (George and Thomas, 2020).

Duman (2020) conducted a study to assess fear of Covid 19 and intolerance of uncertainty among college students. To do this, the researchers applied the Covid-19 Fear Scale (FCV 19S) and the Uncertainty Intolerance Scale 12 (IUS12) to 100 students. The results showed that these college students had a moderate fear of the new coronavirus and a moderate intolerance of uncertainty. In addition, this study found no significant differences in anxiety and insecurity levels based on student gender. Additionally, research shows that students who have lost family members or relatives have significantly higher levels of anxiety than students who have not experienced bereavement. As a result of this study, a correlation between Covid anxiety and intolerance to uncertainty was identified that was positive, highly significant and moderate.

In 2020, a study of 920 students at a private school in Georgia, USA, was conducted to assess the effectiveness of the shift to online learning. Students are divided into 47 classes, which are conducted using Google Hangouts. Some changes have been made to class times and schedules. Additionally, to minimize students' exposure to computers, they reduced their 45 or 35 minutes of face-to-face classes to 30 minutes of online learning. In addition, students have longer breaks between lessons and fewer lessons per day. As a result, lower grade students scored higher on assignments than upper grade students (Basilaia & Kvadze, 2020).

STUDENTS' SATISFACTION WITH ONLINE LEARNING

In March 2020, a group of researchers (Tayyaba, Z.; Fayyaz, Q. & Sarwar K) conducted a study of undergraduates at a private college in southern England. This study was designed to evaluate students' experiences with online learning and virtual courses. 255 students participated in the study, and the results showed that the majority (95%) were using an online platform (Zoom, Microsoft Teams, etc.) for the first time. However, the final results of this study suggest that the decision to switch to online learning immediately was a good one, with the majority of respondents finding online learning to be fun, although they encountered some challenges along the way. In addition, the majority of students want to continue learning online because it is more convenient in terms of displacement and transportation, and provides greater freedom and autonomy.

Jeetendra, P. and Mythili, G. (2021) conducted another study to assess student satisfaction with Open University of India online courses. Conducted through an online survey and collected 269 valid responses, the study focused on student satisfaction with online courses in terms of academic materials, instruction, assignments, exams, and the online assessment process. As part of the results, responses to this question were global levels of "agree" and "strongly agree." Students were satisfied with the quality of the online presentations and the learning materials available both online and in print. In addition, students appreciated the ease of access to study materials in digital form. Furthermore, they expressed satisfaction and satisfaction when asked if the induction training at the research center was worth it.

Another benefit of online courses is that online courses are considered more convenient and less expensive than face-to-face courses. This is because many students are unable to attend classes on Mondays or other times of the day when they normally attend classes. Online courses also allow students to continue their education without having to spend all their time studying. This makes it easy for students to find a balance between completing assignments and participating in class discussions.

Another group of researchers in India (Kumar, et al., 2021) attempted to assess nursing student satisfaction through their study at the All India Institute of Medical Sciences in Jodhpur, Rajasthan Spend. The study was conducted as a result of the Covid-19 pandemic and used quantitative methods from an online survey. A total of 219 students participated in the survey, all female, aged between 21 and 24. The results show that the majority of students (67.6%) are very satisfied with online learning.

In the end, there are many benefits of online education that outweigh limitations such as miscommunication or technical issues.

PROMOTING DIVERSITY IN ONLINE LEARNING ENVIRONMENTS

With the ever-expanding scope of online learning due to the Covid-19 pandemic, finding ways to create a sense of community and shape an inclusive society is critical. This environment should include and accept members of all races, cultures, ethnicities, sexual orientations, religions, and socioeconomic statuses (Biginas, et al., 2020).

To delve deeper into the topic, the University of East London lecturers conducted research for two of the university's undergraduate and postgraduate students. The purpose of this research is to maximize students' learning experience in a virtual environment and give them a sense of community. For this study, a diverse group of students were selected and introduced to some important principles at the beginning of the module. Afterwards, students were given an active voice so that they could easily explain themselves and participate freely in class discussions. The results of this study show that students are very satisfied (90%-100%) with their learning environment. Additionally, students demonstrate high attendance and submit high-quality written assignments in these online courses. The practical implications of this research suggest that students want to combine different activities to guide them in self-discovery and self-reflection activities that allow them to become more aware of their surroundings and the people around them. Another positive result of this research is that students are very willing to diversify and discuss with their peers from different backgrounds and cultures. Therefore, having a good mix of activities in a diverse class is very important for students to achieve better academic and professional performance.

One way to encourage diversity in online learning is to create courses that all students can access. The ability to access education anytime, anywhere makes online learning a great way to reach out to a diverse student body. This provides educational opportunities that are unavailable to many students. It could also help increase the number of students from underrepresented backgrounds taking online courses. By creating courses that all students can access, you open up opportunities for a more diverse student body.

Another way to encourage diversity in online learning is to create courses that incorporate diverse backgrounds and experiences. Many online courses have specific requirements for students as they specialize in specific topics. Creating an inclusive curriculum ensures that students from different backgrounds have the opportunity to learn the same course material as everyone else. It also ensures that teachers have ample opportunity to learn about different perspectives so that they can be better prepared to teach each student's unique needs. This in turn creates a more inclusive environment where everyone has the opportunity to succeed at the college level.

On the other hand, the downside of encouraging diversity in online learning is that trying to create courses with different backgrounds and experiences can be expensive and time-consuming. This requires additional staff and resources, and these types of courses may not be readily available. For example, the use of telepresence robots and web-based communication tools will not have the same costs, impacts and outcomes for schools and students.

A Case Study: Online Education in France During the Pandemic

April 2021, Dr. Fatma Güneri was interviewed by the Turkish State Broadcasting Corporation (TRT). In this interview, she has shared the information about the online teaching experiences in France 2020-221:

"How were the classes organized in France during the Pandemic?

During the first lockdown from March 17 to May 11, 2020, all schools switched to distance learning. This started so quickly and quickly that from one day to the next, all students and teachers encountered by screens on Microsoft Teams and Zoom. I was very lucky. Because the necessary training courses on these topics were immediately put into practice at the university where I work. Unfortunately, this was not possible in all schools. It was a very difficult time for everyone.

In France courses are demonstration and practice oriented. Especially for teachers of application courses, it is very difficult to teach online. However, the fact that students are very accustomed to interacting in social media and other virtual environments makes it easier for them to adjust to this new situation. Unfortunately, while classes brought into classrooms during September-October 2020 were a bit of a relief, interactive instruction with masks was forcing teachers and students to do the impossible.

On the other hand, during the curfew from October 30 to December 15, 2020, only primary and secondary schools were open at specific times. We continued to conduct distance learning at the University. We were exhausted from sitting in front of screens all day because the class intensity this semester was much higher than the spring semester. With social settings such as restaurants, cafes and sports fields closed again, students were more stressed and bored. Because their age means they needed to have fun. The Christmas break was a bit of a relief, but it didn't last long.

How are the classes organized now (on 2021) in France?

We went through our third restricted period from February 26th to April 4th, 2021. During this third period, we began to go to our office at the university more comfortably. Small group teaching in classrooms is possible. The difficulty here is related to class time. Going out after 6:00 pm is banned until the end of March. This is especially difficult for teachers with afternoon and evening classes. Personally, I can go out one day a week as an example. Starting in early April, the restriction was switched to 7 pm.

How did the pandemic process positively and negatively affect the education in France?

If we look at this situation that has been going on for over a year, from a teacher's point of view, it is very difficult for us to do our job well. It's not at all easy to use distance learning to engage students in interactive lessons, understand technology issues and the difficulties they have in empathizing with students. The situation becomes even more difficult for colleagues who have to care for their own children at home. There are times when teachers face unfair criticism. It's not easy to get used to the rules that are updated almost every month. The role of psychologists to remotely support students and teachers is very, very important and valuable these days. As teachers, we talk to our students as much as possible. For them, the situation is depressing to varying degrees. In France, young people are always outside. They like to have fun and to be together. A sudden closure like this creates a huge cultural difference for them. This reduces their motivation. There are also many students who suffer financially. Students living in dorms are struggling to isolate themselves in their rooms.

Students' primary concerns fall into three categories: health, nutrition, and housing. Not all internet connections are of the same quality. Because of this, there are many students who cannot attend classes or actively participate in classes. The total number of students in France is about 2.7 million. Many of these students are foreign students, and the problems they face take on different dimensions. Loneliness, depression, not knowing who to contact when, who to turn to when sick, and language problems make their situation even more difficult. While there are regular updates from the CampusFrance website and their own university, they are very confused. Municipalities also have a lot of support on these issues. They publish the necessary addresses and information in multiple languages.

Local authorities have also given great support to schools. Unfortunately, despite this, Covid continues to spread rapidly. Young people organize entertainment in their studios because they are bored. Unfortunately, they don't want to play by the rules because they want to be close to each other. I know them very well.

A study jointly carried out by some French media agencies summarizes the situation of young people in the 20-year-old group in 2021 using seven indicators: First, 8 out of 10 young people suffer from prejudice. According to the second indicator, one in six young people drop out of school. Third, 21.8% of young people aged 18-25 are unemployed. The fourth indicator is that one in four teens in the 20-year-old group gave up treatment due to health problems. Indicator 5 shows a 31% increase in adolescent addiction problems. According to indicator 6, 33% of young people under the age of 30 consult a psychologist. Finally, there is a 40% increase in calls to the Student Support Line in the evening.

In conclusion, I can summarize the general support of the French government for students as follows: First, the number of student counseling centers is increasing. The dorms provide meals twice a day. The cost of a meal is 1 euro. Face-to-face sessions with students are permitted once per week, provided they do not occupy more than 20% of the teaching area. The national student loan increases from EUR 15,000 to EUR 20,000 per year. Finally, the sanitizing gel is distributed free of charge at the University."

DISCUSSION

With the prevalence of online teaching in higher education, there is a growing need to discuss the challenges and competencies associated with this way of teaching for teachers and students. It has been argued that students taking online courses are less likely to engage in collaborative learning activities, discussions with others, and interactions between students and teachers than their peers in a face-to-face setting. Related to this, the main challenges can be listed as follows: Develop core professional qualities, including communication, interpersonal and practical skills among students, maintain student retention rates, and provide training and support for the effective use of online technologies and overcoming technical issues, and networking Security risks (Norton et al., 2013).

Due to the lack of important social factors such as peer pressure and shared classroom interaction, students in online programs may not receive the same quality of education as traditional schools. By limiting communication between teachers and students, online courses remove some of the most important elements of a successful learning experience. For example, online education is not always effective because the language barriers involved can be difficult for international students. Some students may not understand what they are being taught in class, or fail the class because of this obstacle.

Given the health risks of Covid-19, with the expectation of keeping all classes online, post-pandemic has raised anxiety issues not only related to distance learning, but also the physical and social impact of the virus. International students, in particular, are concerned about their limited resources, being far from home and fraught with obstacles. Some of the ways students relieve stress when they are not face-to-face are chatting online with friends, watching TV shows and movies, and playing video games. However, they have to meet, dance, shop and eat, and engage in physical activity that is inconvenient to do together during the pandemic (Tan et al., 2022.). Like the challenges of online learning, human interaction is the key issue as everything becomes remote.

In conclusion, the challenge with online education is that it is a relatively new way of educating students and has many advantages over traditional methods. Many believe that online education is the future of education and can lead to a better quality of life. However, others argue that online education is less effective than traditional methods because it lacks the human interaction found in other forms of education. Regardless of these opinions, students and professors prefer online education because it is more convenient and affordable than traditional school education.

REFERENCES

Abad-Segura, E., González-Zamar, M. D., Infante-Moro, J. C., & Ruipérez García, G. (2020). Sustainable management of digital transformation in higher education: Global research trends. *Sustainability*, *12*(5), 2107. doi:10.3390u12052107

Adedoyin, O. B., & Soykan, E. (2020). Covid-19 pandemic and online learning: The challenges and opportunities. *Interactive Learning Environments*, 1–13.

Antonina K, Konstantinos B, (2019). Promoting cultural diversity in online learning environments. *Onresearch.*

Basilaia, G., & Kvavadze, D. (2020). Transition to Online Education in Schools during a SARS-CoV-2 Coronavirus (COVID-19) Pandemic in Georgia. *Pedagogical Research*, *5*(4), em0060.

Biginas, K., Sarantinos, V., & Koumproglou, A. (2020). Learning for Organizational Development: How to Design, Deliver and Evaluate Effective L&D. *The Learning Organization*, *27*(3), 273–275. doi:10.1108/TLO-04-2020-252

Bond, M., Marín, V. I., Dolch, C., Bedenlier, S., & Zawacki-Richter, O. (2018). Digital transformation in German higher education: Student and teacher perceptions and usage of digital media. *International Journal of Educational Technology in Higher Education*, *15*(1), 48. doi:10.118641239-018-0130-1

Duman, N. (2020). Covid-19 Fear and Intolerance to Uncertainty In University Students. *The Journal of Social Science*, *4*(8), 426–437.

George, Ginu. & Thomas, Mari Rani. (2021). Quarantined effects and strategies of college students – Covid-19. *Asian Education and Development Studies.*, *10*(4), 565–573.

Güneri, F., Deligny, M. U., & Faye, S. (2022). Telepresence Robots as A Student and As A Teacher in Classrooms. *2022 ACM CHI Conference on Human Factors in Computing Systems*, New Orleans, LA

Jeetendra, P. & G., M. (2021). Investigating Student Satisfaction With Online Courses: A Case Study of Uttarakhand Open University. *International Journal of Information and Communication Technology Education.*

Kumar, A. (2021). Online learning in nursing students: Satisfaction and barriers. *Journal of Education and Health Promotion*. PMID:35071617

Manfuso, L. G. (2020, April 15). How the remote learning pivot could shape Higher Ed IT. *EdTech Magazine.*

Norton, A., Sonnemann, J., & McGannon, C. (2013). *The Online Evolution: When Technology Meets Tradition in Higher Education*. Grattan Institute.

Rosalina, E., Nasrullah, N., & Elyani, E. P. (2020). Teacher's Challenges towards Online Learning in Pandemic Era. LET: *Linguistics. Literature and English Teaching Journal*, *10*(2), 71. doi:10.18592/let.v10i2.4118

Tan, Y. (2022). Influencing Factors of International Students' Anxiety Under Online Learning During the COVID 19 Pandemic: A Cross Sectional Study of 1,090 Chinese International Students. *Frontiers in Psychology*.

Tayyaba, Z., Fayyaz, Q. & Sarwar K. 2020). Mature undergraduate students' satisfaction with online teaching during the covid 19: *European Journal of Education Studies.*

Wenjun, C., & Ziwei, F. (2020). The psychological impact of the COVID-19 epidemic on college students in China. *Psychiatry Research, 287*. PMID:32229390

Chapter 2
Mental Health Post Pandemic:
A Socio-Behavioural Perspective of Change in the Working Class

Bhuvaneswari Mohanraj
Vellore Institute of Technology, India

Aarthi Chandrasantha Singh
Vellore Institute of Technology, India

ABSTRACT

The COVID-19 epidemic has made social isolation the norm. Isolation from society and routines such as hand-washing and wearing masks are examples of necessary lifestyle adjustments. In addition to suffering from pandemic stress, the individual is housebound and able to work remotely. This chapter analyses the effects of behavioural changes, social isolation, a lack of community support, and working from home on mental health in social and professional settings during the pandemic. It also looks at the financial impact of the pandemic on different kinds of workmen. The chapter concludes by discussing how the pandemic's impact affected mental health and how people overcame it.

INTRODUCTION

Coronavirus (COVID-19) is a disease that is extremely contagious and was caused by a strain of the novel coronavirus. When people infected with the pandemic come in contact with one another, they put themselves at risk of developing these serious illnesses, as the disease has a high likelihood of being transmitted from one person to another in close contact with each other. Thus,everyone was given the orders to

DOI: 10.4018/978-1-6684-7221-7.ch002

remain inside their homes throughout the world, and to continue working from where they regularly conduct their duties i.e., their home, and to not go somewhere public at any costuntil further orders were given. People were asked to confine themselves to their houses and remain safe; places that were more populated such as schools, places of worship, social gatherings, industrial workplaces, and offices, as well as any other activities that were capable of accommodating a large number of people, were strictly prohibited. Those individuals who were granted the opportunity to perform their jobs while at home did so within the four walls of their residences. In the name of work-from-home, people were putting in long hours, day and night, no matter what time of day. A significant number of blue-collar workers, migrant workers, and daily wagers lost their jobs and were required to leave the establishments from which they had previously derived their income. The COVID-19 created a substantial deviation from the norm of the day and caused individuals to adopt a broad variety of unusual habits and behaviours. During the time span covered by the pandemic, it made social isolation the norm. People were fully separated from one another, and the practise of quarantining everyone became normal practice rather than the use of sectional medical situations. Trials and tests were being done on new norms and new methods to live one's life while coping with the fatal sickness. Some examples of the essential adaptations to one's way of life that were made to be followed in an obligatory fashion include seclusion from society as well as modifications to everyday rituals such as increased hand-washing and the use of masks. The pandemic stress was tripled and even quadrupled when individuals were given the opportunity to do remote work. Because there were no predetermined parameters to follow and the amount of work pressure was quite high, people in the working class were put through a significant amount of stress by work from home methods. People tended to work over the allotted hours in order to keep their jobs since they were afraid of being fired. Individuals were unable to cope with the stress caused by the unknown financial situations brought on by the epidemic, in addition to the lack of job security. This chapter discusses the working classes of society as well as the adjustments that have been made to their work schedules as a result of the pandemic. The author tries to understand the sudden social and behavioural changes that occurred as a result of the COVID and how those changes have attempted to create an imbalance in mental health. In the end, we can try to relate these social and behavioural changes in society that have affected the working class as a whole and that necessitated the focus on the mental health of the employees. This is something that we can try to do by trying to relate how these changes have affected the working class as a whole.

SOCIAL CHANGES

Aristotle long ago said that "Man is by nature a social animal" (*Man as a Social Animal*, 2012). Humans as a species, have evolved as a result of the flow of cultures, information, trade, language, and methodology that have emerged through the countless years of human colonisation and communication. It has been shown that an individual's mental health can be significantly affected by social norms and beliefs and that social behaviours play an essential part in Indian households. Social dependency is deeply ingrained in Indian culture and society. People have a great sense of connection to the people and groups that they are a part of, including their families, clans, classes, religions, and communities(Jacobson., 2004). People tend to join together to either rejoice or commiserate about significant life events, such as a wedding, the arrival of a new child, or the death of a member of the family. Therefore, attending community events must inevitably become a regular part of one's life. People in society look down on those who don't participate in or host gatherings like this because they think it shows a lack of moral standing. One of the reasons why humans have followed such behaviours is because of the influence of groupthink and social pressure.

The way people think and act are both impacted by social influence, which plays a significant role in the day-to-day activities of people in India. When an individual conforms to the norms of their group, they increase their chances of gaining acceptability within the group as well as importance among its members. For example, in a place where everyone is dressed formally, one might not want to go in casuals and look like an odd man out. Zimbardo et al., (1973) in their classic Stanford Prison Experiment have shown that social roles influence behaviour, humans have a culturally transmitted understanding of how to behave in accordance with the social roles that they play, which allows them to know how to react in any given situation. The social standards of a society decide what kinds of behaviours are acceptable and what kinds of behaviours are unacceptable for each task. In an Indian household the opinions of other individuals are given more importance and as a result, attending social gatherings can occasionally bring about positive mental and health benefits (Griggs, 2014), but the reverse is also true. This sense of identification oneself with the larger community leads to a positive feeling. Researchers have also shown that increased social support has been linked with the ability to cope with difficulties, which reduces stress (Hopkins & Reicher, 2016) is helpful for people to manage their work in demanding jobs (Haslam et al., 2005; Wegge et al., 2006), and more generally among members of local communities (Bakouri & Staerklé, 2015; Khan et al., 2014). This epidemic has posed a significant threat to the mental health and social interactions of humans. Isolation and restricted community mobility have become the norm. Numerous studies (Bonanno et al., 2007; Makwana, 2019; Pitanatri et al.,

2022) have shown that it is challenging to get back to normal life after a natural or man-made disaster and that memories of the event tend to stick around for a long time. The inability of a population to participate in social gatherings and informal interactions has had a huge impact on their mental schemas of events, which has led to increased levels of stress and a desire for the support of others.

BEHAVIOURAL CHANGES

According to psychologists, changes in behaviour can be beneficial; yet, a behavioural shift brought on by a change in the environment as a response to a cue in the environment might cause the individual greater and more severe harm (Rogers et al., 2010). The current epidemic has spurred a lot of behavioural modifications, such as frequently washing one's hands, regularly sanitising one's hands, consistently cleaning surfaces and things that are routinely used, and other similar practises. The behaviour of often washing one's hands and using hand sanitizer is closely linked to the psychological issues associated with obsessive-compulsive disorder (OCD), (https://www.anxiety.org/does-excessive-hand-washing-mean-obsessive-compulsive-disorder) which can cause anxiety and worry in people. It is possible for someone to develop paranoid thoughts, a sort of anxious thought, if they have self-doubts over whether or not they have properly washed and sanitised their hands in order to safeguard their loved ones from illness. Roy et al., (2020) performed an online poll in India and discovered, based on the 662 replies, that 80% of the respondent population was preoccupied with COVID – 19 and 72% felt the necessity to use gloves and sanitizers. High anxiety levels were reported in the study. In addition, sleep difficulties and worry of contracting COVID-19 were mentioned. More than 80% of the population surveyed in the study felt a need for mental health treatment.

Fear of a pandemic caused people more likely to develop the obsessive-compulsive disorder than they had ever been before. The development of obsessive-compulsive disorder has been linked to several different types of repeated behaviours, including routinely monitoring the news for new virus outbreaks and washing one's hands multiple times a day. Even when conditions are normal, the majority of persons who have OCD have profound anxiety around the possibility of contamination. People who suffer from OCD have a very difficult time overcoming this anxiety, and given the circumstances of the pandemic, everyone was scared of becoming infected with the virus. This worry increased the possibility that everyone will develop OCD as a learned behaviour at least once in their lives. According to Mowrer's Two Process Theory(1947), the obsessive-compulsive disorder can be brought on by learned behaviours, as per his hypothesis, classical conditioning has the effect of creating anxiety by causing a non-reactive stimulus to become linked with a frightening concept or event. For instance, the idea of contamination might be linked to touching a doorknob or shaking hands, after being constantly reminded of this connection, the individual will make an effort to alleviate some of their anxiety by regularly doing hand hygiene practises such as washing and sanitising their hands. When frequent handwashing and anxiety reduction are combined, the response of increased handwashing becomes more habitual and consistent. In the future, it will be more probable to occur if a situation causes people to anticipate infection. It is quite improbable that these trained avoidance reflexes will become nonexistent after they have been learnt (Marakas, 2013), thus people are going to great lengths to ensure the well-being of their family by complying to all of the safety regulations.

Physical separation and extended periods spent at home are two factors that have contributed to shifts in lifestyle that have had a negative impact on mental health. Alterations in lifestyle, such as changes in sleeping habits, home boredom, loss of interest in work due to no external stimuli, reduced energy levels due to cutting off or reducing outdoor activities, overeating, and other such alterations, have been linked with mood and associated disorders. A survey of the general population in India found that anxiety and problems in sleeping were substantially more common than in the past and that the epidemic had a considerable impact on the participants' mental health (Chakraborty & Chatterjee, 2020). In the aftermath of the pandemic, it was seen that the present shifts in lifestyle, when combined with any pre-existing mental problems, led to a worsening of symptoms (Van Rheenen et al., 2020). Alterations to one's way of life might render an otherwise healthy person extremely susceptible to mood and other problems.

COVID-19 AND ITS IMPACT ON VARIOUS SECTORS OF THE WORKING CLASS

Primary sector industries in India include industries like agriculture, mining, fishing, forestry, and dairy production, amongst others. Even though it might appear to be the industry that would have been least affected by the COVID-19 pandemic lockdown, the reality is that it was harmed just as much as any other industry because of its smooth operation is dependent on the proper functioning of other industries. People like farmers and farm workers were unable to bear the burden because there were no trade exchanges. Transportation, intrastate and interstate services, market locations, and shopping malls were all tightly regulated and monitored for their transport movements. This made it impossible for people like farmers and farm workers to thrive.Many Indian farmers have committed suicide in the past for a variety of reasons, including crop failure, financial difficulties, the marriage of a daughter, the strain of mounting debt, falling prices, and so on; covid made it even worse as the prices of agricultural goods dropped by 20% after the COVID-19 epidemic (Bhosale, 2020). Suicide the act of intentionally ending one's own life is a significant factor in all types of depression. Even though the specific circumstances that push a person over the edge to take their own life can take on a wide variety of forms, it is pretty apparent that suicidal behaviour is linked to unfortunate occurrences such as major setbacks in one's financial situation, detainment, and various types of interpersonal conflicts. After the financial crisis began to take hold in 2007, for instance, the rate of suicide increased dramatically (i.e., it quadrupled) in the United States, Great Britain, and Hong Kong between the years 2008 and 2010.The vulnerabilities and power inequalities in the Indian agricultural system have been brought to light by COVID-19, which will facilitate learning and the building of resilience against future shocks. The epidemic brought to light the differences in income discrepancies that exist across the country, which were manifested in the response to various social strata. It is essential and of the utmost importance to find short-term solutions, as the pandemic, despite appearing to be on the decline, could very well reassert itself, having a negative impact not only on the economy but also on mental health, thereby threatening both food security and people's livelihoods.

Manufacturing and other types of production units, including as textile production, handicraft production, manufacturing of raw materials, manufacture of finished products, manufacturing of automobiles, and so on, are included in the secondary sector of the economy. Due to the fact that the vast majority of businesses operating in this industry are production units that are dependent on functioning at the source location, the COVID-19 pandemic made it difficult to continue working. As a result, this industry was considered to be the one that was impacted the hardest. The production schedules and supply networks were disrupted, which led to a significant increase in worldwide demand and shortages of supply. Earlier during the pandemic for the units that were given permission to work with a smaller staff, the government stipulated a number of precautionary measures that had to be adhered to, such as the use of masks and gloves, the maintenance of an appropriate social distance, and the application of sanitizers at regular intervals. These ritualistic behaviour as discussed earlier have OCD forming habits and anxiety issues in the long run(Kluger, 2022).The pandemic was seen as a broad stressor and it is common knowledge that stress can exacerbate psychiatric symptoms, including generalised increases in anxiety(Grant et al., 2022).

During the pandemic, many businesses in the tertiary sector, such as hotels, restaurants, dining establishments, logistics, communication, investment firms, insurance, online platforms, private and social services, educational services, and others, were either completely shut down or operated on a limited scale from a remote location. People who worked in these industries saw significant changes in both their financial situations and their day-to-day lives as a result of the recession (Nicola et al., 2020). All levels of education, from elementary schools to universities, were disrupted since schools across the board were forced to close until further notice. Because education moved online, teachers and professors found themselves under more pressure to engage their students in meaningful ways through the medium of online learning.A lack of motivation on the part of students to attend online classes, feedback responses from students, and interactions with students face to face were some of the key pressures that educators experienced when taking online classes. In comparison to the rest of the world's teachers, those working in the education sector in India were overworked and poorly compensated which causes burnout and job distress(Punit, 2020).

The Information Technology sector was seen as the most benefitted one from the Covid-19 pandemic due to the work from home option provided as there was a significant rise in the number of people working remotely. Before the crisis, it was common knowledge that workers who did their jobs from home put in longer hours than those who did their jobs in offices; this was a pattern that was also consistently seen throughout the COVID-19 crisis. Though it may look lucrative to work remotely, telework can have a number of negative effects on mental health, including the overlapping of boundary lines between work and home life, the contribution of extended working hours, and the result of a sense of detachment from one's place of employment. Despite the fact that telework can have a number of positive effects, such as more flexible working arrangements, it can also impact on one's mental health (Oakman et al., 2020).No defined working guidelines, timings, zero to limited work life balance have taken immense toll on the employees, there are no weekdays or weekends when working from home. Overwork, tiredness, stress, insomnia, and anxiety become the norm (Times, 2020).

The Financial Impact of Covid in Working Sector

Covid had a great implication of the financial aspect on the working class.61% of working men maintained their employment status throughout the lockdown and in the months that followed, whereas 7% of working men were laid off and did not find new employment. During the lockdown, just 19% of women kept their jobs, while 47% of women experienced a permanent loss of employment and did not return to work until at least the end of the year 2020(Azim Premji University, 2021).It has been discovered that women are more likely to have bad mental health due to financial difficulties, whilst men are more likely to experience poor mental health due to unemployment. This study is consistent with the findings of a systematic review, which indicated that men were more likely than women to experience poor mental health due to unemployment (Paul & Moser, 2009).According to other research, in comparison to males, women are more likely to experience mental health problems in the absence of adequate social support when confronted with adverse life circumstances such as unemployment or other setbacks(Dalgard et al., 2006; Leana & Feldman, 1991). Six months after the initial lockdown in India, during the COVID-19 pandemic, researchers investigated the connection between financial difficulty, job loss, and mental health symptoms in a rural area of Maharashtra. They discovered that women reported more severe new-onset mental health symptoms than men (Chatterji et al., 2021).Three systematic reviews found that people who lost their jobs during a recession and/or experienced financial crises had a higher risk of reporting poor health, increased stress, depression, mental hardship, anxiety, and suicidal behaviours, these studies included both longitudinal and cohort designs (Frasquilho et al., 2016; Margerison-Zilko et al., 2016; Modrek et al., 2013).

Agriculture, construction, and retail trade have all developed as potentially viable standby industries in recent years. The highest number of employees left the education, healthcare, and professional services sectors to work in other types of businesses. It is estimated that approximately 18% of workers in the education sector are now employed in agriculture, while an equivalent percentage of people in the healthcare sector are engaged in petty trade.Many industries have taken out short-term bank loans to survive the current economic downturn as a result of a decline in revenue. Numerous small- and large-scale enterprises have received huge economic aid packages from the Indian government to help them survive and overcome this emergency. Yet, those in the low-income bracket with unpredictable employment, contract employees, and micro-business owners have reported increased levels of depression and anxiety post-lockdown, with the loss of revenue being the primary stressor(Alradhawi et al., 2020).

MENTAL HEALTH POST PANDEMIC

Post the COVID-19 pandemic there was a sharp increase in stress, anxiety, sleep disturbances, and panic among individuals (Das, 2020). The dreadful outbreak resulted in unprecedented nationwide lockdowns in numerous nations, including India.The abrupt changes in everyday life brought after the pandemic clubbed with the on and off lockdowns caused psychological discomfort in people to a great extent (Tanoue et al., 2020). People became irritated due to the isolation and confinement as they feel constrained. People who knew someone in their family who has COVID-19 and who were experiencing major problems experienced anticipatory grieving (Zhai & Du, 2020). Students and office workers have been found to exhibit increased depression symptoms than before the lockdown, presumably due to house confinement, stress, and anxiety(Majumdar et al., 2020). Since the epidemic, the Indian Psychiatry

Society recorded a 20% increase in mental disease cases (Kumar & Nayar, 2020). The rate of suicide increased due to the fear of infection and a sense of helplessness (Dsouza et al., 2020).

In the midst of the epidemic, numerous social networking platforms rather than promoting, actually endangered the mental health of persons living in the community. People have their own unique ways of dealing with stressful situations, and not everyone is able to view the pandemic lockdown as an effective learning environment. During the lockdown, several messages were circulated asking individuals come out with new skills, which has further exacerbated the psychological pressure and emotional stress that people were already experiencing. Because of this pressure, people have had feelings of remorse and shame, as well as overpowering emotions and bad thoughts. Their self-esteem also plummeted, and needed to addressed to prevent a mental collapse (Mukhtar, 2020).

CONCLUSION

According to the ancient Greek philosopher Heraclitus "change is the only constant in life," (Graham, 2021) which means that nothing is permanent other than change, and we shall experience change whenever we seek permanence. The covid epidemic has resulted in multiple rapid developments that have left little time to adapt or comprehend them. These modifications were so profound that they brought about a dramatic shift in lifestyle, behaviour, cognitive process, and cultural events. There was no time for individuals to contemplate what caused them to become used to the changes. The pandemic introduced hybrid approaches of work and learning into the standard system, and working from home and online education became popular. Individuals feel anxious when confronted with abrupt onsets of change; hence, alterations in mental health are unavoidable. Beginning with social changes such as not meeting other people, connecting with them, and not having a social life during the pandemic, India's peer support system for mental health balance was impaired for many individuals. The hygienic habits formed during the covid, including as washing hands and wearing masks, are all linked to a fear of contamination, resulting in compulsive behaviours. People who worked during the peak phase of the epidemic were subjected to all of these changes, including isolation, adherence to cleanliness practises, and working in a remote place, rendering them susceptible to mental health problems. However, these reforms did attempt to unbalance the working class, but they adapted magnificently. The rapid adjustments have now become permanent due to the pandemic's official persistence in its spread. Individuals have marvellously adapted to the societal and behavioural changes in accordance with the criteria of the contemporary society. The alterations in behaviour have gradually become a part of one's daily routine. Changes brought about by the covid, which were first somewhat stressful and disruptive to people's lives, have been handled well by humans, indicating that life continues on.

REFERENCES

Alradhawi, M., Shubber, N., Sheppard, J., & Ali, Y. (2020). Effects of the COVID-19 pandemic on mental well-being amongst individuals in society. In International Journal of Surgery, 78, 147–148. Elsevier Ltd. doi:10.1016/j.ijsu.2020.04.070

Azim Premji University. (2021). State of Working India 2021. Azim Premji University.

Bakouri, M., & Staerklé, C. (2015). Coping with structural disadvantage: Overcoming negative effects of perceived barriers through bonding identities. *British Journal of Social Psychology, 54*(4), 648–670. doi:10.1111/bjso.12102 PMID:25683895

Bhosale, J. (2020). *Prices of agricultural commodities drop 20% post COVID-19 outbreak.* Economic Times. https://economictimes.indiatimes.com/news/economy/agriculture/prices-of-agricultural-commodities-drop-20-post-covid-19-outbreak/articleshow/74705537.cms

Bonanno, G. A., Galea, S., Bucciarelli, A., & Vlahov, D. (2007). What Predicts Psychological Resilience After Disaster? The Role of Demographics, Resources, and Life Stress. *Journal of Consulting and Clinical Psychology, 75*(5), 671–682. doi:10.1037/0022-006X.75.5.671 PMID:17907849

Chakraborty, K., & Chatterjee, M. (2020). Psychological impact of COVID-19 pandemic on general population in West Bengal: A cross-sectional study. *Indian Journal of Psychiatry, 62*(3), 266–272. doi:10.4103/psychiatry.IndianJPsychiatry_276_20 PMID:32773869

Chatterji, S., McDougal, L., Johns, N., Ghule, M., Rao, N., & Raj, A. (2021). COVID-19-Related Financial Hardship, Job Loss, and Mental Health Symptoms: Findings from a Cross-Sectional Study in a Rural Agrarian Community in India. *International Journal of Environmental Research and Public Health, 18*(16), 8647. doi:10.3390/ijerph18168647 PMID:34444394

Dalgard, O. S., Dowrick, C., Lehtinen, V., Vazquez-Barquero, J. L., Casey, P., Wilkinson, G., Ayuso-Mateos, J. L., Page, H., & Dunn, G. (2006). Negative life events, social support and gender difference in depression. *Social Psychiatry and Psychiatric Epidemiology, 41*(6), 444–451. doi:10.1007/s00127-006-0051-5

Das, N. (2020). Psychiatrist in post-COVID-19 era – Are we prepared? *Asian Journal of Psychiatry*, *51*, 102082. doi:10.1016/j.ajp.2020.102082 PMID:32283513

Dsouza, D. D., Quadros, S., Hyderabadwala, Z. J., & Mamun, M. A. (2020). Aggregated COVID-19 suicide incidences in India: Fear of COVID-19 infection is the prominent causative factor. *Psychiatry Research*, *290*, 113145. doi:10.1016/j.psychres.2020.113145 PMID:32544650

Frasquilho, D., Matos, M. G., Salonna, F., Guerreiro, D., Storti, C. C., Gaspar, T., & Caldas-De-Almeida, J. M. (2016). Mental health outcomes in times of economic recession: A systematic literature review. *BMC Public Health*, *16*(1), 115. Advance online publication. doi:10.118612889-016-2720-y PMID:26847554

Graham, D. W. (2021). Heraclitus. In E. N. Zalta (Ed.), Stanford Encyclopedia of Philosophy (Summer2021 ed.). Metaphysics Research Lab, Stanford University.

Grant, J. E., Drummond, L., Nicholson, T. R., Fagan, H., Baldwin, D. S., Fineberg, N. A., & Chamberlain, S. R. (2022). Obsessive-compulsive symptoms and the Covid-19 pandemic: A rapid scoping review. *Neuroscience and Biobehavioral Reviews*, *132*, 1086–1098. doi:10.1016/j.neubiorev.2021.10.039 PMID:34740755

Griggs, R. A. (2014). Coverage of the Stanford Prison Experiment in Introductory Psychology Textbooks. *Teaching of Psychology*, *41*(3), 195–203. doi:10.1177/0098628314537968

Haslam, S. A., O'Brien, A., Jetten, J., Vormedal, K., & Penna, S. (2005). Taking the strain: Social identity, social support, and the experience of stress. *British Journal of Social Psychology*, *44*(3), 355–370. doi:10.1348/014466605X37468 PMID:16238844

Hopkins, N., & Reicher, S. (2016). The psychology of health and well-being in mass gatherings: A review and a research agenda. In Journal of Epidemiology and Global Health, 6(2), 49–57). Elsevier Ltd. doi:10.1016/j.jegh.2015.06.001

Jacobson, D. (2004). Indian Society and Ways of Living. *Asia Society*. https://asiasociety.org/education/indian-society-and-ways-living

Khan, S. S., Hopkins, N., Tewari, S., Srinivasan, N., Reicher, S. D., & Ozakinci, G. (2014). Efficacy and well-being in rural north India: The role of social identification with a large-scale community identity. *European Journal of Social Psychology*, *44*(7), 787–798. doi:10.1002/ejsp.2060 PMID:26160989

Kluger, J. (2022). Pandemic Anxiety Is Fueling a Rise in OCD Symptoms. *Time Magizine*. https://time.com/6140256/ocd-covid-19-anxiety/

Kumar, A., & Nayar, K. R. (2020). COVID 19 and its mental health consequences. doi:10.1080/09638237.2020.1757052

Leana, C. R., & Feldman, D. C. (1991). Gender differences in responses to unemployment. *Journal of Vocational Behavior*, *38*(1), 65–77. doi:10.1016/0001-8791(91)90018-H

Majumdar, P., Biswas, A., & Sahu, S. (2020). COVID-19 pandemic and lockdown: Cause of sleep disruption, depression, somatic pain, and increased screen exposure of office workers and students of India. *Chronobiology International*, *37*(8), 1191–1200. doi:10.1080/07420528.2020.1786107 PMID:32660352

Makwana, N. (2019). Disaster and its impact on mental health: A narrative review. *Journal of Family Medicine and Primary Care*, *8*(10), 3090. doi:10.4103/jfmpc.jfmpc_893_19 PMID:31742125

Man as a social animal. (2012). The Hindu. https://www.thehindu.com/features/education/research/man-as-a-social-animal/article2988145.ece

MarakasG. M. (2013). *Abnormal Psych*.

Margerison-Zilko, C., Goldman-Mellor, S., Falconi, A., & Downing, J. (2016). Health Impacts of the Great Recession: A Critical Review. *Current Epidemiology Reports*, *3*(1), 81–91. doi:10.100740471-016-0068-6 PMID:27239427

Modrek, S., Stuckler, D., McKee, M., Cullen, M. R., & Basu, S. (2013). A Review of Health Consequences of Recessions Internationally and a Synthesis of the US Response during the Great Recession. *Public Health Reviews, 35*(1), 1–33. doi:10.1007/BF03391695

Mowrer, O. H. (1947). On the dual nature of learning—A re-interpretation of "conditioning" and "problem-solving.". *Harvard Educational Review*, *17*, 102–148.

Mukhtar, S. (2020). Psychological health during the coronavirus disease 2019 pandemic outbreak. *The International Journal of Social Psychiatry*, *66*(5), 512–516. doi:10.1177/0020764020925835 PMID:32434402

Nicola, M., Alsafi, Z., Sohrabi, C., Kerwan, A., Al-Jabir, A., Iosifidis, C., Agha, M., & Agha, R. (2020). The socio-economic implications of the coronavirus pandemic (COVID-19): A review. In International Journal of Surgery, 78, 185–193. Elsevier Ltd. doi:10.1016/j.ijsu.2020.04.018

Oakman, J., Kinsman, N., Stuckey, R., Graham, M., & Weale, V. (2020). A rapid review of mental and physical health effects of working at home: How do we optimise health? *BMC Public Health*, *20*(1), 1–13. doi:10.118612889-020-09875-z PMID:33256652

Paul, K. I., & Moser, K. (2009). Unemployment impairs mental health: Meta-analyses. *Journal of Vocational Behavior*, *74*(3), 264–282. doi:10.1016/j.jvb.2009.01.001

Pitanatri, P. D. S., Pitana, I. G., & Valeri, M. (2022). Natural and Man-Made Crisis Management in a Small Island Tourism Destination: The Case of Bali. *Tourism Risk*, 61–79. doi:10.1108/978-1-80117-708-520221005

Punit, I. S. (2020). India school teachers grapple unruly online classes amid lockdown. *Quartz India*. https://qz.com/india/1851939/india-school-teachers-grapple-unruly-online-classes-amid-lockdown/

Rogers, Y., Hazlewood, W. R., Marshall, P., Dalton, N., & Hertrich, S. (2010). Ambient influence: Can twinkly lights lure and abstract representations trigger behavioral change? *UbiComp'10 - Proceedings of the 2010 ACM Conference on Ubiquitous Computing*, (pp. 261–270). ACM.10.1145/1864349.1864372

Roy, D., Tripathy, S., Kar, S. K., Sharma, N., Verma, S. K., & Kaushal, V. (2020). Prevalence of stress, anxiety, depression among the general population during the COVID-19 pandemic: A systematic review and meta-analysis. *Asian Journal of Psychiatry*, *51*, 102083. doi:10.1016/j.ajp.2020.102083 PMID:32283510

Tanoue, Y., Nomura, S., Yoneoka, D., Kawashima, T., Eguchi, A., Shi, S., Harada, N., & Miyata, H. (2020). Mental health of family, friends, and co-workers of COVID-19 patients in Japan. *Psychiatry Research*, *291*, 113067. doi:10.1016/j.psychres.2020.113067 PMID:32535504

Times, T. E. (2020). Work from home burnout: Stress, insomnia, anxiety becoming the new normal. *The Economic Times*. https://economictimes.indiatimes.com/magazines/panache/work-from-home-burnout-stress-insomnia-anxiety-becoming-the-new-normal/articleshow/75425733.cms

Van Rheenen, T. E., Meyer, D., Neill, E., Phillipou, A., Tan, E. J., Toh, W. L., & Rossell, S. L. (2020). Mental health status of individuals with a mood-disorder during the COVID-19 pandemic in Australia: Initial results from the COLLATE project. *Journal of Affective Disorders*, *275*, 69–77. doi:10.1016/j.jad.2020.06.037 PMID:32658826

Wegge, J., Van Dick, R., Fisher, G., Wecking, C., & Moltzen, K. (2006). Work motivation, organisational identification, and well-being in call centre work. *Work and Stress*, *20*(1), 60–83. doi:10.1080/02678370600655553

Zhai, Y., & Du, X. (2020). Loss and grief amidst COVID-19: A path to adaptation and resilience. *Brain, Behavior, and Immunity*, *87*, 80–81. doi:10.1016/j.bbi.2020.04.053 PMID:32335197

Zimbardo, P. G., Haney, C., Banks, W. C., & Jaffe, D. (1973). Interpersonal dynamics in a simulated prison. *International Journal of Criminology and Penology*, *1*, 69–97.

Chapter 3
Women and Mental Health Concerns in the New Normal

Dharti Parikh
Navrachana University, India

Niyati Patel
Navrachana University, India

ABSTRACT

Women have been hit harder than men by the Covid-19 pandemic, both on the job and at home. Women's transition to a new normal is influenced by biological, social, psychological, and economic factors. One of the main concerns when it comes to psychological elements is mental health. This had an impact on sadness, anxiety, posttraumatic stress, losing a loved one, and having inadequate coping mechanisms. As a result, it is critical to examine the impact of COVID-19 on the mental health of working women in terms of challenges and concerns as the pandemic transitions to the new normal. The primary goal of this research is to identify factors influencing women's mental health as they move from the COVID-19 pandemic to the new normal. Hence, the authors consolidated the research with the aid of secondary data and to examine the effects of COVID 19 on working women's mental health in terms of difficulties and worries during the transition from the COVID-19 paradigm to the new normal. Stress, anxiety, depression, insomnia, denial, anger, and fear were the most commonly reported mental health issues.

DOI: 10.4018/978-1-6684-7221-7.ch003

INTRODUCTION

It has been seen over the past few months that the routine health services, including mental health care, are adversely affected in many countries, including India. At the same time, several lay media reports are suggesting an increase in mental health issues such as anxiety, depression, posttraumatic stress-like symptoms, insomnia, and anger among the general population, health workers, as well as people who are kept in isolation (due to infection with coronavirus or contact with infected persons) (Roy et al., 2020). Women who are pregnant, postpartum, miscarrying, or experiencing intimate partner violence are at especially high risk for developing mental health problems during the pandemic. Proactive outreach to these groups of women and enhancement of social supports could lead to prevention, early detection, and prompt treatment. Social support is a key protective factor. Similarly, parenting may be substantially more stressful during a pandemic. Gender disparities may be accentuated, particularly for employed women or single parents, as women are disproportionately responsible for the bulk of domestic tasks, including childcare and eldercare (Almeida et al., 2020). Due to a large population, equity issues, gender issues, a lack of positive deviance at the community level, illiteracy, socioeconomic factors, migration from rural to urban areas, the inability to access legal assistance, and of course many other factors, the protection of women is of the utmost importance and a top concern in India (Kumar, 2021).

The primary aim of this chapter is to identify factors affecting women's mental health during the transition from the COVID-19 pandemic to the new normal. A secondary aim is to review the impact of COVID-19 on the mental health of working women in terms of challenges and concerns during the transition from the COVID-19 pandemic to the new normal.

HEALTH: PHYSICAL AND MENTAL AND WOMEN MENTAL HEALTH

Every family is being impacted both emotionally and financially by the 2019 coronavirus (COVID-19). Around the world, a panicky scenario is present. Numerous flaws and alterations in everyone's regular daily activities as well as other leisure activities exist as a result of Novel Coronavirus existence. For older persons in middle- and low-income countries like India, adjusting to this new normal existence is a serious struggle. Indians are dealing with a wide range of psychological issues as they adjust to the modern lifestyles and their dread of illness. Domestic abuse against women has grown following the subsequent lockdowns. (Lokeshvar et al., 2021).

Mental health is an essential component of overall health; it is more than the absence of illness, and it is inextricably linked to physical health and behavior. According to the World Health Organization, mental health is "a state of well-being in which the individual realizes his or her own abilities, can cope with the normal stresses of life, can work productively and fruitfully, and is able to contribute to his or her community." In this sense, mental health is the foundation for an individual's and a community's well-being and effective functioning. It is more than just the absence of mental illness, because the states and capacities mentioned in the definition are valuable in and of themselves. (WHO, 2004).

A level of cognitive or emotional well-being or the absence of a mental condition are both referred to as having good mental health. According to positive psychology or holistic viewpoints, a person's ability to enjoy life and strike a balance between daily activities and endeavors to develop psychological resilience may be considered a sign of mental health. A mental disease or mental illness, on the other hand, is an uncontrollable psychological or behavioral pattern that affects a person and is believed to cause distress or incapacity and is not expected as a natural component of development or culture. The patterns of psychiatric disease and psychological discomfort among women are distinct from those seen among men, according to analysis of mental health indices and data. (Malhotra & Shah, 2015).

Men and women's ability to influence the factors that determine their health, such as their economic standing, social standing, access to resources, and treatment in society, is influenced by their gender. (WHO, 2004). Women have, however, been more severely impacted by the COVID-19 pandemic than males in several ways, including at work (particularly in the health and social sector) and at home, where lockdown and quarantine procedures have increased the workload. Women make about 70% of the health workforce globally, and they frequently work as front-line healthcare providers (nurses, midwives, and community health workers). Similarly, women make up most of the workforce working in health facilities (cleaners, laundry, and catering). In contrast to males at the time of COVID, females had significantly worse mental health (Venugopal et al., 2022). Men and women's ability to influence the factors that determine their health, such as their economic standing, social standing, access to resources, and treatment in society, is influenced by their gender. (Thibaut & van Wijngaarden-Cremers, 2020).

Factors Affecting Women's Mental Health

Because of the large proportion of socially and economically vulnerable people in India, mental health issues are more complicated in the context of the COVID-19 pandemic. Women's mental health are affected by variety of factors named:

Biological

During the period of Pre covid, the general health score for men was higher than the score for women, indicating that women may be more susceptible to developing mental disorders (Venugopal et al., 2022). community pressure regarding stereotypical social roles based on gender may impact mental health responses differently in women. domestic violence and abuse toward women related to the greater prevalence of mental illness among women. Gender disparities in depressive disorders may be significantly impacted by social factors, particularly gender inequality (Yu, 2018). women make up the majority of those who are impacted by the COVID-19 in terms of their physical condition, emotional reaction, and effect on recovery. Trauma and mental illnesses are now more likely to occur as a result of the lockdown, sluggish economic growth, financial insecurities, and health problems (Malik & Naeem, 2020).

Social

Women who are in a more vulnerable position in the household are more likely to suffer from mental health problems and to be concerned about their safety. While potentially important for public health, containment is associated with significant negative consequences for both standard socioeconomic outcomes and outcomes that are more difficult to observe and measure, such as mental health (Bau et al., 2022).

Psychological

The most prevalent psychological factors affecting women's mental health are: Anxiety, depression, and post-traumatic stress disorder. Female patients and those admitted to intensive care reported higher levels of fatigue, pain, anxiety, and depression. Up to three months after COVID-19, there was an overall decline in quality of life. Women are more susceptible to the effects of traumatic events and to stress from the many roles they play at home and at work, which can be one reason for the high rates of psychological disorders in women (Semo & Frissa, 2020; Shanbehzadeh et al., 2021).

Economical

The most vital economic factors influencing women's mental health are: poor economic conditions, job loss or potential job loss, and economic uncertainty (Dalal et al., 2020). Broad-based macro-level determinants of mental health include by the Human Development Index (HDI), which was examined. The HDI was created as a performance indicator that highlights both human outcomes and a nation's economic performance. Other examples of macro-level national indicators include the Gender-related Development Index (GDI) and the Gender Empowerment Index (GEI). They provide measurements of mental health with an appropriate context by describing some fundamental aspects of human development. Pidemiological studies of mental health, cross-national studies of quality of life, conclusions about the link between social determinants and inequalities and health and mental health outcomes, psychometric studies, and findings from health surveillance and monitoring (WHO, 2004).

Mode of Working

During the lockdown, the physical and mental demands on the women who work from home and for themselves are substantially heightened. Due to the pandemic and the burden of working from home and household duties, the mental health of women who do so is substantially harmed during the national lockdown (work for home). The emergence of musculoskeletal issues has a negative impact on health as well (Sharma & Vaish, 2020).

Challenges, Concerns, and Problems Faced by Women on Their Mental Health During Covid-19

Physical Challenges

During the lockdown caused by the corona pandemic, it is crucial to take precautions for women who work from home and for the home to prevent any physical problems and mental illness. (Sharma & Vaish, 2020). Women's health services are provided by healthcare professionals from various disciplines and specialties who provide care to girls and women throughout their lives, including sexual and reproductive health, pregnancy, childbirth, and lactation. (Ramirez et al., 2020). Although child care, senior care, and housework traditionally fall to women, households are under pressure. There is growing concern regarding the rise in domestic violence (Lancet, 2020).

Gender Discrimination

It is commonly known that women in academics confront difficulties in non-pandemic eras. These obstacles include institutional cultures that are controlled by men, a dearth of female mentors, conflicting family duties brought on by gendered domestic work, and implicit and unconscious biases in hiring, research allocation, peer review results, and citation count. In contrast to COVID-19, women bear a different kind of burden. During lockdowns, inequities have a disproportionately negative impact on their well-being and economic resilience. Prenatal and postpartum care for women, as well as sexual and reproductive health services, are disrupted due to overburdened health systems and underfunded charities (Lancet, 2020) .

WOMEN AND MENTAL HEALTH: PRE COVID-SCENARIO

Broad-based macro-level determinants of mental health include by the Human Development Index (HDI), which was examined by the UN in 2000. The HDI was created as a performance indicator that highlights both human outcomes and a nation's economic performance. Other examples of macro-level national indicators include the Gender-related Development Index (GDI) and the Gender Empowerment Index (GEI). They provide measurements of mental health with an appropriate context by describing some fundamental aspects of human development. Epidemiological studies of mental health, cross-national studies of quality of life, conclusions about the link between social determinants and inequalities and health and mental health outcomes, psychometric studies, and findings from health surveillance and monitoring (WHO, 2004).

In India, domestic abuse affected almost two-thirds of married women. Consolidated initiatives on the social, political, economic, and legal levels can transform the lives of Indian women and help to enhance their mental health. As per the report of WHO 2001, Nearly 41.9% of the disability caused by neuropsychiatric diseases in women is attributable to depressive disorders, compared to 29.3% in males. In order to address the mental health of women, education, training, and interventions aimed at the social and physical environment are essential. Identification of significant individuals within government agencies and other pertinent groups in the community is essential in order to collect and document data on the scope of women's problems, the burden associated with those problems, and the development of policies to safeguard and advance women's mental health. The prevalence and course of mental disorders in female sufferers are determined by social and gender-specific factors (Malhotra & Shah, 2015).

Gender inequality and gender differences in mental health are significantly correlated. A population's income distribution is measured by the Gini index which has a strong correlation with male, but not female, prevalence of depressive disorders. There are differences between men and women in depressive illnesses according to a nation's affluence. Social injustices were shown to have varied effects on men's and women's mental health. Also, social factors, particularly gender inequality, may have a significant impact on gender disparities in depressive disorders. The regional effects on gender differences related to depressive illnesses varied across different geographic areas. Community pressure regarding stereotypical social roles based on gender may impact mental health responses differently in women. domestic violence and abuse toward women related to the greater prevalence of mental illness among women (Yu, 2018).

WOMEN AND MENTAL HEALTH: DURING COVID-19 PANDEMIC

Stigma is something that is connected to everyone's worldviews and fosters a particular attitude about the phenomenon. It had been connected to destruction and death from the start of COVID-19. This received a very unfavorable global impression. There are just a few explanations for the COVID-19 controversy. The extremely contagious nature of the illness, laborious preventative measures, social isolation, the lack of specific treatment options, prolonged quarantine, and the possibility of catastrophic consequences and/or death are the elements that contribute to the heightened stigma associated with COVID-19 (Dalal et al., 2020).

The appearance and spread of COVID19, a new disease with the most destructive effects globally, according to the WHO report for the year 2020, has left the general population confused, alarmed, and afraid. Hatred and stigma grow in a climate of fear. As a result of specific communities (those from the north-east of India) being blamed for the outbreak, social stigma has emerged. Women are not exempt from this scenario. Every individual is affected by society's worries and anxieties to varying degrees on a worldwide scale. According to recent research, those who are placed in isolation or quarantine suffer from severe suffering, including anxiety, rage, bewilderment, and post-traumatic stress symptoms. The public's attitudes and understanding are anticipated to have a significant impact on the level of adherence to personal preventive measures and, ultimately, the clinical outcome. Due to COVID 19, people began working remotely, and women were able to work both remotely and at home. One study looked at how women professionals' physical and emotional health were affected by the COVID-19 lockout. According to a recent piece of Indian literature, rumors can encourage people to adopt a variety of undesirable lifestyle and nutritional changes, which can have a negative influence on mental health (Roy et al., 2020).

According to research, when there is a national lockdown because of the pandemic plus other stresses from their jobs, housework, and working from home, it has a significant negative impact on the mental health of women (Sharma & Vaish, 2020). WHO noted that social media is one of the key sources of worry, fear, and stigma, which feed rumors and false information. A recent study found that during the COVID-19 outbreak, there was a significant prevalence of mental health issues that are positively correlated with regular social media use (Gao et al., 2020).

Women complained of pain in their necks, backs, legs, and arms as well as eye strain, and more than 50% of them showed a tendency to overreact in the given circumstance. Research suggests that characteristics related to psychosocial work, such as excessive job stress, poor job control, and psychosocial job expectations, may also be predictors or risk factors for musculoskeletal illnesses (Sharma & Vaish, 2020). The psychological anguish brought on by a situation that is thought to be uncontrollable might result in persistent suffering feelings, which therefore have an impact on health. Musculoskeletal problems may develop from increased muscle tension brought on by psychological discomfort (Roy et al., 2020).

Women who are in a more vulnerable position in the household are more likely to suffer from mental health problems and to be concerned about their safety. While potentially important for public health, containment is associated with significant negative consequences for both standard socioeconomic outcomes and outcomes that are more difficult to observe and measure, such as mental health. A significant phone poll was conducted using India's geographically diverse containment strategies to calculate the relationship between the epidemic, containment strategies, and indicators of women's wellbeing, such as food security and mental health. As a result, there was a 38% rise in the risk that people would report increased despair, a 73% increase in fatigue, and a 44% increase in anxiety. Even more severe reductions in mental health occur in women whose social standing may make them more vulnerable, such as those who have daughters and those who live in households where women are the head of household (Bau et al., 2022).

WOMEN AND MENTAL HEALTH: POST COVID SCENARIO

The perceived threat of the pandemic has a negative impact on mental health. The activation of future anxiety can explain this process, which is moderated by resilience as a personality trait. Individuals with higher levels of resilience are less vulnerable to the pandemic's negative psychological consequences because they experience a lower increase in future anxiety than those with lower levels of resilience. Mental health intervention strategies aimed at strengthening resilience and preventing future anxiety have a significant potential to mitigate the negative impact on mental well-being of the Covid-19 pandemic and the social measures put in place to combat it (Almeida et al., 2020).

In the fight against COVID-19, the female paramedic crew is actively involved. In the global health sector, women make up over 70% of the workforce (Boniol et al., 2019). Evidence suggests that the bulk of them are fighting the virus from the front lines in nursing professions. 90% of the paramedic crew in China are women (Wenham et al., 2020). Despite their active roles and duties, global health organisations in virus-affected nations have not yet conducted a gender analysis of this epidemic. COVID-19 has dealt a severe blow to the informal economy of two billion workers worldwide. Because of their high employment share, female workers are expected to be hit the hardest. For example, the United Nations Women reported that globally, 65 percent of women work in the informal sector and are more vulnerable to economic insecurity (Haldevang, 2020). According to Ministry of Human Rights 2020, an analysis of home-based workers (HBWs), currently 12 million HBWs with an average income of PKR 3,000 to 4,000 will face multidimensional uncertainties due to the lack of social protection schemes for them, financial insecurity, and unprecedented economic vulnerability during the lockdown (Malik & Naeem, 2020).

There was an overall decline in quality of life up to three months after COVID-19. Anxiety (range: 6.5% to 63%), depression (4% to 31%), and post-traumatic stress disorder (12.1% to 46%) were the three most prevalent mental health issues. Female patients and those admitted to intensive care reported higher levels of exhaustion, pain, anxiety, and sadness. Fatigue (range 28% to 87%), pain (myalgia 4.5% to 36%), arthralgia (6.0% to 27%), decreased physical capacity (six-minute walking test range 180 to 561 m), and declines in physical role functioning, usual care, and daily activities (reduced in 15% to 54% of patients) were the most frequently reported physical health issues. Compared to men, women typically suffer exhaustion to a larger degree. This is in line with females being more likely than males to experience chronic fatigue syndrome, which has been associated with stress-related issues. Females were more likely to experience signs of mental illness. This might be because women are more vulnerable to stressors, but more likely it's because more women report experiencing psychological problems (Shanbehzadeh et al., 2021).

COMPARATIVE ANALYSIS OF WOMEN'S MENTAL HEALTH

COVID-19 has affected people of all ages, including children, men, and women. COVID may have different effects on men and women. This book chapter has analyzed the factors, problems and its implications of COVID -19 on women and their mental health. Table 1 provides an overview of the comparative analysis of women's mental health pre, during, and post the COVID scenario.

Table 1. Comparative analysis of women's mental health: Pre, during and post COVID scenario (2000-2018, 2019-2021, 2021 & 2022)

	Pre – COVID (2000-2018)	During COVID (2019 - 2021)	Post - COVID (2021 & 2022)
Factors	Biological – gender disparities, family history of psychiatric illness, inherited conditions and genetic make-up. Social - low socioeconomic status Economical - poor economic condition, poverty	Biological – physical comorbidities, family history of psychiatric illness Psychological - Anxiety, depression, and poor mental health status Economical - loss or potential loss of job, uncertainties regarding economic conditions Mode of working – work from home	Social - low socioeconomic status, living alone Psychological – Quality of Life, post-traumatic stress disorder, work life balance Economical – uncertainties regarding economic conditions, fear of layoff Mode of working – hybrid mode
Challenges/ Concerns/Problems	Domestic abuse Gender inequality Social injustices and stereotypes	Physical Challenges Gender Discrimination Social isolation Emotional health Balancing work for and from home	Mental illness and well-being Economic and Financial insecurity Lack of social protection Physical capacity

SUGGESTIVE MEASURES TO OVERCOME WOMEN'S MENTAL HEALTH CHALLENGES

The preceding discussion clearly calls for gender-based policies to address their vulnerabilities and protect them economically, psychologically, and physically during and post pandemic. National coordination in service delivery is critical. The pandemic response must include both mental health and psychosocial support. Treatment efforts should be accompanied by a response to patients' and their families' psychosocial needs. Coordination of training for facility and community-based health workers is required, as are guidelines for mental health support during outbreaks, which must be made available and disseminated to all service providers. Lockdown and physical separation measures should be contextualized, while cultural characteristics and resources that provide social support and resilience should be utilized. To combat misinformation and fear-based behaviors, strong communication and community engagement are critical. Government has to provide financial health aid to citizens of the country by making effective health policy specifically in India, it's a need of an hour.

FINDINGS AND CONCLUSION

Data collected here is from the various literature, interprets numerous factors that women have faced pre, during and post the Covid-19 time and how it affects her daily life. In this, factors include social, biological, psychological, economical, and physical. The critical challenges faced by working-women is to manage both work and life from Home only, adoption of innovative technology, time dedicated to work may disturb because of family priority, depression towards loosing of job because of gender bias and so on. Women in the category of Work for home face the challenge related to work load as helping hand are now no more available, depression, stress, anxiety, taking care of all family members 24*7 including physical task related to home cleaning and making up a food. Working women's concerns have been identified as children's online education, loneliness at work, isolation at work, overwork, balancing work and life. The major mental health issues reported were stress, anxiety, depression, insomnia, denial, anger, and fear. The community's mental health issues can be diverse and segregated as per the specific group of population. Mental health-related initiatives include mental health and psychosocial considerations during the COVID-19 outbreak, as well as a series of messages that can be used in communications to support mental and psychosocial well-being in different target groups during the outbreak.

REFERENCES

Al-Ali, N. (2020). Covid-19 and feminism in the Global South: Challenges, initiatives and dilemmas. *European Journal of Women's Studies*, *27*(4), 333–347. doi:10.1177/1350506820943617

Almeida, M., Shrestha, A. D., Stojanac, D., & Miller, L. J. (2020). The impact of the COVID-19 pandemic on women's mental health. *Archives of Women's Mental Health*, *23*(6), 741–748. doi:10.100700737-020-01092-2 PMID:33263142

Basak, S. (2021). Factors affecting work-life balance of women in Bangladesh: A study during COVID-19 pandemic. *Canadian Journal of Business and Information Studies*, *3*(3), 38–48.

Bau, N., Khanna, G., Low, C., Shah, M., Sharmin, S., & Voena, A. (2022). Women's Well-being During a Pandemic and its Containment. *Journal of Development Economics*, *156*, 102839. doi:10.1016/j.jdeveco.2022.102839 PMID:35221446

Boniol, M., McIsaac, M., Xu, L., Wuliji, T., Diallo, K., & Campbell, J. (2019). *Gender equity in the health workforce: analysis of 104 countries.* World Health Organization.

Cousins, S. (2020). COVID-19 has "devastating" effect on women and girls. *Lancet, 396*(10247), 301–302. doi:10.1016/S0140-6736(20)31679-2 PMID:32738942

Dalal, P. K., Roy, D., Choudhary, P., Kar, S. K., & Tripathi, A. (2020). Emerging mental health issues during the COVID-19 pandemic: An Indian perspective. *Indian Journal of Psychiatry, 62*(9, Suppl 3), S354. doi:10.4103/psychiatry.IndianJPsychiatry_372_20 PMID:33227050

de Haldevang, M. (2020). *Coronavirus has crippled global protest movements.* Quartz.

Gao, J., Zheng, P., Jia, Y., Chen, H., Mao, Y., Chen, S., Wang, Y., Fu, H., & Dai, J. (2020). Mental health problems and social media exposure during COVID-19 outbreak. *PLoS One, 15*(4), e0231924. doi:10.1371/journal.pone.0231924 PMID:32298385

Horesh, D., Kapel Lev-Ari, R., & Hasson-Ohayon, I. (2020). Risk factors for psychological distress during the COVID-19 pandemic in Israel: Loneliness, age, gender, and health status play an important role. *British Journal of Health Psychology, 25*(4), 925–933. doi:10.1111/bjhp.12455 PMID:32656926

Kumar, D. (2021). What Impact Have SARS-CoV-2/Covid-19 Pandemic on domestic violence against women in India? *How Covid-19 Pandemic Induced Lockdown Influence Mental Health of Women in India.*

Lai, J., Ma, S., Wang, Y., Cai, Z., Hu, J., Wei, N., Wu, J., Du, H., Chen, T., Li, R., Tan, H., Kang, L., Yao, L., Huang, M., Wang, H., Wang, G., Liu, Z., & Hu, S. (2020). Factors associated with mental health outcomes among health care workers exposed to coronavirus disease 2019. *JAMA Network Open, 3*(3), e203976–e203976. doi:10.1001/jamanetworkopen.2020.3976 PMID:32202646

The Lancet. (2020). The gendered dimensions of COVID-19. *Lancet, 395*(10231), 1168. doi:10.1016/S0140-6736(20)30823-0 PMID:32278370

Lokeshvar, R., Deepa, N., Madhivadhani, K., Divya, P., & Asuvathaman, M. (2021). Evaluating the Impact of COVID-19 on Mental Health problems in Indian context. *J Pharm Adv Res, 4*(6), 1296–1301.

Malhotra, S., & Shah, R. (2015). Women and mental health in India: An overview. *Indian Journal of Psychiatry, 57*(6, Suppl 2), S205. doi:10.4103/0019-5545.161479 PMID:26330636

Malik, S., & Naeem, K. (2020). *Impact of COVID-19 Pandemic on Women: Health, livelihoods & domestic violence.*

Maunder, R., Hunter, J., Vincent, L., Bennett, J., Peladeau, N., Leszcz, M., Sadavoy, J., Verhaeghe, L. M., Steinberg, R., & Mazzulli, T. (2003). The immediate psychological and occupational impact of the 2003 SARS outbreak in a teaching hospital. *Canadian Medical Association Journal, 168*(10), 1245–1251. PMID:12743065

WHO. (2004). *Promoting mental health: Concepts, emerging evidence, practice: Summary report.* World Health Organization.

Ramirez, P. T., Chiva, L., Eriksson, A. G. Z., Frumovitz, M., Fagotti, A., Martin, A. G., Jhingran, A., & Pareja, R. (2020). COVID-19 global pandemic: Options for management of gynecologic cancers. [). BMJ Specialist Journals.]. *International Journal of Gynecological Cancer, 30*(5), 561–563. doi:10.1136/ijgc-2020-001419 PMID:32221023

Roy, A., Singh, A. K., Mishra, S., Chinnadurai, A., Mitra, A., & Bakshi, O. (2021). Mental health implications of COVID-19 pandemic and its response in India. *The International Journal of Social Psychiatry, 67*(5), 587–600. doi:10.1177/0020764020950769 PMID:32873106

Roy, D., Tripathy, S., Kar, S. K., Sharma, N., Verma, S. K., & Kaushal, V. (2020). Study of knowledge, attitude, anxiety & perceived mental healthcare need in Indian population during COVID-19 pandemic. *Asian Journal of Psychiatry, 51*, 102083. doi:10.1016/j.ajp.2020.102083 PMID:32283510

Roy, D., Tripathy, S., Kar, S. K., Sharma, N., Verma, S. K., & Kaushal, V. (2020). Study of knowledge, attitude, anxiety & perceived mental healthcare need in Indian population during COVID-19 pandemic. *Asian Journal of Psychiatry, 51*, 102083. doi:10.1016/j.ajp.2020.102083 PMID:32283510

Semo, B., & Frissa, S. M. (2020). The mental health impact of the COVID-19 pandemic: Implications for sub-Saharan Africa. *Psychology Research and Behavior Management, 13*, 713–720. doi:10.2147/PRBM.S264286 PMID:32982500

Shanbehzadeh, S., Tavahomi, M., Zanjari, N., Ebrahimi-Takamjani, I., & Amiri-Arimi, S. (2021). Physical and mental health complications post-COVID-19: Scoping review. *Journal of Psychosomatic Research, 147*, 110525. doi:10.1016/j.jpsychores.2021.110525 PMID:34051516

Sharma, N., & Vaish, H. (2020). Impact of COVID–19 on mental health and physical load on women professionals: An online cross-sectional survey. *Health Care for Women International*, *41*(11–12), 1255–1272. doi:10.1080/07399332.2020.1825441 PMID:33021925

Thibaut, F., & van Wijngaarden-Cremers, P. J. M. (2020). Women's mental health in the time of Covid-19 pandemic. *Frontiers in Global Women's Health*, *1*, 588372. doi:10.3389/fgwh.2020.588372 PMID:34816164

Venugopal, V. C., Mohan, A., & Chennabasappa, L. K. (2022). Status of mental health and its associated factors among the general populace of India during COVID-19 pandemic. *Asia-Pacific Psychiatry*, *14*(2), e12412. doi:10.1111/appy.12412 PMID:32830876

Wenham, C., Smith, J., & Morgan, R. (2020). COVID-19: The gendered impacts of the outbreak. *Lancet*, *395*(10227), 846–848. doi:10.1016/S0140-6736(20)30526-2 PMID:32151325

Yu, S. (2018). Uncovering the hidden impacts of inequality on mental health: A global study. *Translational Psychiatry*, *8*(1), 1–10. doi:10.103841398-018-0148-0 PMID:29777100

Chapter 4
Well-Being of Organizational Leaders in the New Normal

Rahul Paul Gaddam
Vellore Institute of Technology, India

Syed Khalid Perwez
Vellore Institute of Technology, India

ABSTRACT

This chapter discusses that well-being is a skill that has to be mastered by every professional by practicing meditation, sleep, exercise, nutrition, belonging to a community, a spiritual connection, and other factors such as mindfulness training, maintaining the positive psychological capital, and psychological contract in our day-to-day life. This chapter focuses on the impact of mindfulness, psychological capital, and psychological contract on the well-being of organisational leaders. It concludes with the impact of mindfulness, psychological capital, and psychological contract on the well-being of organisational leaders in the new normal.

INTRODUCTION

The pandemic, Covid-19, has changed many organizations to go through a transition as a result of a series of disturbances that helped pave the way for a "new normal". They have been impacted as a result of the introduction of new business models, the rapid acceptance of new technologies, the rise of hybrid and remote work modes, and the workers' ever-shifting requirements and objectives (Krippendorff, 2005). These seismic shifts have also left corporate leaders to struggle with a new challenge in developing meaningful engagement mechanisms that improve both leader's

DOI: 10.4018/978-1-6684-7221-7.ch004

and employee well-being within the context of the new normal (Jena et al., 2018; Oladapo, 2014). For any organization, it is essential that leader play a major role in increasing the positive psychological aspects of an employee (Park et al., 2017).

In the new normal, businesses are fighting a losing battle to maintain employee engagement and motivation (Bhatnagar, 2007; Mulliner, 2018; Rust & Koketso, 2012). While this can be accomplished in a number of different ways, the essential change needs to take place in the mindsets of today's leaders in an organization. It is imperative that leaders move away from viewing employees as merely instruments to be used in the pursuit of organizational goals and instead focus on appreciating and acknowledging the value that employees bring to the workplace. Employees should be viewed as the organization's primary source of strength by its leaders. However, this cannot occur unless management considers the health and engagement of leaders and employees to be essential business priorities rather than merely "nice to have" characteristics (A. Sharma, 2021; Travis et al., 2019).

WELL-BEING IS A SKILL TO BE LEARNED

Well-being as a skill is a daily intention that can be increased by aspects such as meditation, sleep, exercise, nutrition, belonging to a community, a spiritual connection, and other factors (Ayala et al., 2017; Herholdt, 2008). Having a daily intention to be well is a skill. Companies with a forward-thinking mindset will embrace wellness not as a nebulous term but rather as an index of behaviours that can be learned and daily practice. These can be trained in the leaders and also employees by supporting them with mindfulness training and increasing their hope, efficacy, resilience, and optimism (Charoensukmongkol & Suthatorn, 2018).

Just like any other talent, well-being requires consistent, daily practice. Employers who want to develop a workplace that places an emphasis on well-being will treat it as a growth priority by implementing self-assessment activities and assessing improvement in relation to the skills required to attain well-being in the workplace (Grossmeier et al., 2016; Mellor & Webster, 2013). Both leaders and employees are able to track their own growth as a result of this, as well as identify their beginning places and uncover the building pieces that make up their work. Every one of them will have a unique combination of behaviours and experiences that, on the one hand, contribute to a pleasant sense of well-being, and, on the other, lead to feelings of tension, worry, or discomfort. It is essential to acknowledge this fact and make conscious efforts to acquire the qualities that contribute to improved health.

Organisations with a vision towards the future will enable and empower their leaders and employees to select the appropriate combination of tools and experiences to meet their unique requirements. Taking the time to recharge might mean different things to different people. For others, it means making sure they get enough sleep, exercise, or diet. Some people may place more importance on making time for mindfulness practises, stepping away from technological distractions, or reengaging with their communities.

Employees will look for leaders who not only make a commitment to promoting employee health and wellness, but also provide clear and easy access to assistance for workers who may require it, as well as the ability to tailor their methods to the specific needs of individual workers. This will boost the loyalty and psychological contract of the employees towards the leaders and their organisation.

CULTIVATING WELL-BEING SKILLS FOR THE BETTER FUTURE

Through mentoring of the employees and participation in formal learning opportunities, leaders will be able to strengthen their skills in areas such as problem-solving, communicating, efficacy, resilience and taking the lead at work (Basadur, 2004; Steinke et al., 2015). In the same vein, taking care of one's health and wellness ought to be regarded as a mission-essential talent that may be enhanced through various training and development programmes.

It is essential for leaders to place equal importance on the professional and personal well-being of their subordinates and peers (Plomp et al., 2016; Schabracq, 2003). It is also the leaders' duty to serve as a positive example for their subordinates and give priority by assisting their subordinates in their own endeavours. It may be as easy as incorporating well-being into the agenda of team meetings and making sure that essential resources, such as self-help tools, are within easy reach. Leaders can eliminate a work culture that implies work should come before personal needs and empower employees to invest in themselves so that they can be at their best for others by having open conversations about the importance of self-care and backing up those conversations with significant action. This will eliminate a work culture that suggests work should come before personal needs.

Leaders needs to be equipped with the skills necessary to create a secure environment that allows the employees to discuss on their mental health. It is impossible to attain well-being without first building work environments in which individuals are given the authority to prioritise themselves and openly discuss their mental health, in the same way that they might discuss a broken arm. The employees must get the early intervention support to those who are experiencing psychological distress and should provide the resources that will assist employees in the development of skills that will nurture their well-being and build emotional flexibility. At this day, when technology enables the demands of work to penetrate our lives every second, there is a clear case for businesses to acquire the skills necessary for their employees to maintain their health and well-being. As leaders work through the difficulties of the present, the extent to which they are able to promote well-being despite the unpredictability of the future will define the efficacy of the leadership.

IMPACT OF MINDFULNESS ON THE WELL-BEING OF LEADERS

Mindfulness can be regarded as an important psychological concept that leaders are required to consider in regard to the process of managing their responsibilities. It is a fact that psychologists have scant knowledge regarding the factors that can make life worth living (Seligman & Csikszentmihalyi, 2014). They have been able to understand a bit about how people are surviving and enduring under conditions of adversity. In this regard, it is important to state that mindfulness is an important psychological concept that helps them to survive and it can also provide a significant effect on the well-being of leaders. Mindfulness can be regarded as a type of meditation in which people focus on being intensively aware of what they are sensing and of what they are feeling in a moment.

In this regard, they do not get judgmental or do not try to interpret their feeling rather than trying to feel their actual sense. In order to survive in the dynamic and ever-changing world where people can face dilemmatic situation anytime, being mindfulness and less judgmental becomes necessary as it helps people to get a clear perception regarding the situation of the world around. Apart from that, through mindfulness, a person can be highly able to explore own qualities and self-awareness is something that can enable a person to become more suitable for the dilemmatic world and mindfulness is something that can enhance the self-awareness of people. In order to be successful in professional and personal life, being mindful is highly important.

Productivity can be increased through the cultivation of managerial skills (Konte, 2021; Venturella et al., 2018). These skills include personality (Khan et al., 2010), emotional maturity (Jalili Nikoo et al., 2018; Kulkarni et al., 2021; Saadatkhah et al., 2021), and self-reflection (Ardelt & Grunwald, 2018; Knapp et al., 2017). Achieving stronger leadership abilities, such as performance, group cohesion, and decision-making intelligence can be accomplished through cultivating mindfulness, which has a positive effect on performance (Carleton et al., 2018). This direct influence is made possible by the aspects of mindfulness that enable a company to effectively communicate information; have a greater attentiveness to social relations; have a perspective that assists in making decisions in the present moment; have the resilience to deal with challenges; and have overall good health. (Glomb et al., 2011; Kotzé,

2021; Malinowski & Lim, 2015; Wells & Klocko, 2018) Research has shown that practicing mindfulness can improve both leadership and employee performance. This is accomplished by enhancing psychological well-being and building resilience, both of which lead to more effective performance.

Research has shown that practicing mindfulness can help relieve stress, stimulate sluggish areas of the brain, and improve creative thinking and problem-solving abilities (Al-Shargie & GOH, 2019; Hassed & Chambers, 2014; Nayak & Shenoi, 2013; Norris & Currieri, 1999; Reiner, 2019; Stinson & Arthur, 2013; Wells & Klocko, 2018). The most considerable proof would be the indirect influence of attention being paid to skill in transformational leadership in intervention initiatives employing qualitative methodologies (Rahman et al., 2017). Because therapies for web-based awareness only require a few minutes over the course of many days for modest research efficiency, the negative impact that awareness has on genuine, ethical leadership should be investigated further.

According to the viewpoint of (Brown et al., 2007; Brown & Ryan, 2003; Frisch, 2005; Hyland, 2015, 2016; Vohra & Pandey, 2018; Wise et al., 2012), it can be stated that many philosophical, spiritual, and psychological traditions place a strong emphasis on the value of consciousness as a quality for the preservation and improvement of well-being. The practice of mindfulness is something that is quite important in this regard. When the perspectives of these authors are taken into consideration, it is possible to assert that attention and awareness can be seen of as being an essential component of regular functioning.

Mindfulness, on the other hand, has been shown to significantly boost people's attention and awareness, which in turn can result in a more effective way of dealing with challenging situations. Leaders play a very important part in the accomplishment of goals and processes (al Khajeh, 2018). Awareness and attention are two attributes that one must possess in order for one to be successful in their career. Mindfulness is the most important idea that people must think about in a concrete way if they want to make major use of these qualities. Without sufficient mindfulness, it is impossible for a leader to be extremely attentive and aware of the needs of the circumstance. It is impossible for a leader to handle situational deals in an appropriate manner if they do not have this knowledge or attentiveness (Gonzalez, 2012; Mahfouz, 2018).

Awareness and attention in relation to psychological and behavioral functioning have been examined in a number of different theories that are relevant to self-regulation. In this regard, the self-regulation theory is the one that ought to be taken into consideration as an explanation. In light of this notion, having an open awareness may be of great help in influencing the selection of behaviors that are consistent with one's requirements and principles. In an ideal world, leaders will be able to alter their behaviors to better suit their requirements, which will, in the end, contribute to their overall sense of well-being. The upshot of practicing mindfulness is open awareness, and it is in this area that the obvious effect on the well-being of leaders can be observed (Brown et al., 2007; Brown & Ryan, 2004, 2015; de Bruin et al., 2014; Glomb et al., 2011; Lyvers et al., 2014; Parto & Besharat, 2011; Rigby et al., 2014; Schultz & Ryan, 2015; Snyder et al., 2012).

By taking into account the idea of mindfulness, (Brown & Ryan, 2003) researchers have been able to evaluate day-to-day self-regulatory and emotional well-being. According to the findings of the research, practicing mindfulness confers the ability to forecast more autonomous activities in day-to-day life and can control the adverse impacts of stressful situations. A person's level of self-assurance increases when they experience fewer negative impacts as a result of their actions and discover that those actions are very effective in meeting the requirements of the scenario. As a consequence of this, the person becomes more aware of the success, and as a result of this, the person's degree of confidence also gets strengthened, which ultimately results in the process of the leader's well-being improving. In light of all of these considerations, it is possible to assert that a leader has to practice mindfulness in order to become more effective and to ensure their mental and emotional well-being.

IMPACT OF PSYCHOLOGICAL CAPITAL ON THE WELL-BEING OF LEADERS

Psychological capital is nothing other than the set of resources that an individual can use in order to improve their performance on the job and in order to ensure their success. By considering the viewpoint of (Gupta & Singh, 2014), it can be stated that psychological capital is found affecting a variety of variables that include the performance of employees, job satisfaction, and organizational commitment. It is a fact that earlier studies have been able to document a positive relationship between psychological capacities and creativity in non-R and D contexts. On the other hand, by going through the article written by these authors, it has also been possible to understand that the capacities that are included in psychological capital are considered as states rather than traits and they are highly open to development. The resources that fall under the psychological capital concept are self-efficiency, optimism, resilience, and hope. In this regard, it is important to state that it is possible to coach and train psychological capitals. In order to work in an effective manner, the importance of having all of these resources is important. On the other hand, leaders face the requirement to have the ability to improve these particular resources of employees. Here, the importance of the concept in regard to the field of leadership can be found. In the following section of the study paper, a detailed discussion regarding the concept in regard to the well-being of leadership is going to be illustrated by considering the viewpoint of different authors.

The researchers investigated the potential mediating mechanism of the well-known constructive multi-model of PsyCap, focusing on the negative link between leaders' awareness and a variety of dysfunctional outcomes (King & Haar, 2017; Roche et al., 2014). PsyCap is an employee's positive state of mind of progress that is characterized by having credibility (efficacy), generating important cognitions and possessing brighter future preconceptions (optimism); persisting toward objectives and, when required, diverting pathways to aspirations (hope); and jumping back from failure (resilience). PsyCap is also characterized by an employee's ability to bounce back from a setback. Additionally, it is distinguished by positive psychology and positive organizational behavior (resilience), all of which contribute to its overall success (Luthans, Avey, & Patera, 2008; Luthans, Avey, et al., 2006; Luthans, Avolio, et al., 2007; Luthans, Youssef, et al., 2007; Magnano et al., 2016).

PsyCap has been found to have a positive association with favorable attitudes, behaviors, actions, effectiveness, and mental and emotional well-being of staff members, as well as a potential conflict with skepticism, intentions to turn over, and employee absenteeism, according to the findings of the most recent thematic analysis (Arghode et al., 2021; Darr & Johns, 2008; B.-J. Kim, 2019; Riasudeen & Singh, 2021; Tanjung et al., 2021). In addition to this, as was said earlier, mindfulness has been found to be a vital component in the process of cultivating knowledgeable and self-determined behavioral autonomy and independence related to psychological health (Roche et al., 2014).

(Avey, Reichard, et al., 2011; Kappagoda et al., 2014; Newman et al., 2014) have said that PsyCap, also considered as PsyCap, has been conceptually identified by Luthans and colleagues. Hope, resilience, optimism, and a sense of one's own efficacy are the four positive psychological resources that make up the notion, when their respective conceptual standpoints are taken into consideration. As soon as it is possible to unite all of these different aspects, it will then be possible to identify it as the second-order core construct. It is essential to state that a second-order construct is a variance among the four first-order constructs; hope, optimism, resilience, and efficacy (Hizam-Hanafiah et al., 2017; Jones et al., 2013; Kotzé, 2018; Mathe et al., 2017; Wernsing, 2014). This is because it becomes essential to state that a second-order construct is a variance among the four first-order constructs.

There has been supplied here a definition of PsyCap that is both unambiguous and all-encompassing. According to the definition, it is considered to be the favorable psychological condition of an individual that is related with the individual's progression. It is considered a personal asset that can contribute to an increase in the efficiency of one's work(Kappagoda et al., 2014; Kotzé, 2018; Newman et al., 2014). Taking into account the definition of the idea, it is possible to assert that PsyCap operates in a variety of modes. It helps people develop a positive belief in their ability to succeed both now and in the future by pursuing their goals, and it gives people the assurance they need to put forth the necessary effort to prevail in trying circumstances. Considering the necessity of situational requirements can help people redirect the path toward their goals (Baluku et al., 2016; du Plessis & Barkhuizen, 2012; Luthans, Avey, & Patera, 2008; Luthans, Avolio, et al., 2007; Luthans et al., 2010; Luthans, Vogelgesang, et al., 2006).

Apart from them, other researchers (Britt et al., 2016; Luthans, Avey, Clapp-Smith, et al., 2008; Luthans, Vogelgesang, et al., 2006; Luthans, Youssef, et al., 2007; Luthans & Broad, 2022; Patnaik et al., 2021; Rabenu & Tziner, 2021; S. Sharma & Sharma, 2016) have stated that, it's helpful for an individual to learn how to deal with the requirements of different situations. When one considers the obligations of a leader, it is possible to state that a leader confronts the complete circumstance. For instance, facing challenges, dealing with the dynamic situation by taking into account the actual requirements of the situation, managing challenges with confidence, and being committed to goals are all factors that can be regarded as some important responsibilities of a leader, and in order for a leader to be able to handle all of these responsibilities, they need to have PsyCap (Chully et al., 2022; M. Kim et al., 2019; Malik & Dhar, 2017; Walumbwa et al., 2011).

According to the findings of a number of studies, the psychological well-being of employees, their level of job satisfaction, and their PsyCap score all play an important part in the human resources of an organization (Kurt & Demirbolat, 2018). PsyCap is built on a number of fundamental pillars, one of which is efficacy, which focuses on having confidence. A leader will never achieve success in their endeavors if they do not have sufficient self-assurance. Because of the challenges they confront, even effective leaders are susceptible to experiencing mental and emotional breakdowns (Chemers et al., 2000; "Leader Self-Regulation: The Role of Self-Efficacy and Multiple Intelligences," 2021; Lee et al., 2017; Luthans, 2002; Murphy & Ensher, 2008). Efficacy, on the other hand, enables a leader to maintain control over both their mental and emotional condition in any given circumstance, in addition to helping them achieve a high level of confidence. This demonstrates the significance of effectiveness with regard to the mental well-being of leaders (Armour, 2020; Broad & Luthans, 2017; Luthans & Avolio, 2003).

On the other side, a positive attribution is necessary for a leader in order to be able to cope with challenges. However, with the optimism that one gains from PsyCap, one becomes capable of dealing with any kind of challenging circumstance with the maximum level of positivity (Avey, Avolio, et al., 2011; Humphrey, 2002; Luthans & Avolio, 2003; A. Rego et al., 2012; Steinberg & Elmer, 2022). The significance of this component with regard to the functioning of a leader, as well as the health and happiness of a leader, can be shown here.

PsyCap is built on a number of foundational ideas, one of which being hope. It provides assistance to leaders in coping with any form of unfavorable situation in the interest of achieving something positive in the future. It makes a good impact on the leaders' mental state while also assisting them in maintaining a positive emotional condition (Avey, Reichard, et al., 2011; Avolio & Gardner, 2005; Luthans, 2002; Park et al., 2017; Peterson & Luthans, 2003; P. Rego et al., 2016). The mental and emotional factors significantly affect the well-being of leaders, and here their relationship is evident (Bernerth & Hirschfeld, 2016; Roche et al., 2014; Zineldin & Hytter, 2012).

It is generally acknowledged that leadership is one of the most significant things that can successfully increase the performance of employees (Demir & Budur, 2019). Resilience is yet another crucial aspect of this equation that must be taken into consideration. Considering the discussion made in the above-stated passages, it can be stated that resilience is nothing other than a person's ability to be beset by problems and adversity and having the ability to sustain and bounce and even beyond to attain success (Luthans et al., 2010). It is possible for the functioning of an organization as a whole to be disrupted if its leaders lose their patience in maintaining the status quo and begin to give up readily. Aside from that, having less patience than is required for a task can hinder a leader's chances of being promoted to a higher position. It has the potential to put them in a condition of frustration as well as another mental estate, both of which have the potential to destroy their mental strength and emotional capabilities. Additionally, it may have an effect on their physical health. The calming effect of resilience, which assists leaders in avoiding such repercussions, is one manner in which resilience positively influences the well-being of leaders (Athota, 2021; Dimas et al., 2018; Ihme & Sundstrom, 2021; Koprowski et al., 2021; Spialek et al., 2016).

IMPACT OF PSYCHOLOGICAL CONTRACT ON THE WELL-BEING OF LEADERS

It is a fact that in this changing world everything has become more formal. Now, people trust others by considering the written deals that have been developed among them. However, the matter is that in such a dilemmatic situation, a psychological contract is something that can strengthen the trust among people, mainly employees, and employers. It can be regarded as the unwritten and intangible agreement that is developed among employees and their employers. It describes the informal commitment, expectations, and related understanding that can strengthen their relationship. Though this contract is mainly applicable in the case of employees and employees, the application of it in regard to other relationships is also evident. It is a fact that the world is getting more and more challenging and diplomatic. In this world, people do not trust others just by considering their words. It becomes important to develop written agreements in order to develop a relationship of trust. However, the matter is that beyond written agreements, there are soothing that people want to trust. For instance, there are many things that employers do not read in the agreement that they developed when they give joining to someone. They trust their employees that they would work by considering the requirements of the business in the best possible manner. On the other hand, without having a written explanation, employees develop an understanding of the requirements of employers. They understand what employers are expecting from them and they also develop an effective perception regarding the benefits or obligations that they can experience from the side of employers. This kind of relationship can be regarded as the outcome of a psychological contract. Employee loyalty can be regarded as a psychological condition and it describes the relationship between employees and the organization. This contract can boost loyalty effectively. It undoubtedly strengthens a relationship while developing a mental bridge between employees and employers. It is a fact that agreements and written contracts are important. However, it is also important to mention that it is impossible for employers or employees to express all of their expectations through agreements. On the other hand, it is also impossible to express the ways through which they should understand each other just by writing some agreements and contracts. In order to be successful in this regard, they have to develop a psychological contract with their employees first.

Organizations are actively successful in protecting their managerial leadership incentives at the workplace and maximising staff retention in every feasible way (Rothwell, 2010). As a consequence of this, the state in question places a strong focus on the requirement of a psychological contract being in place between employees and employers in order to raise the level of employee engagement in firms (Naidoo et al., 2019). In particular, interpersonal connections are comprised not just of the responsibilities that employees believe their employer owes them, but also of the responsibilities that individuals believe they ought to perform for their employer in return. The research on emotional commitment has uncovered two fundamental components: procedural contracts, which are centred on the concept of work-reward, and relational contracts, which are not predicated on monetary rewards or empathic contracts. Both of these components are equally important (Antoinette Bargagliotti, 2012; Rifai, 2005). Additionally, the social learning theory provides support for the interpersonal psychological contract, which is necessary for establishing long-term employee engagement and productivity (Peng et al., 2016; Rayton et al., 2015).

In recent decades, scholars have devoted a significant amount of attention to investigating the psychological contract theory (Caldwell & Hasan, 2016; Chen et al., 2008; Henderson et al., 2008). The psychological contract focuses mostly on the behaviours that are appropriate within the context of a relationship between two people. These duties are frequently unspoken, mutual, and hazy, and the resolutions to them depend on the actions taken by both employers and employees (Cullinane & Dundon, 2006; Fehr & Falk, 2002; Walker & Hutton, 2006). It is also possible to categorise it as a relationship and as transformative in the context of a psychological contract. The transaction contract is just for a limited time and is primarily concerned with the financial and economic benefits, whereas the relationship contract is for the longer term and takes into account the social, economic, and financial context (Baec & Shin, 2017; Epitropaki, 2013; Goodwin et al., 2001; McDermott et al., 2013).

Within this context, a conversation about the psychological contract has already taken place. Now, it is essential to have a conversation about the significance of it in the context of the area of leadership that will be detailed. The success of a group is directly correlated to the quality of its leaders (Densten, 2005; Howell & Shamir, 2005; Joseph, 2016; Koning & van Kleef, 2015). They are accountable for handling a number of different works. Leaders are required to manage a wide range of activities, including hiring personnel, providing them with equipment, and directing them in their work (Blanchard & Hodges, 2008). However, the fact of the problem is that in order for them to handle all of these activities in a significant method, they are going to be required to establish productive relationships with members of the team. It is impossible to establish the relationship while taking into consideration certain agreements or contracts because there needs to be a good understanding between the leaders and the members (Ahmad et al., 2018). The idea of the psychological contract served as the foundation for the development of these comprehensions.

It is necessary for leaders to make efficient use of this notion in order to gain a deeper understanding of the people who work for them. It is a well-established truth that employee engagement can be conceptualised as a state of mind on the part of the workforce (Luthans & Peterson, 2002; Truss et al., 2013). However, the fact of the issue is that it becomes hard for a leader to increase the level of engagement that employees have towards the work they do without first gaining a proper understanding of those individuals. Leaders can gain an understanding of the employees working under their control by utilising psychological contracts (Caron et al., 2019; Low et al., 2016). It is much simpler for a leader to be effective in their role when they are able to comprehend the needs and desires of the people they are responsible for leading. In the end, it has an effect on the well-being of the leader by having a beneficial influence on the person's mental fortitude and degree of confidence (Erkutlu & Chafra, 2013).

Psychological contracts will help the leaders to understanding their employees by making simpler for a leader to be effective in their role when they are able to comprehend the needs and desires of the people they are responsible for leading. The beneficial influence on the person's mental fortitude and degree of confidence will positively affect the well-being of the leader.

CONCLUSION

Leaders need more resources to protect themselves against the ever-increasing pressures of professional growth and day-to-day operations. Mindfulness has recently seen a resurgence as a potential positive addition to the cognitive defensive systems of leaders, as well as a constructive and proactive commitment to the emotional well-being of those leaders. Excitement always overcomes the truth when it comes to any new idea whose early prominence may be termed a trend; this is especially true regarding awareness and its stated leadership advantages. In situations like these, the scientific enterprise fulfils a function that is entirely unique.

Better PsyCap and job performance are either overtly or implicitly associated, with the decreasing features of mindfulness including psychological weariness, anxiety, sadness, and the harmful effect. The study topic was taken into consideration, which led to the generation of topics, and a debate was produced by taking into consideration the themes as well as the points of view of the authors of existing literary pieces. Through the examination of a variety of written works, it has been feasible to gain an understanding of how mindfulness, PsyCap, and the psychological contract can have a substantial impact on the well-being of leaders. In addition to this, it has the potential to effectively motivate subordinates to achieve the greatest possible performance for the organisation.

Theorists from a number of different schools of personality and psychology have, it is a well-established fact, explored the significance of open awareness, observance, and attention in relation to the enhancement of self-regulation and overall well-being. The job of a leader is extremely challenging since they are required to interact with people who come from a variety of backgrounds and have a variety of perspectives. In order to deal with them appropriately while also taking into consideration their own well-being, the first thing that they need to do is become adequately informed of both them and their suitability in relation to a work. It has the potential to make them more effective participants in the process of resolving the crisis. When a leader is able to handle challenging events with the appropriate level of confidence, awareness, and attention, a positive outcome is produced as a result. It has a beneficial effect on the psychological condition of a leader, which in turn has an impact on their mental well-being.

REFERENCES

Ahmad, I., Donia, M. B. L., Khan, A., & Waris, M. (2018). Do as I say, and do as I do? The mediating role of psychological contract fulfillment in the relationship between ethical leadership and employee extra-role performance. *Personnel Review*.

al Khajeh, E. H. (2018). Impact of leadership styles on organizational performance. *Journal of Human Resources Management Research, 2018*, 1–10. doi:10.5171/2018.687849

Al-Shargie, F., & GOH, C. M. (2019). Cognitive Enhancement Techniques and Their Impact on Performance Improvements. *RE:view*.

Antoinette Bargagliotti, L. (2012). Work engagement in nursing: A concept analysis. *Journal of Advanced Nursing*, *68*(6), 1414–1428. doi:10.1111/j.1365-2648.2011.05859.x PMID:22044047

Ardelt, M., & Grunwald, S. (2018). The importance of self-reflection and awareness for human development in hard times. *Research in Human Development*, *15*(3–4), 187–199. doi:10.1080/15427609.2018.1489098

Arghode, V., Lathan, A., Alagaraja, M., Rajaram, K., & McLean, G. N. (2021). Empathic organizational culture and leadership: Conceptualizing the framework. *European Journal of Training and Development*.

Armour, R. (2020). *Transformational versus servant leadership: Their role on employee eudaimonic well-being*.

Athota, V. S. (2021). Lessons from failures. In *Mind over Matter and Artificial Intelligence* (pp. 49–56). Springer. doi:10.1007/978-981-16-0482-9_5

Avey, J. B., Avolio, B. J., & Luthans, F. (2011). Experimentally analyzing the impact of leader positivity on follower positivity and performance. *The Leadership Quarterly*, *22*(2), 282–294. doi:10.1016/j.leaqua.2011.02.004

Avey, J. B., Reichard, R. J., Luthans, F., & Mhatre, K. H. (2011). Meta-analysis of the impact of positive psychological capital on employee attitudes, behaviors, and performance. *Human Resource Development Quarterly*, *22*(2), 127–152. doi:10.1002/hrdq.20070

Avolio, B. J., & Gardner, W. L. (2005). Authentic leadership development: Getting to the root of positive forms of leadership. *The Leadership Quarterly*, *16*(3), 315–338. doi:10.1016/j.leaqua.2005.03.001

Ayala, E. E., Omorodion, A. M., Nmecha, D., Winseman, J. S., & Mason, H. R. C. (2017). What do medical students do for self-care? A student-centered approach to well-being. *Teaching and Learning in Medicine*, *29*(3), 237–246. doi:10.1080/10401334.2016.1271334 PMID:28632007

Baec, C.-Y., & Shin, J.-G. (2017). The Differential Effects of Transformational Leadership and Organizational Justice on Work Engagement: The Mediating Role of Psychological Contract Breach. *The Journal of The Korea Contents Association, 17*(1), 299–336. doi:10.5392/JKCA.2017.17.01.299

Baluku, M. M., Kikooma, J. F., & Kibanja, G. M. (2016). Psychological capital and the startup capital–entrepreneurial success relationship. *Journal of Small Business and Entrepreneurship, 28*(1), 27–54. doi:10.1080/08276331.2015.1132512

Basadur, M. (2004). Leading others to think innovatively together: Creative leadership. *The Leadership Quarterly, 15*(1), 103–121. doi:10.1016/j.leaqua.2003.12.007

Bernerth, J. B., & Hirschfeld, R. R. (2016). The subjective well-being of group leaders as explained by the quality of leader–member exchange. *The Leadership Quarterly, 27*(4), 697–710. doi:10.1016/j.leaqua.2016.04.003

Bhatnagar, J. (2007). Talent management strategy of employee engagement in Indian ITES employees: Key to retention. *Employee Relations, 29*(6), 640–663. doi:10.1108/01425450710826122

Blanchard, K., & Hodges, P. (2008). *Lead like Jesus: Lessons from the greatest leadership role model of all time*. Thomas Nelson.

Britt, T. W., Shen, W., Sinclair, R. R., Grossman, M. R., & Klieger, D. M. (2016). How much do we really know about employee resilience? *Industrial and Organizational Psychology: Perspectives on Science and Practice, 9*(2), 378–404. doi:10.1017/iop.2015.107

Broad, J. D., & Luthans, F. (2017). Leading and developing health and safety through collective psychological capital. *Leading to Occupational Health and Safety: How Leadership Behaviours Impact Organizational Safety and Well-Being, 255.*

Brown, K. W., & Ryan, R. M. (2003). The Benefits of Being Present: Mindfulness and Its Role in Psychological Well-Being. In Journal of Personality and Social Psychology, 84(4). doi:10.1037/0022-3514.84.4.822

Brown, K. W., & Ryan, R. M. (2004). Fostering healthy self-regulation from within and without: A self-determination theory perspective. *Positive Psychology in Practice*, 105–124.

Brown, K. W., & Ryan, R. M. (2015). A self-determination theory perspective on fostering healthy self-regulation from within and without. *Positive Psychology in Practice: Promoting Human Flourishing in Work, Health, Education, and Everyday Life, 2*, 139–157. doi:10.1002/9781118996874.ch9

Brown, K. W., Ryan, R. M., & Creswell, J. D. (2007). Mindfulness: Theoretical foundations and evidence for its salutary effects. *Psychological Inquiry*, *18*(4), 211–237. doi:10.1080/10478400701598298

Caldwell, C., & Hasan, Z. (2016). Covenantal leadership and the psychological contract: Moral insights for the modern leader. *Journal of Management Development*, *35*(10), 1302–1312. doi:10.1108/JMD-02-2016-0027

Carleton, E. L., Barling, J., & Trivisonno, M. (2018). Leaders' trait mindfulness and transformational leadership: The mediating roles of leaders' positive affect and leadership self-efficacy. *Canadian Journal of Behavioural Science/Revue Canadienne Des Sciences Du Comportement, 50*(3), 185.

Caron, J., Asselin, H., Beaudoin, J.-M., & Muresanu, D. (2019). Promoting perceived insider status of indigenous employees: A review within the psychological contract framework. *Cross Cultural & Strategic Management*, *26*(4), 609–638. doi:10.1108/CCSM-02-2019-0031

Charoensukmongkol, P., & Suthatorn, P. (2018). Salespeople's trait mindfulness and emotional exhaustion: The mediating roles of optimism, resilience, and self-efficacy. *International Journal of Services. Economics and Management*, *9*(2), 125–142.

Chemers, M. M., Watson, C. B., & May, S. T. (2000). Dispositional affect and leadership effectiveness: A comparison of self-esteem, optimism, and efficacy. *Personality and Social Psychology Bulletin*, *26*(3), 267–277. doi:10.1177/0146167200265001

Chen, Z. X., Tsui, A. S., & Zhong, L. (2008). Reactions to psychological contract breach: A dual perspective. *Journal of Organizational Behavior: The International Journal of Industrial. Occupational and Organizational Psychology and Behavior*, *29*(5), 527–548. doi:10.1002/job.481

Chully, A. A., Jose, J., & Luthufi, M. (2022). Authentic leadership in a pandemic world: an exploratory study in the Indian context. *Journal of Management Development*.

Cullinane, N., & Dundon, T. (2006). The psychological contract: A critical review. *International Journal of Management Reviews*, *8*(2), 113–129. doi:10.1111/j.1468-2370.2006.00123.x

Darr, W., & Johns, G. (2008). Work strain, health, and absenteeism: A meta-analysis. *Journal of Occupational Health Psychology*, *13*(4), 293–318. doi:10.1037/a0012639 PMID:18837626 de Bruin, E. I., Zijlstra, B. J. H., & Bögels, S. M. (2014). The meaning of mindfulness in children and adolescents: Further validation of the Child and Adolescent Mindfulness Measure (CAMM) in two independent samples from the Netherlands. *Mindfulness*, *5*(4), 422–430.

Demir, A., & Budur, T. (2019). Roles of leadership styles in corporate social responsibility to non-governmental organizations (NGOs). *International Journal of Social Sciences & Educational Studies*, *5*(4), 174–183.

Densten, I. L. (2005). The relationship between visioning behaviours of leaders and follower burnout. *British Journal of Management*, *16*(2), 105–118. doi:10.1111/j.1467-8551.2005.00428.x

Dimas, I. D., Rebelo, T., Lourenço, P. R., & Pessoa, C. I. P. (2018). Bouncing back from setbacks: On the mediating role of team resilience in the relationship between transformational leadership and team effectiveness. *The Journal of Psychology*, *152*(6), 358–372. doi:10.1080/00223980.2018.1465022 PMID:30089085

du Plessis, Y., & Barkhuizen, N. (2012). Psychological capital, a requisite for organisational performance in South Africa. *Suid-Afrikaanse Tydskrif vir Ekonomiese en Bestuurswetenskappe*, *15*(1), 16–30. doi:10.4102ajems.v15i1.122

Epitropaki, O. (2013). A multi-level investigation of psychological contract breach and organizational identification through the lens of perceived organizational membership: Testing a moderated–mediated model. *Journal of Organizational Behavior*, *34*(1), 65–86. doi:10.1002/job.1793

Erkutlu, H., & Chafra, J. (2013). Effects of trust and psychological contract violation on authentic leadership and organizational deviance. *Management Research Review*, *36*(9), 828–848. doi:10.1108/MRR-06-2012-0136

Fehr, E., & Falk, A. (2002). Psychological foundations of incentives. *European Economic Review*, *46*(4–5), 687–724. doi:10.1016/S0014-2921(01)00208-2

Frisch, M. B. (2005). *Quality of life therapy: Applying a life satisfaction approach to positive psychology and cognitive therapy*. John Wiley & Sons.

Glomb, T. M., Duffy, M. K., Bono, J. E., & Yang, T. (2011). Mindfulness at work. In *Research in personnel and human resources management*. Emerald Group Publishing Limited. doi:10.1108/S0742-7301(2011)0000030005

Gonzalez, M. (2012). *Mindful leadership: The 9 ways to self-awareness, transforming yourself, and inspiring others*. John Wiley & Sons.

Goodwin, V. L., Wofford, J. C., & Whittington, J. L. (2001). A theoretical and empirical extension to the transformational leadership construct. *Journal of Organizational Behavior: The International Journal of Industrial. Occupational and Organizational Psychology and Behavior*, *22*(7), 759–774. doi:10.1002/job.111

Grossmeier, J., Fabius, R., Flynn, J. P., Noeldner, S. P., Fabius, D., Goetzel, R. Z., & Anderson, D. R. (2016). Linking workplace health promotion best practices and organizational financial performance. *Journal of Occupational and Environmental Medicine*, *58*(1), 16–23. doi:10.1097/JOM.0000000000000631 PMID:26716844

Gupta, V., & Singh, S. (2014). Psychological capital as a mediator of the relationship between leadership and creative performance behaviors: Empirical evidence from the Indian R&D sector. *International Journal of Human Resource Management*, *25*(10), 1373–1394. doi:10.1080/09585192.2013.870311

Hassed, C., & Chambers, R. (2014). *Mindful Learning: Reduce stress and improve brain performance for effective learning* (Vol. 3). Exisle Publishing.

Henderson, D. J., Wayne, S. J., Shore, L. M., Bommer, W. H., & Tetrick, L. E. (2008). Leader—member exchange, differentiation, and psychological contract fulfillment: A multilevel examination. *The Journal of Applied Psychology*, *93*(6), 1208–1219. doi:10.1037/a0012678 PMID:19025243

Herholdt, M. D. (2008). An integrated approach to human existence with spirituality as a facet of wellness: spirituality and well-being. *Practical Theology in South Africa= Praktiese Teologie in Suid-Afrika, 23*(1), 183–200.

Hizam-Hanafiah, M., Yousaf, S. U., & Usman, B. (2017). The influence of psychological capital on the growth intentions of entrepreneurs: A study on Malaysian SME entrepreneurs. *Business and Economic Horizons (BEH), 13*(1232-2019–722), 556–569.

Howell, J. M., & Shamir, B. (2005). The role of followers in the charismatic leadership process: Relationships and their consequences. *Academy of Management Review*, *30*(1), 96–112. doi:10.5465/amr.2005.15281435

Humphrey, R. H. (2002). The many faces of emotional leadership. *The Leadership Quarterly*, *13*(5), 493–504. Advance online publication. doi:10.1016/S1048-9843(02)00140-6

Hyland, T. (2015). On the contemporary applications of mindfulness: Some implications for education. *Journal of Philosophy of Education*, *49*(2), 170–186. doi:10.1111/1467-9752.12135

Hyland, T. (2016). The limits of mindfulness: Emerging issues for education. *British Journal of Educational Studies*, *64*(1), 97–117. doi:10.1080/00071005.2015.1051946

Ihme, K. R. M., & Sundstrom, P. (2021). The mindful shield: The effects of mindfulness training on resilience and leadership in military leaders. *Perspectives in Psychiatric Care*, *57*(2), 675–688. doi:10.1111/ppc.12594 PMID:32740947

Jalili Nikoo, S., Ghasemi Jobaneh, R., & Taghvaeinia, A. (2018). Effectiveness of Mindfulness Training on Emotional Maturity and Occupational Stress of Nurses. *Reviews in Health Care*, *4*(1), 20–25.

Jena, L. K., Pradhan, S., & Panigrahy, N. P. (2018). Pursuit of organisational trust: Role of employee engagement, psychological well-being, and transformational leadership. *Asia Pacific Management Review*, *23*(3), 227–234. doi:10.1016/j.apmrv.2017.11.001

Jones, C. N., You, S., & Furlong, M. J. (2013). A preliminary examination of covitality as integrated well-being in college students. *Social Indicators Research*, *111*(2), 511–526. doi:10.100711205-012-0017-9

Joseph, T. (2016). Developing the Leader-Follower Relationship: Perceptions of Leaders and Followers. *Journal of Leadership, Accountability and Ethics*, *13*(1).

Kappagoda, U., Othman, P., Zainul, H., & Alwis, G. (2014). Psychological capital and job performance: The mediating role of work attitudes. *Dr. Hohd. Zainul and Alwis, Gamini, Psychological Capital, and Job Performance: The Mediating Role of Work Attitudes (June 27, 2014). Journal of Human Resource and Sustainability Studies.*

Khan, N., Ahmad, N., Beg, A. H., Ismail, E. I., Abd Alla, A. N., & Nubli, M. (2010). Epilepsy control by prayer type Yoga exercise. *2010 Second International Conference on Computer Research and Development*, 391–395. 10.1109/ICCRD.2010.61

Kim, B.-J. (2019). Unstable jobs cannot cultivate good organizational citizens: The sequential mediating role of organizational trust and identification. *International Journal of Environmental Research and Public Health*, *16*(7), 1102. doi:10.3390/ijerph16071102 PMID:30934804

Kim, M., Kim, A. C. H., Newman, J. I., Ferris, G. R., & Perrewé, P. L. (2019). The antecedents and consequences of positive organizational behavior: The role of psychological capital for promoting employee well-being in sport organizations. *Sport Management Review*, *22*(1), 108–125. doi:10.1016/j.smr.2018.04.003

King, E., & Haar, J. M. (2017). Mindfulness and job performance: A study of Australian leaders. *Asia Pacific Journal of Human Resources*, *55*(3), 298–319. doi:10.1111/1744-7941.12143

Knapp, S., Gottlieb, M. C., & Handelsman, M. M. (2017). Enhancing professionalism through self-reflection. *Professional Psychology, Research and Practice*, *48*(3), 167–174. doi:10.1037/pro0000135

Koning, L. F., & van Kleef, G. A. (2015). How leaders' emotional displays shape followers' organizational citizenship behavior. *The Leadership Quarterly*, *26*(4), 489–501. doi:10.1016/j.leaqua.2015.03.001

Konte, A. G. (2021). Mindfulness and its impacts on managers: A pilot study. *Human Systems Management*, *40*(4), 605–617. doi:10.3233/HSM-201016

Koprowski, K., Meyer, D., Stanfill, T., & Tivis, L. J. (2021). Cultivating joy: Improving nurse resilience through use of a practice playbook. *Applied Nursing Research*, *62*, 151484. doi:10.1016/j.apnr.2021.151484 PMID:34814992

Kotzé, M. (2018). The influence of psychological capital, self-leadership, and mindfulness on work engagement. *South African Journal of Psychology. Suid-Afrikaanse Tydskrif vir Sielkunde*, *48*(2), 279–292. doi:10.1177/0081246317705812

Kotzé, M. (2021). The relationship between public service employees' personal resources and psychological well-being. *International Review of Administrative Sciences*, 0020852320985926.

Krippendorff, K. (2005). *The semantic turn: A new foundation for design*. CRC Press.

Kulkarni, C. A., Telang, P., & Wane, M. (2021). Efficacy of Mindfulness Meditation on Emotional Maturity of Mothers of Cerebral Palsy Children. *Journal of Pharmaceutical Research International*, 615–622.

Kurt, N., & Demirbolat, A. O. (2018). Investigation of the Relationship Between Psychological Capital Perception, Psychological Well-Being and Job Satisfaction of Teachers. *Journal of Education and Learning*, *8*(1), 87. doi:10.5539/jel.v8n1p87

Lee, D., Choi, Y., Youn, S., & Chun, J. U. (2017). Ethical Leadership and Employee Moral Voice: The Mediating Role of Moral Efficacy and the Moderating Role of Leader–Follower Value Congruence. *Journal of Business Ethics*, *141*(1), 47–57. doi:10.100710551-015-2689-y

Low, C. H., Bordia, P., & Bordia, S. (2016). What do employees want and why? An exploration of employees' preferred psychological contract elements across career stages. *Human Relations*, *69*(7), 1457–1481. doi:10.1177/0018726715616468

Luthans, F. (2002). Positive organizational behavior: Developing and managing psychological strengths. *The Academy of Management Perspectives*, *16*(1), 57–72. doi:10.5465/ame.2002.6640181

Luthans, F., Avey, J. B., Avolio, B. J., Norman, S. M., & Combs, G. M. (2006). Psychological capital development: toward a micro-intervention. *Journal of Organizational Behavior: The International Journal of Industrial. Occupational and Organizational Psychology and Behavior*, *27*(3), 387–393. doi:10.1002/job.373

Luthans, F., Avey, J. B., Avolio, B. J., & Peterson, S. J. (2010). The development and resulting performance impact of positive psychological capital. *Human Resource Development Quarterly*, *21*(1), 41–67. doi:10.1002/hrdq.20034

Luthans, F., Avey, J. B., Clapp-Smith, R., & Li, W. (2008). More evidence on the value of Chinese workers' psychological capital: A potentially unlimited competitive resource? *International Journal of Human Resource Management*, *19*(5), 818–827. doi:10.1080/09585190801991194

Luthans, F., Avey, J. B., & Patera, J. L. (2008). Experimental analysis of a web-based training intervention to develop positive psychological capital. *Academy of Management Learning & Education*, *7*(2), 209–221. doi:10.5465/amle.2008.32712618

Luthans, F., & Avolio, B. J. (2003). Authentic leadership development. *Positive Organizational Scholarship*, *241*, 258.

Luthans, F., Avolio, B. J., Avey, J. B., & Norman, S. M. (2007). Positive psychological capital: Measurement and relationship with performance and satisfaction. *Personnel Psychology*, *60*(3), 541–572. doi:10.1111/j.1744-6570.2007.00083.x

Luthans, F., & Broad, J. D. (2022). Positive psychological capital to help combat the mental health fallout from the pandemic and VUCA environment. *Organizational Dynamics*, *51*(2), 100817. doi:10.1016/j.orgdyn.2020.100817 PMID:35719171

Luthans, F., & Peterson, S. J. (2002). Employee engagement and manager self-efficacy. *Journal of Management Development*, *21*(5), 376–387. doi:10.1108/02621710210426864

Luthans, F., Vogelgesang, G. R., & Lester, P. B. (2006). Developing the psychological capital of resiliency. *Human Resource Development Review*, *5*(1), 25–44. doi:10.1177/1534484305285335

Luthans, F., Youssef, C. M., & Avolio, B. J. (2007). Psychological capital: Investing and developing positive organizational behavior. *Positive Organizational Behavior*, *1*(2), 9–24. doi:10.4135/9781446212752.n2

Lyvers, M., Makin, C., Toms, E., Thorberg, F. A., & Samios, C. (2014). Trait mindfulness in relation to emotional self-regulation and executive function. *Mindfulness*, *5*(6), 619–625. doi:10.100712671-013-0213-y

Magnano, P., Craparo, G., & Paolillo, A. (2016). Resilience and Emotional Intelligence: Which role in achievement motivation. *International Journal of Psychological Research*, *9*(1), 9–20. doi:10.21500/20112084.2096

Mahfouz, J. (2018). Mindfulness training for school administrators: Effects on well-being and leadership. *Journal of Educational Administration*, *56*(6), 602–619. doi:10.1108/JEA-12-2017-0171

Malik, N., & Dhar, R. L. (2017). Authentic leadership and its impact on extra role behaviour of nurses: The mediating role of psychological capital and the moderating role of autonomy. *Personnel Review*, *46*(2), 277–296. doi:10.1108/PR-05-2015-0140

Malinowski, P., & Lim, H. J. (2015). Mindfulness at work: Positive affect, hope, and optimism mediate the relationship between dispositional mindfulness, work engagement, and well-being. *Mindfulness*, *6*(6), 1250–1262. doi:10.100712671-015-0388-5

Mathe, K., Scott-Halsell, S., Kim, S., & Krawczyk, M. (2017). Psychological capital in the quick service restaurant industry: A study of unit-level performance. *Journal of Hospitality & Tourism Research (Washington, D.C.)*, *41*(7), 823–845. doi:10.1177/1096348014550923

McDermott, A. M., Conway, E., Rousseau, D. M., & Flood, P. C. (2013). Promoting effective psychological contracts through leadership: The missing link between HR strategy and performance. *Human Resource Management*, *52*(2), 289–310. doi:10.1002/hrm.21529

Mellor, N., & Webster, J. (2013). Enablers and challenges in implementing a comprehensive workplace health and well-being approach. *International Journal of Workplace Health Management*, *6*(2), 129–142. doi:10.1108/IJWHM-08-2011-0018

Mulliner, J. (2018). *Employee engagement, motivation, resilience, and leadership: An exploration of relationships within a higher education institution.*

Murphy, S. E., & Ensher, E. A. (2008). A qualitative analysis of charismatic leadership in creative teams: The case of television directors. *The Leadership Quarterly*, *19*(3), 335–352. doi:10.1016/j.leaqua.2008.03.006

Naidoo, V., Abarantyne, I., & Rugimbana, R. (2019). The impact of psychological contracts on employee engagement at a university of technology. *SA Journal of Human Resource Management*, *17*. doi:10.4102ajhrm.v17i0.1039

Nayak, S., & Shenoi, S. (2013). Synopsis of training programme for dermatologists in non-pharmacological (Psychological) interventions in dermatology. *Indian Journal of Dermatology, Venereology and Leprology*, *79*(2), 275.

Newman, A., Ucbasaran, D., Zhu, F. E. I., & Hirst, G. (2014). Psychological capital: A review and synthesis. *Journal of Organizational Behavior*, *35*(S1), S120–S138. doi:10.1002/job.1916

Norris, S. L., & Currieri, M. (1999). Performance enhancement training through neurofeedback. In *Introduction to quantitative EEG and neurofeedback* (pp. 223–240). Elsevier. doi:10.1016/B978-012243790-8/50011-0

Oladapo, V. (2014). The impact of talent management on retention. *Journal of Business Studies Quarterly*, *5*(3), 19.

Park, J. G., Kim, J. S., Yoon, S. W., & Joo, B.-K. (2017). The effects of empowering leadership on psychological well-being and job engagement: The mediating role of psychological capital. *Leadership and Organization Development Journal*.

Parto, M., & Besharat, M. A. (2011). Mindfulness, psychological well-being, and psychological distress in adolescents: Assessing the mediating variables and mechanisms of autonomy and self-regulation. *Procedia: Social and Behavioral Sciences*, *30*, 578–582. doi:10.1016/j.sbspro.2011.10.112

Patnaik, S., Mishra, U. S., & Mishra, B. B. (2021). Can psychological capital reduce stress and job insecurity? An experimental examination with indian evidence. *Asia Pacific Journal of Management*, 1–26.

Peng, J. C., Jien, J.-J., & Lin, J. (2016). Antecedents and consequences of psychological contract breach. *Journal of Managerial Psychology*, *31*(8), 1312–1326. doi:10.1108/JMP-10-2015-0383

Peterson, S. J., & Luthans, F. (2003). The positive impact and development of hopeful leaders. *Leadership and Organization Development Journal*, *24*(1), 26–31. doi:10.1108/01437730310457302

Plomp, J., Tims, M., Akkermans, J., Khapova, S. N., Jansen, P. G. W., & Bakker, A. B. (2016). Career competencies and job crafting: How proactive employees influence their well-being. *Career Development International*, *21*(6), 587–602. doi:10.1108/CDI-08-2016-0145

Rabenu, E., & Tziner, A. (2021). Back to routine after the coronavirus pandemic lockdown: A proposal from a psychological perspective. *Industrial and Organizational Psychology: Perspectives on Science and Practice*, *14*(1–2), 178–183. doi:10.1017/iop.2021.23

Rahman, U. U., Rehman, Ch. A., Imran, M. K., & Aslam, U. (2017). Does team orientation matter? Linking work engagement and relational psychological contract with performance. *Journal of Management Development*, *36*(9), 1102–1113. doi:10.1108/JMD-10-2016-0204

Rayton, B. A., Brammer, S. J., & Millington, A. I. (2015). Corporate social performance and the psychological contract. *Group & Organization Management*, *40*(3), 353–377. doi:10.1177/1059601114561476

Rego, A., Sousa, F., Marques, C., & Cunha, M. P. (2012). Optimism predicting employees' creativity: The mediating role of positive affect and the positivity ratio. *European Journal of Work and Organizational Psychology*, *21*(2), 244–270. doi:10.1080/1359432X.2010.550679

Rego, P., Lopes, M. P., & Nascimento, J. L. (2016). Authentic leadership and organizational commitment: The mediating role of positive psychological capital. [JIEM]. *Journal of Industrial Engineering and Management*, *9*(1), 129–151. doi:10.3926/jiem.1540

Reiner, M. (2019). Emerging technologies for sport performance enhancement: Embodied cognition and manipulation of brain rhythms. Handbook of Embodied Cognition and Sport Psychology, 333–355.

Riasudeen, S., & Singh, P. (2021). Leadership effectiveness and psychological well-being: The role of workplace spirituality. *Journal of Human Values*, *27*(2), 109–125. doi:10.1177/0971685820947334

Rifai, H. A. (2005). A test of the relationships among perceptions of justice, job satisfaction, affective commitment, and organizational citizenship behavior. *Gadjah Mada International Journal of Business*, *7*(2), 131–154. doi:10.22146/gamaijb.5574

Rigby, C. S., Schultz, P. P., & Ryan, R. M. (2014). Mindfulness, interest-taking, and self-regulation. The Wiley Blackwell Handbook of Mindfulness, 1, 216–235.

Roche, M., Haar, J. M., & Luthans, F. (2014). The role of mindfulness and psychological capital on the well-being of leaders. *Journal of Occupational Health Psychology, 19*(4), 476–489. doi:10.1037/a0037183 PMID:24933594

Rothwell, W. (2010). *Effective succession planning: Ensuring leadership continuity and building talent from within*. Amacom.

Rust, A. A., & Koketso, L. P. (2012). *Perceived challenges to talent management in the South African public service: An exploratory study of the City of Cape Town municipality*.

Saadatkhah, M., Narimani, M., Mousazadeh, T., & Varniyab, S. T. (2021). *Comparison of the efficacy of mindfulness-based cognitive therapy and acceptance and commitment therapy on emotional maturity in people with substance abuse disorders*.

Schabracq, M. J. (2003). What an organisation can do about its employees' well-being and health: An overview. The Handbook of Work and Health Psychology, 585.

Schultz, P. P., & Ryan, R. M. (2015). The "why,""what," and "how" of healthy self-regulation: Mindfulness and well-being from a self-determination theory perspective. In *Handbook of mindfulness and self-regulation* (pp. 81–94). Springer. doi:10.1007/978-1-4939-2263-5_7

Murphy, S. (2021). The Role of Self-Efficacy and Multiple Intelligences. In Multiple Intelligences and Leadership. doi:10.4324/9781410606495-18

Seligman, M. E. P., & Csikszentmihalyi, M. (2014). Positive psychology: An introduction. In *Flow and the foundations of positive psychology* (pp. 279–298). Springer. doi:10.1007/978-94-017-9088-8_18

Sharma, A. (2021). Retention and Engagement of Human Capital: Causal Contribution of Perceived Organi/alional Prestige and Job Characteristics. *The Journal of Applied Business and Economics, 23*(2), 68–82.

Sharma, S., & Sharma, S. K. (2016). Team resilience: Scale development and validation. *Vision (Basel), 20*(1), 37–53. doi:10.1177/0972262916628952

Snyder, R., Shapiro, S., & Treleaven, D. (2012). Attachment theory and mindfulness. *Journal of Child and Family Studies, 21*(5), 709–717. doi:10.100710826-011-9522-8

Spialek, M. L., Czlapinski, H. M., & Houston, J. B. (2016). Disaster communication ecology and community resilience perceptions following the 2013 central Illinois tornadoes. *International Journal of Disaster Risk Reduction, 17*, 154–160. doi:10.1016/j.ijdrr.2016.04.006

Steinberg, A., & Elmer, J. (2022). Public perceptions on post-cardiac arrest care and outcomes. In Resuscitation (Vol. 170). doi:10.1016/j.resuscitation.2021.11.011

Steinke, J., Bolunmez, B., Fletcher, L., Wang, V., Tomassetti, A. J., Repchick, K. M., Zaccaro, S. J., Dalal, R. S., & Tetrick, L. E. (2015). Improving cybersecurity incident response team effectiveness using teams-based research. *IEEE Security and Privacy, 13*(4), 20–29. doi:10.1109/MSP.2015.71

Stinson, B., & Arthur, D. (2013). A novel EEG for alpha brain state training, neurobiofeedback and behavior change. *Complementary Therapies in Clinical Practice, 19*(3), 114–118. doi:10.1016/j.ctcp.2013.03.003 PMID:23890456

Tanjung, S. R., Syahrizal, & Abror. (2021). *The Influence of Organizational Climate Support on Psychological Well-Being and Employee Loyalty with Psychological Capital as Mediating Variables.* Proceedings of the Sixth Padang International Conference On Economics Education, Economics, Business and Management, Accounting and Entrepreneurship (PICEEBA 2020). Atlantis Press. 10.2991/aebmr.k.210616.078

Travis, D. J., Nugent, J. S., & Lengnick-Hall, R. (2019). Cultivating healthy, inclusive workplaces: Why it matters and how organizations make progress. In *Creating psychologically healthy workplaces*. Edward Elgar Publishing. doi:10.4337/9781788113427.00029

Truss, C., Delbridge, R., Alfes, K., Shantz, A., & Soane, E. (2013). *Employee engagement in theory and practice*. Routledge London. doi:10.4324/9780203076965

Venturella, I., Crivelli, D., Fronda, G., & Balconi, M. (2018). Neurocognitive enhancement: mindfulness practices applied to management. *10th International Scientific Conference on Neuroethics and 5th Conference of the Italian Society for Neuroethics*. N-A.

Vohra, M., & Pandey, N. (2018). Effects of mindfulness on psychological well-being among school going children. *IAHRW International Journal of Social Sciences Review*, *6*(5), 952–954.

Walker, A., & Hutton, D. M. (2006). The application of the psychological contract to workplace safety. *Journal of Safety Research*, *37*(5), 433–441. doi:10.1016/j.jsr.2006.06.001 PMID:17125794

Walumbwa, F. O., Luthans, F., Avey, J. B., & Oke, A. (2011). Retracted: Authentically leading groups: The mediating role of collective psychological capital and trust. *Journal of Organizational Behavior*, *32*(1), 4–24. doi:10.1002/job.653

Wells, C. M., & Klocko, B. A. (2018). Principal well-being and resilience: Mindfulness as a means to that end. *NASSP Bulletin, 102*(2), 161–173. doi:10.1177/0192636518777813

Wernsing, T. (2014). Psychological capital: A test of measurement invariance across 12 national cultures. *Journal of Leadership & Organizational Studies, 21*(2), 179–190. doi:10.1177/1548051813515924

Wise, E. H., Hersh, M. A., & Gibson, C. M. (2012). Ethics, self-care, and well-being for psychologists: Reenvisioning the stress-distress continuum. *Professional Psychology, Research and Practice, 43*(5), 487–494. doi:10.1037/a0029446

Zineldin, M., & Hytter, A. (2012). Leaders' negative emotions and leadership styles influencing subordinates' well-being. *International Journal of Human Resource Management, 23*(4), 748–758. doi:10.1080/09585192.2011.606114

ADDITIONAL READING

Bassarear, T., Byrnes, K., Cherkowski, S., Hanson, K., Kelly, J., Latta, M. M., Mackenzie, E., & Soloway, G. (2015). *Mindful teaching and learning: developing a pedagogy of well-being*. Lexington Books.

Compton, W. C., & Hoffman, E. (2019). *Positive psychology: The science of happiness and flourishing*. Sage Publications.

Gregory, E. M., & Rutledge, P. B. (2016). *Exploring Positive Psychology: The Science of Happiness and Well-Being: The Science of Happiness and Well-Being*. ABC-CLIO.

Guest, D. E., Isaksson, K., & De Witte, H. (Eds.). (2010). *Employment contracts, psychological contracts, and employee well-being: an international study*. Oxford University Press. doi:10.1093/acprof:oso/9780199542697.001.0001

Ivtzan, I., & Lomas, T. (Eds.). (2016). *Mindfulness in positive psychology: The science of meditation and wellbeing*. Routledge. doi:10.4324/9781315747217

Kashdan, T. B., & Ciarrochi, J. V. (Eds.). (2013). *Mindfulness, acceptance, and positive psychology: The seven foundations of well-being*. New Harbinger Publications.

KEY TERMS AND DEFINITIONS

Mindfulness: Maintaining awareness of our thoughts, emotions, bodily sensations, and immediate environment on a moment-by-moment basis is known as mindfulness.

Optimism: Hopefulness and conviction on the success of something in the future.

Psychological Capital: A person's psychological potential that can be developed and organised for performance enhancement.

Psychological Contract: The expectations, convictions, goals, and duties of an individual as seen by the employer and the employee.

Psychological Well-Being: The overall functioning and emotional health of an individual.

Resilience: The ability to bounce back rapidly from setbacks.

Self-Efficacy: A person's confidence in their ability to carry out the actions required to achieve performance goals.

Chapter 5
Mental Health Education:
A Pathway for Entrepreneurial Readiness

Smita Panda
Vellore Institute of Technology, India

Rishwin Lal Thayat
Vellore Institute of Technology, India

Rakshan Vaishnav S.
Vellore Institute of Technology, India

ABSTRACT

The pandemic has brought about hitherto unimaginable transformations. Anxiety, loss, and sadness have taken their toll resulting in various frightening results, such as disruptive conduct in younger children and aggression and bullying tendencies in older people. Thus, mental health education is essential. However, mental health education not only helps combat the different challenges in our society but also contributes to many sectors that are not always evident to the human eye and are sometimes overlooked. This chapter addresses how mental health education might help students create their businesses. Through an appended assessment of existing research, this chapter covers the components of mental health education and the various linked dimensions of entrepreneurial readiness/competencies. A thorough examination of present and possible ways for providing adequate mental health education has allowed this chapter to offer explicit content. The chapter concludes with a review of the relationships and alignments shared by the areas of mental health education and entrepreneurship.

DOI: 10.4018/978-1-6684-7221-7.ch005

INTRODUCTION

The word Education has its roots buried deep in the dead language of Latin. It comes from the Latin word 'Educare,' meaning - to rear or bring up. Since the world's inception in the 16th century, over the past 600 years, the word has seen many interpretations according to the various situations and circumstances it has been used in. In the relatively immediate past, majorly in the 20th century, education addressed almost everything but the domain of mental health. Statistics show that about 12-13% of school students in India suffer from mental, emotional, and communicative problems. Fifty million children in India had mental health issues with no support howsoever. These statistics and the numbers they bring into the picture are often downplayed and not treated with adequate seriousness, leading to catastrophic consequences.

Nevertheless, that is not the case now. These numbers have brought about a change in the way people perceive mental well-being. Humans are now more cautious about the same. It has proved to change the education being imparted around us as we breathe. This word might not have seen a more significant change in its entire history than it has started to see in the 21st century.

Education is no longer seen as the exclusive means of imparting predefined skills to students. Now the range and scope being considered are beyond just academic and physical education. In the twenty-first century, our educational system has started emphasizing mental health education more. This has ensured overall development in numerous ways. Mentally healthy individuals are more excited to learn new things, actively participate in various extracurricular activities, have excellent interpersonal relationship skills with adults and people younger than them, and display enhanced problem-solving and risk-taking. Decision-making skills, have non-aggressive and composed behavioral patterns, and always add positivity wherever and whenever they interact.

Yet, it has never been more significant than in the face of terrible socioeconomic situations such as Covid-19. The pandemic has resulted in changes hitherto undreamt of. The anxiety, grief, and depression have taken a toll on almost all individuals, leading to various scary outcomes like crying and disruptive behavior in younger kids, and increased probabilities of violence and bullying tendencies in older individuals. Hence, mental health education is the need of the hour.

However, imparting mental health education does not just serve to overcome the various issues in our society but also contributes to many essential realms that are often not so visible to the naked eye and often looked past. One of those realms is among the most sought-after fields, i.e., entrepreneurship. In the simplest way possible, entrepreneurship is the process of setting up a business to make a profit.

Entrepreneurship, in the language engineers, love to describe, is directly proportional to communal economic growth. The more the number of entrepreneurs in a system, the better the economy and welfare of it. But apart from this direct proportionality, entrepreneurial readiness is another element worth looking at. In layperson's terms, entrepreneurial enthusiasm refers to an individual's mental state related to the entrepreneurship domain. The main factor influencing the mentioned readiness is an individual's ability to appropriately use his entrepreneurial potential, explore the available opportunities and use all the resources at hand.

The definition itself tells us it is no surprise that entrepreneurship is one of the most mentally demanding fields. Uncertainty, responsibility, balance, and loneliness are some of the critical aspects of an entrepreneur's voyage and are all extremely exhaustive as far as the mental game is concerned. Hence, enlightening individuals who are related to the field of entrepreneurship with the correct form of mental health education could go on to give them a healthy edge over their peers.

This chapter discusses how mental health education may enable students to start their entrepreneurial journey. Through a review of existing research, this chapter outlines the many facets of mental health education and the various related dimensions of entrepreneurial readiness/competencies through the literature review that has been appended. A detailed study of existing and potential methods to carry out proper mental health education has enabled this chapter to share explicit content. The chapter culminates with a discussion of the relations and alignments shared by mental health education and entrepreneurship domains. In addition, an empirical study has also been conducted on technical and professional students to understand better the influence of Mental Health Education on entrepreneurial preparation. This chapter develops a detailed framework related to this and many more. Something also worth mentioning is that the studies are not region-specific, as current mental health education scenarios in India and across the globe have been considered.

LITERATURE REVIEW

Mental Health Education

Mental health is the well-being of human beings on aspects of cognitive, behavioral, and emotional patterns. It affects our characteristics, mannerisms, way of thinking, and emotions. Mental health differs and varies from individual to individual. It includes psychological, emotional, and social well-being. It is essential to ensure and maintain good mental health from childhood to adolescence. When people are exposed to different conditions of a pressurized environment, harsh experiences, and desperate situations, they tend to undergo mental health disorders. These include various factors like frequent panic attacks, frequent anxiety, depression, mood swings, etc. The way of pursuing things, improving mental health, importance, and role in achieving entrepreneurial readiness are discussed briefly. Modern research revealed that student-centered self-narratives helped them improve their mental state and voice their opinions. (Yang et al.,2018)

Education, the key to success, also elucidates mental health as an essential element. The role and importance of mental health in students and adult groups and its relationship with entrepreneurship quality are deeply analyzed. Mental health is an essential key element for self-growth. The range and scope of education are beyond just academic and physical education. A study on attitudes toward mental illness and its influence on education has revealed a significant result. The nursing students who completed their experimental and instructional programs were compared to those who joined the same course. Their perceptions, beliefs, and ideas are analyzed by asking them to fill out a questionnaire with their concern. The results were analyzed and found no difference in their attitudes towards the mentally ill, and the groups shared optimism about prognosis.

As conclusive evidence, a comparison of two groups of nursing students revealed that direct exposure to a psychiatrist and instructional education has minimal impact on influencing their ability to perceive the presence of mental illness. The training program also showed little influence on their desire to increase or decrease the social distance from someone they perceive as mentally ill (Malla & Shaw, 1987). Experiments reveal that graduate students are more than six times more likely to experience depression and anxiety than the general population (Evans et al., 2018). This creates a link between education and mental health, how mental health is affected by education, and how mental health education helps in improvising the readiness of entrepreneurship quality in an individual.

Mental health is strongly linked with an individual's behavioral aspects and growth. Poor mental health in childhood can severely impact the chances of life. Mental health in childhood also affects the future, like employment, behavioral problems, professional skills, income, and other sources (Cornaglia et al., 2015). Entrepreneurship is the quality of making a profit by setting up a business. It requires higher skills, good cognitive thinking ability, and the capability to perceive things. Emotional Quotient plays a vital role in organizational behavior and entrepreneurial readiness, including self-awareness, motivation, empathy, social skills, and self-regulation.

Entrepreneurial education refers to entrepreneurship by establishing a start-up perspective focussed on the specific context of venture creation and an enterprising attitude focussing more broadly on personal development, mindset, emotional skills, mental skills, and abilities. The collection of literature reviews provides knowledge of how the concept of enterprising, beyond starting up a new venture, is related to different entrepreneurial education objectives and outcomes. (Hagg & Gabrielsson, 2019; Erkkila,2000; Greene et al, 2004)

Entrepreneurial education has witnessed a high level of teaching to reach the goal of progress and facilitate learning. The analysis and evidence prove that entrepreneurship quality and readiness are greatly affected by mental health. "Mental health is a resource in the entrepreneurial process, together with a stream of research that focuses on mental health conditions as a strength in entrepreneurship" (Hatak, 2021). This defines the importance of representing the link and relationship between mental health and its impact on entrepreneurship.

(Cathy, 2003) stated that Entrepreneurship education is not just about teaching people how to run a business but also about enlightening students on creating a business. The learning entrepreneur education helps gather core knowledge on recognizing opportunities and reaching out to the possibilities. (Burleson, 2005) Besides expertise and skill, entrepreneurial education is about developing beliefs, values, mental perseverance, and moral and ethical relationships. (Hasan and Nabi, 2017)

Mental health is defined by the World Health Organisation (WHO) as not merely the absence of mental health problems but as a "state of well-being in which every individual realizes his or her potential, can cope with the normal stresses of life, can work productively and fruitfully, and can contribute to her or his community" (Mental Health, 2014). Therefore, as a part of social and emotional skills are a prerequisite of entrepreneurial skills, we need to understand the role and importance of mental health and its impact.

The entrepreneurial environment directly impacts the psychological stress rate of young entrepreneurs. Young entrepreneurs undergo such situations of stress rates which relates to the concept of mental health. Therefore, a proper and good entrepreneurial environment can effectively alleviate entrepreneurs' psychological anxiety, and it also has a chain impact on the entrepreneurial performance of young entrepreneurs (Zhao et al., 2022). Thus, with the help of the segregation of conclusive shreds of evidence from collective research articles and studies, it is apparent to understand the roles and importance of communication, its impact on entrepreneurial quality and readiness, and the social and mental prerequisites of entrepreneurship.

Current Mental Health Education in India

India was never known for its mental health education provisions owing to no such thought processes for a very long time in the country. However, the year 2010 saw a huge change in this long-standing trend. To increase the availability of people who are trained in the field of mental health education, a lot of initiatives were taken. 7 Regional institutes were funded, and 9 institutes supported 9 PG departments for manpower development. A sum of 150 crores was approved for various mental health programs. This kind of value, importance, and fiscal support to the largely ignored mental health domain was never seen before in India. This kind of situation demands appreciation because it occurred, as mentioned before, in a situation that has never been seen before. For context, during the time of independence, India's population stood over 300 million but had just around 10,000 psychiatric beds, whereas the UK, with around 10% of India's population, had over 1,50,000 psychiatric beds. This shows that although India might be late to the party, it has started making steps in the right direction (Murthy, 2014).

For the first 2 decades after independence, the focus was on increasing the psychiatric beds 2-fold. India, since prehistoric times, has been known for its highly rational and superior way of thought processes. One such instance related to the theme of mental health took place around this time in India. All over the world, the general education of mental health assumed that families were toxic to mentally unfit patients and hence keeping them far away from their family members was necessary. But India took a stand on this theme that was unheard and unseen. An initiative started at Amritsar by Vidya Sagar was far ahead of its time, where they educated people to facilitate the presence of family members near mentally sick patients. It was observed that this boosted their morale and enabled them to get free of their mental issues. There have been various programs that have tried to tackle the problem of mental health education in India as of today. One such program is the school mental health program (SMHP)

SMHP has proven to be very efficient when it comes to the all-round development of children. The most important factors that determine how well students can react to mental health issues are their resilience and stress tolerance. These two factors are among the primary focus of SMHP, and in addition, it also takes care that by addressing these factors, the psychological problems that children face are tackled when and where they face them. Moving on to the secondary focus of SMHP, bully control and training people for suicide prevention is something that SMHP has put its time into as well. This facilitates the avoidance of undesirable outcomes of psychological issues. This is of vital importance in India as there is a very high number of cases when it comes to violence and suicide among school children. Unfortunately, however SMHP speed is terribly ignored in India. There are a lot of cases where the school administrations have expressed their concern regarding the mental health and mental health education of children. However, these issues are rarely taken up seriously, and it's very frequent that there is no logical outcome or solution provided to these problems. As a result of this constant failure as far as the implementation of a systematic framework for nationwide SMHP is concerned, mental health education in India is still a dream unachieved. (Kumar, 2021)

India is the 7th largest country geographically and 2nd largest in terms of population. Even if we keep the sheer area aside, each part of the country displays distinct socioeconomic conditions. Hence this explicitly means that schools, by a huge margin, differ in terms of the available resources, the background of children, the educational and financial abilities of parents, and so on. If we talk about the technical aspects, schools also differ in terms of the board that they come under, like The Central board of education, State board of education, international board of education, etc. Moreover, the political divisions also play a role as the various ministries that are associated with the different states play a role in deciding the kind of educational curriculum that the schools there will have. Keeping all of this in mind, it is safe to say that establishing a program for mental health education in a vast country like India is extremely difficult. But history is proof of the fact that no task is impossible. It has been just over 75 years since India gained its independence and detached itself from the deeply hooked claws of the British. It is only fair for us to be patient and continue having faith in our country as far as mental health education is concerned because, as much as the current situation seems worrisome, the future certainly does hold better times.

Current Mental Health Education Across the Globe

It is very often said by learned men and women worldwide that there has never been a better time to be alive. Life expectancy has increased in the last 5 decades faster than it has in the past 500 decades; Medical advancement is at an all-time high with the cure for illnesses that were once thought to be incurable; The average education right now is far better than it ever was; the living conditions for the average population has never been better. After taking all of this into consideration, it can be assumed that this era is among the best eras for human beings. But what if we bring Mental Health into the picture?

Mental health, as a topic, has never seen more open discussions than it is being subjected to now. People have started realizing and acknowledging the important role that mental health education plays, both personally and communally. This kind of importance being given to mental health education is totally required and valid. Depression is among the highest leading causes of disabilities. In the age group of 15- to 29-year-olds, suicide ranks number 4 as far as the leading causes of death are concerned. One in seven 10–19-year-olds suffers from a mental health disorder, accounting for 13% of diseases globally. Untreated mental health issues go on to cause physical and mental health issues in adulthood as well, which restricts the ability to live free, happy, and fulfilling lives.

Statistics tell us that people, irrespective of their age group, who suffer from severe mental health conditions die as much as two decades early compared to those who are mentally fit due to avoidable physical conditions. Although it can be said that there has been significant progress in some countries as compared to the situation about a century ago, we still have a long way to go. The mentally affected community often faces severe violation and discrimination as far as their human rights are concerned and are very often stigmatized. It is understandably assumed that mental health education is a very complex process with a very complicated framework, but that is a huge misconception. Most mental health issues can significantly be treated at relatively low costs. But the major issue is the enormous gap between the people who need help and those with access to proper care.

The question that arises after all these superficially difficult issues is how to tackle mental health illnesses and how to bring about the education required to address mental health. The solution is simple. Anything and everything that starts from a young age shapes the lives of human beings and determines a huge portion of who and what they become in the future. Keeping this in mind, mental health education needs to be primarily brought in the early school years. This is when children form their first bonds, i.e., with their teachers, their friends, and all those around them. School is where teenagers first come face to face in realizing their self-worth and self-esteem. Challenges like being excluded, conflicts with those around you, conflict with oneself, and poor self-confidence are all first faced in the teenage years. If children and teenagers are not educated to tackle these seemingly small issues, they might never properly understand how to stand the challenges and successfully go past them. Later in life, when these small issues take the shape of actual life-threatening situations, people find themselves down on their knees. As mentioned before, this humongous task can easily be contained within the domain of parents, teachers, students, and, if required, professionals.

The World Health Organisation (WHO) has suggested a 4-level framework for mental health education.

The first level involves proper education on the interrelation of various social factors and personal behavior and thoughts, which essentially needs to be added as a part of the education curriculum. The second level focuses on mental health education as a concept and needs to be put in the general health curriculum. The third level goes beyond the range of normal students and focuses more on those students who need extra psychosocial help in school. The final level, i.e., level 4, is exclusively for those students who need professional intervention and help from skilled personnel for their mental health issues. All in all, this multi-level program urges that.

1. The program should cover each and every student in schools and not just those who are affected by mental health issues.

2. The activities that mental health education fields undertake should not just be restricted to its domain and should rather be made a part of the school system.

To summarize, what the World Health Organisation says is that a successful Mental Health Education Program in each education system will follow an approach to public health based on the Promotion, Prevention, and Early Intervention (PPEI) model. To elaborate, the PPEI model for the schools is required to establish an environment that can facilitate the enhancement of resilience, cooperation, resistance, and other such skills that are required to combat mental health issues. Life skills are another such important skill that would include developing all-around creative thinking, critical thinking, empathy, problem-solving abilities, healthy interpersonal relationships, effective communication, etc. In short, all the daily activities that occur, like teaching, fun activities, playground time, curriculum, etc., should go about in a way where mental health education is imbibed in it both directly and indirectly. Overall, a world where human beings support each other and mental health is treated as normally as any other subject is far from reality. But the distance is measurable now. With the right kind of steps in the right direction, we can turn that dream into reality.

Methods of Mental Health Education

Mental health is the state of well-being of an individual in aspects of emotional, psychological, and social skills. Mental health is essential to overcoming stress, leading a positive life, and making meaningful contributions to your community. In addition, mental health education is critical to enhancing the value of society by teaching individuals how their perceptions impact culture and social and entrepreneurial aspects. Some methods of mental health educational development are discussed below:

Inculcating Knowledge Through Awareness

Knowledge of mental health and its importance must be understood by the commoners of society, which is a significant base for the welfare of society. This act of awareness can be reached the public through various means, like awareness programs, media, mass media, and social media.

Positive Approach to Coping Skills

It is imperative to understand the coping skills to use during pressurized conditions. This helps to a great extent in handling problems and acting.

Methods of mental health provide us with a massive scope of reference and approaching a stable mental health condition. In defining methods of mental health education, the factors included were mental health workforce, school-based mental health, suicide prevention, peer workforce, criminal justice, mental health, and supported housing. (Walker et al., 2021)

Mental health education must be valued more than just curriculum and academics. The mental health of each student can be significantly influenced by the school and décor random of the institutions. The research team has conducted a complete analysis, and it has been evident that the school environment, the part of the curriculum, the entire school community, student-teacher interaction, and accommodation of different cultural students could significantly affect the intensity of impact upon mental health. The condition of creating an environment conducive to promoting psycho-socio competence and well-being can lead to an impact on mental health education upon knowledge, attitude, and behavior. The way of treating psycho-social interventions and problems of students is now a need of an hour. The professional approach of treating mental illness through therapy sessions can be a resolving factor of such hindrance. The ways to improve the mental health level of students by understanding students requiring general help in school and students requiring additional mental health intervention must be determined. (Wyn et al.,2000)

Mental health in childhood is a significant concern that also impacts later stages of life. (Weist et al.,2005; Paternite, 2005) Provided a few methods to enhance mental health education which included

- Ensuring strong coordination and collaboration among families, school leaders, and mental health program leaders as programs are being planned.
- Ensuring that school mental health providers are well trained, closely supervised, and socially skilled and that they understand the culture of schools and how to work as collaborative partners in them. Thus, mental health education, in general, is treated with high importance, and its methods and ways of implementation are discussed.

Role and Importance of Mental Health Education During the Pandemic

The global pandemic, covid-19, has created a huge impact on individuals in the country. It affected the whole economic, social, and mental conditions worldwide. The evidence and supporting events on mental health during the pandemic have been collected and portrayed.

"In the context of Covid-19, these mental health implications may be amplified by factors such as increased uncertainty related to an individual's health because of the exposure to a new highly infectious disease, the profound economic consequences of the pandemic in the US, and globally, the implementation of lockdown measures, resulting in the practice of prolonged social distancing" (Kampfen et al.,2020)

People were stuck at home during the pandemic with obsessing thoughts and engaging themselves with online resources. This is the time the members of the family get to understand each other by spending quality time. In contrast, people also showed anxiety, depression, and stress due to high levels of online activities, screen timing, and lockdown. Mental health education is very important to understand their moods and behavior. The mental health of many individuals was affected, and they are seemingly stressed, in outbursts, and irritable. Fatigue, laziness, and loss of interest are other factors that hugely impact mental health and productivity at work.

The disruption in the healthcare system from COVID-19 impacts the care of other patients with chronic illnesses who need to visit healthcare facilities for chronic care. It is believed that high-stress levels due to the inability to access timely care can cause mental illness. Psychiatric patients were noted to have higher rates of depression, anxiety, stress, and intense suicidal ideation. (Li & Gang, 2021)

Mental health has been imparted to individuals' behavior and mental ability. During Covid-19, many people were jobless, including vendors, daily workers, and artisans. Such people, especially those working daily, faced a substantial economic hit during this difficult period, and, due to this, their mental health has been affected.

Covid-19 created a significant impact on the mind of patients who had undergone different reactions, mood swings, and behaviors, as mental health issues of social isolation, social disconnectedness, loneliness, anxiety, depression, phobia, fear of getting the infection, etc. (Brooks et al.,2020) Though mental wellness sessions and the welfare of human mental health have been developed in our modern society, it requires an understanding of people to vent their emotions and express them in the right way. The condition worsens when people undergo mental illness and are not treated properly. It is not essentially a requisite that illnesses are complex and occur only in emotionally weak people. It also refers to depressive feelings, overstressed conditions, anger, and irritability, even under normal conditions. These feelings are not only undergone by an employer at work or a person working with heavy loads. This was the condition during the pandemic when people were struggling to spend time over long internet sessions, high screen time, sleeplessness, eye irritability, and mental illness.

Despite being poor and rich, mental illness can be undergone by any individual, and it is imperative to analyse how to overcome obstacles caused due to mental trauma and illness. So, it is important to understand the need for mental health education and how to reach a mentally stabilized condition. Mental health education helps us understand how to revive various mental illnesses such as depressed conditions, trauma, anxiety, and fear. It becomes the responsibility of everyone to understand this situation and act wisely on improving mental health and helping others create a change.

Role and Importance of Mental Health Education During Post-Pandemic

International bodies such as the United Nations (UN), the World Health Organisation (WHO), the International Labour Organisation (ILO), and the Organisation for Economic Co-operation and Development (OECD) have commented that the pandemic has made the earth a hard place to live. (Berry, 2021). The case was true where covid had killed lots of citizens, not only physically but mentally as well. People who were victims of covid witnessed a lot of mental health issues and underwent a depressive state of mind. As discussed in previous scenarios during covid, people during post covid were reviving and reconditioning their mental health.

The pandemic has shown that people could accept policies where necessary. The majority of people wanted mental peace and climatic change after covid. Mental health recovery through education also requires Interest, optimism, confidence, and energy in young people. (Berry, 2021). People's mental health was remarkably under consideration by the government before and after the disposal of Lockdown conditions. People were subjected to lots of mixed emotions in the period of post-covid conditions.

The mentality of students after covid was a challenging thing to recover. The mandatory presence of online sessions during covid created a lethargic mentality during post covid conditions. Experimental research had been conducted on students who investigated whether the imposition of lockdown could aggravate other mental health problems: anxiety symptoms, as measured by the Beck Anxiety Inventory, and obsessive-compulsive symptoms, as measured by the Obsessive-Compulsive Inventory. The research team surveyed questionnaires before and after covid with students and found that the scores of kids were low on questionnaires conducted during post-covid situations. (Meda et al.,2021)

Recent reports and surveys taken during the pandemic have provided us with the facts regarding how students cope with and adapt to physical distancing, school closures, and quarantining time at home. Reports have been published that food insecurity, lacking literacy skills, unreliable internet access, and precarious housing situations are a new reality (Van Lancker & Parolin, 2020), while others anticipate that children and youth may experience increased stress and anxiety related to the COVID-19 pandemic (Kelly et al., 2021)

The pandemic not only left a significant impact on history but also on people's mental health. The post covid period was challenging for people, especially of the working class, to revive back into active life after a long period of inactivity. Many of them required time to adapt to mental conditions after post covid.

During a child's formative years, when their personalities are shaped, parents are in regular contact with paediatricians, as parents reach out to their local paediatricians whenever they encounter health/Behavioral complaints associated with their children. The methods suggested to improve the mental health of students during post-covid scenarios were:

- The workers of Mental health care should focus on the main task of constructing and administering online questionnaires to detect psychological distress
- Psychiatrists had to carefully weigh the risks and benefits of psychotropic medications for children and adolescents. e.g., antidepressant
- Coordinated and innovative mental health care are essential for growth. For improving mental health, coordination among people who play a crucial role in the mental health care of children and adolescents is essential, e.g., parents, paediatricians, teachers, etc.
- Usage of contingency management, providing psychological first aid, referring to mental health care professionals to create material for schools for mental health promotion and management of behavior problems (Singh et al., 2020).

The improvement in the advancement of technology, along with the practical usage of resources, has brought a new change in individuals. The online resources that have been popularly bloomed during the pandemic are still in use, and people have started to adopt an adaptive mindset and improve their mental mindset.

MENTAL HEALTH EDUCATION AND ENTREPRENEURIAL EDUCATION

Entrepreneurship as a field has gained a lot of popularity in the 21st century. With the kind of technological advancement and change in mindset, gone is the time when getting into the field of entrepreneurship was limited to just certain specific individuals. Now, this field has seen a lot of people, especially young minds turn to it. However, a select few success stories have created an incorrect impression of this highly challenging domain. (Sharma, 2019) By sharing the experiences of a very small proportion of successful entrepreneurs, a false image of this mentally, physically, and emotionally draining venture has been created. This erroneous image has invariably led the people in discussion to feel that they are supposed to put up and not speak or express the challenges that they face in this journey. This ecosystem that has been created poses huge threats to both the person and those around him/her. It has become increasingly difficult for them to accept the fact that they are normal human beings as well who have the basic right to express themselves mentally.

The most basic definition of entrepreneurship would be the activity of developing, organizing, and running a business enterprise and facing all the uncertainties associated with it to go forward and make a profit. In this process, people's psychological qualities are put to an extremely difficult test. The performance of individuals in this field is directly proportional to their mental health and their ability to overcome challenges. Psychological qualities will determine if people can successfully go from being just potential entrepreneurs to real entrepreneurs.

If we consider the case of students who are about to enter the real world, we will observe that a lot of them pass out of their education phase with a lot of new ideas. Many of them may take solid steps toward shaping those ideas into reality. But the harsh truth of the real world is that a very small proportion of these people and their ideas make it past all the obstacles that are waiting to pull them down. Facing these hindrances, i.e., the change in environment and self-identity, requires people to be ready. This readiness cannot be achieved within a single night. Schools, colleges, and universities must take the initiative to conduct second-degree activities that focus on cultivating determination, perseverance, and resistance to stress in the face of difficulties, and they should be able to fill themselves with logical positivity and optimism to get out of the depths of these setbacks. Tagging those who express their mental vulnerabilities as weaklings must immediately cease. Mentally healthy entrepreneurs will always result in increased productivity (Cao, 2022).

CONCLUSION

Maintaining a good level of mental health has never been more important. The era we live in has demanded the strongest of us to bow down to the never-ending process of life, and in doing so, it has tested our abilities to withstand Mental health issues. Stabilization of behaviors that can be constructive, thoughts, and emotions depends not only on how well we can maintain an optimistic mental health state but also on how well we can treat mental health illnesses. Paying basic attention to mental health care can enhance our self-confidence, self-esteem, and productivity and improve interpersonal relationships.

Maintaining and nurturing mental health doesn't just improve our day-to-day functioning, but it can also help us keep a check and even combat some of the physical health issues that share a link with mental health issues. For instance, the heart diseases that we might have, and their deterioration is related to our stress level. Hence managing stress levels could help us in a positive way and alleviate our heart condition. (Mental Health, 2019)

Apart from this, as far as the close link that entrepreneurship and mental health education share is concerned, it goes without saying that both go hand and hand. They're both two sides of the same coin and hence need to be taken care of simultaneously. Entrepreneurship is probably one of the most challenging fields in the world right now, and as much as the field seems rewarding, a major portion of receiving those rewards depends on how well we combat mental health issues. Entrepreneurial readiness, which in layman's terms refers to an individual's mental state, is related to the domain of entrepreneurship. It is one of the factors that decide how well an entrepreneur performs. This highly demanding task and the uncertainty, responsibility, balance, and loneliness related to it can only and only be handled if the correct kind of mental health education is imparted, that too preferably at a young age. Hence mental health education, for the umpteenth time, plays a major role in navigating entrepreneurs.

The world, as mentioned before, has never been a better place to live in. It is without a doubt important that we focus on the areas that require changes to be inculcated. However, it is equally important to acknowledge and appreciate the efforts that have already been taken/are being taken as we speak. Only a positive mindset can help us combat this very sensitive topic. But it goes without saying that although the sporadic nature of efforts (such as conducting various programs in educational institutions) is praiseworthy, they are miles away from making a comprehensive and sustainable process. Consistent and unwavering efforts are required to destigmatize and revolutionize the world.

Case Study

Harry was 31 at the time of the interview. His first breakdown was two years previously. He had been admitted to a psychiatric unit twice, both voluntarily for around one week. The interview begins with the interviewer asking Harry about his involvement with psychiatry. Harry had been attending the psychiatry sessions continuously and found a significant change in his negative aspects.

Harry lets the psychiatrists identify a problem through the things he says. He found that his active strategy to access psychiatric services is to become a passive repository of pathology. Rather than drawing directly from the patient discourse, Harry appears to be endorsing the patient discourse. He found improvements in mental health through various methods suggested by psychiatrists and improved his knowledge of mental health education. His paranoia was not caused by socially constructed hatred but by his perception. It is essential to understand the medical model and passivity that hold sway about treatment. He relates the different conceptions that psychoanalysis and psychiatry had of his pathology.

Harry's social contact with mental health education was good, and his talk about psychotherapy was positive. It is essential to understand the social and psychological factors contributing to mental health and mental illness. This case study on Harry, his breakdown during different pressurized situations, and his revival positively impact us in understanding the importance and role of mental health education. (Ewen, 2006).

REFERENCES

Berry, H. L. (2021). Enabling a youth-and mental health-sensitive greener post-pandemic recovery. *World Psychiatry; Official Journal of the World Psychiatric Association (WPA)*, *20*(2), 152–153. doi:10.1002/wps.20843 PMID:34002504

Burleson, W. (2005). Developing creativity, motivation, and self-actualization with learning systems. *International Journal of Human-Computer Studies*, *63*(4), 436–451. doi:10.1016/j.ijhcs.2005.04.007

Cao, J. (2022). Exploration on the Cultivation of Undergraduates' Entrepreneurship Ability from the Perspective of Mental Health Education. *Journal of Healthcare Engineering*, *2022*, 1–9. doi:10.1155/2022/9668220 PMID:35340258

Cathy, A. (2003). *The consortium for entrepreneurship education.*

Cornaglia, F., Crivellaro, E., & McNally, S. (2015). Mental health and education decisions. *Labour Economics*, *33*, 1–12. doi:10.1016/j.labeco.2015.01.005

Duan, L., & Zhu, G. (2020). Psychological interventions for people affected by the COVID-19 epidemic. *The Lancet. Psychiatry*, *7*(4), 300–302. doi:10.1016/S2215-0366(20)30073-0 PMID:32085840

Erkkilä, K. (2000). Entrepreneurial education: mapping the debates in the United States, the United Kingdom, and Finland. Taylor & Francis.

Evans, T. M., Bira, L., Gastelum, J. B., Weiss, L. T., & Vanderford, N. L. (2018). Evidence for a mental health crisis in graduate education. *Nature Biotechnology*, *36*(3), 282–284. doi:10.1038/nbt.4089 PMID:29509732

Greene, P. G., & Brush, C. (2014a). *Teaching entrepreneurship: A practice-based approach*. Edward Elgar Publishing.

Grover, S., Dua, D., Sahoo, S., Mehra, A., Nehra, R., & Chakrabarti, S. (2020). Why all COVID-19 hospitals should have mental health professionals: The importance of mental health in a worldwide crisis! *Asian Journal of Psychiatry*, *51*, 102147. doi:10.1016/j.ajp.2020.102147 PMID:32473537

Hägg, G., & Gabrielsson, J. (2019). A systematic literature review of the evolution of pedagogy in entrepreneurial education research. *International Journal of Entrepreneurial Behaviour & Research*, *26*(5), 829–861. doi:10.1108/IJEBR-04-2018-0272

Hasan, S. M., Khan, E. A., & Nabi, M. N. U. (2017). Entrepreneurial education at university level and entrepreneurship development. *Education + Training*, *59*(7/8), 888–906. doi:10.1108/ET-01-2016-0020

Hatak, I. (2021). *Mental health in entrepreneurship. In the World Encyclopaedia of Entrepreneurship*. Edward Elgar Publishing.

Kämpfen, F., Kohler, I. V., Ciancio, A., Bruine de Bruin, W., Maurer, J., & Kohler, H. P. (2020). Predictors of mental health during the Covid-19 pandemic in the US: Role of economic concerns, health worries, and social distancing. *PLoS One*, *15*(11), e0241895. doi:10.1371/journal.pone.0241895 PMID:33175894

Kumar, D. (2021). School mental health program in India: Need to shift from a piecemeal approach to a long-term comprehensive approach with strong intersectoral coordination. *Indian Journal of Psychiatry*, *63*(1), 91. doi:10.4103/psychiatry.IndianJPsychiatry_204_20 PMID:34083828

Malla, A., & Shaw, T. (1987). Attitudes towards mental illness: The influence of education and experience. *The International Journal of Social Psychiatry*, *33*(1), 33–41. doi:10.1177/002076408703300105 PMID:3583603

Meda, N., Pardini, S., Slongo, I., Bodini, L., Zordan, M. A., Rigobello, P., Visioli, F., & Novara, C. (2021). Students' mental health problems before, during, and after the COVID-19 lockdown in Italy. *Journal of Psychiatric Research*, *134*, 69–77. doi:10.1016/j.jpsychires.2020.12.045 PMID:33360865

Murthy, R. S. (2014). Mental health initiatives in India (1947-2010). *Social Work in Mental Health: Contexts and Theories for Practice*, *5*, 28.

Paternite, C. E. (2005). School-based mental health programs and services: Overview and introduction to the special issue. *Journal of Abnormal Child Psychology*, *33*(6), 657–663. doi:10.100710802-005-7645-3 PMID:16328742

Singh, S., Roy, D., Sinha, K., Parveen, S., Sharma, G., & Joshi, G. (2020). Impact of COVID-19 and lockdown on mental health of children and adolescents: A narrative review with recommendations. *Psychiatry Research*, *293*, 113429. doi:10.1016/j.psychres.2020.113429 PMID:32882598

Speed, E. (2006). Patients, consumers, and survivors: A case study of mental health service user discourses. *Social Science & Medicine*, *62*(1), 28–38. doi:10.1016/j.socscimed.2005.05.025 PMID:15993529

Walker, E. R., Moore, E., Tapscott, S., Alperin, M., Cummings, J. R., & Druss, B. G. (2021). Developing Regional Mental Health Priorities: Mixed-Methods Needs Assessment of Eight States in the Southeastern United States. *Psychiatric Services (Washington, D.C.)*, *72*(3), 358–361. doi:10.1176/appi.ps.202000141 PMID:33234050

Wyn, J., Cahill, H., Holdsworth, R., Rowling, L., & Carson, S. (2000). MindMatters, a whole-school approach promoting mental health and well-being. *The Australian and New Zealand Journal of Psychiatry*, *34*(4), 594–601. doi:10.1080/j.1440-1614.2000.00748.x PMID:10954390

Yang, J., Lopez Cervera, R., Tye, S. J., Ekker, S. C., & Pierret, C. (2018). Adolescent mental health education InSciEd Out: A case study of an alternative middle school population. *Journal of Translational Medicine*, *16*(1), 1–10. doi:10.118612967-018-1459-x PMID:29615090

Zhao, X., Lin, X., Chen, M., & Mahmood, S. (2022). Research on the influence mechanism of entrepreneurial environment on college students' entrepreneurial performance based on psychology. *Psychiatria Danubina*, *34*(suppl 2), 319–319.

Chapter 6
Mental Health Challenges of Higher Education Students During the COVID-19 Pandemic:
Concerns and Considerations in the New Normal

Akhil M. P.
Alliance University, India

ABSTRACT

Higher education is affected by the COVID-19 outbreak, which forced thousands of schools and educational institutions to close in a short amount of time in order to enact social segregation measures. Educational institutions, particularly in India, face considerable challenges in their system of planning, implementing, and assessing. The main purpose of the study was to gather qualitative data about the pandemic-related worries of college students from various part of the country. Education, personal and public safety, mental health, job security and financial instability, future uncertainty, pandemic's effects on social relationships, misleading news and information, politics, the economy, and travel were among the main topics of concern. Universities must seize the potential to enhance their evidence-based practices, provide readily accessible mental health therapies, and modify their courses to meet the needs of the contemporary world.

DOI: 10.4018/978-1-6684-7221-7.ch006

INTRODUCTION

The World Health Organization (WHO) proclaimed COVID-19 a global epidemic in March 2020, which has caused unrest across(A. Sharma et al., 2020). In an effort to stop the spread of the virus, various lockdown measures were implemented by countries, disrupting educational institutions throughout(N. Sharma & Vaish, 2020). Universities all over the world have generally switched to online teaching to protect student health and follow legislative guidelines and some were also able to shift student support services online throughout the academic year(De' et al., 2020). Educational institutions have also introduced safety measures like alternating the occupancy of residence halls and changing dining halls to only allow takeout(Ronchi et al., 2020).

For college students, the abrupt switch from in-person instruction to online learning has had a significant impact on their mental health(Barrot et al., 2021). The interruption of routine that occurred during lockdowns and quarantines also made the symptoms of mental illnesses more severe among(Lekamwasam & Lekamwasam, 2020). Although not limited to college students, COVID-19 has had a negative impact on society at large, including job loss, uncertainty in the economy and politics, difficulties in relationships, and confusion brought on by the overabundance of information on social media(Acuti Martellucci et al., 2020).

The mental health of college and university students was already an important topic of study before the COVID-19 pandemic. Since 2010, there was a considerable increase in the number of mental health diagnoses and services used among college students (Hager et al., 2020). Students in higher education have been observed to suffer from increased levels of stress, depression, anxiety, and other typical mental problems globally(Scheier & Carver, 1992). Colleges and universities frequently provide assistance with student mental health, but when campuses were evacuated, these assistance programmes had to immediately move online(Zhao et al., 2020). Some colleges found it difficult to adjust to the online environment, particularly when addressing the requirements of vulnerable students.

All of these problems have made it more difficult and diverse for educational institutions to respond to crises like the COVID-19 epidemic. The boundary spanning theory, which examines the barriers and connections between organisations and their surrounding environment, is one framework for comprehending the lessons learnt from previous emergencies and disasters(Nüchter et al., 2021). Indeed, communication between campus stakeholders has been identified as a crucial requirement in previous research on universities' disaster preparedness. Communication between important academic, support, and faith-based student services during an emergency might be hampered by the division of university departments and organisational structures. Insufficient post-disaster communication led to students' uncertainty about the continuity of their education(Schwartz & Graham, 2020). Despite the fact that many students think they are in charge of their own readiness, they frequently hold colleges accountable for educating them and providing emergency response guidance. Unsurprisingly, colleges with a specialized emergency management role tend to be the best equipped. However, universities and colleges with various sizes and focuses may encounter risk and liability in various ways (Naser et al., 2020).

The current study was conducted among currently enrolled undergraduate and graduate students in India. For this study, qualitative concerns related to the COVID-19 pandemic were examined.

Figure 1. Higher education scenario during Covid-19 pandemic (blogs.sap.com)

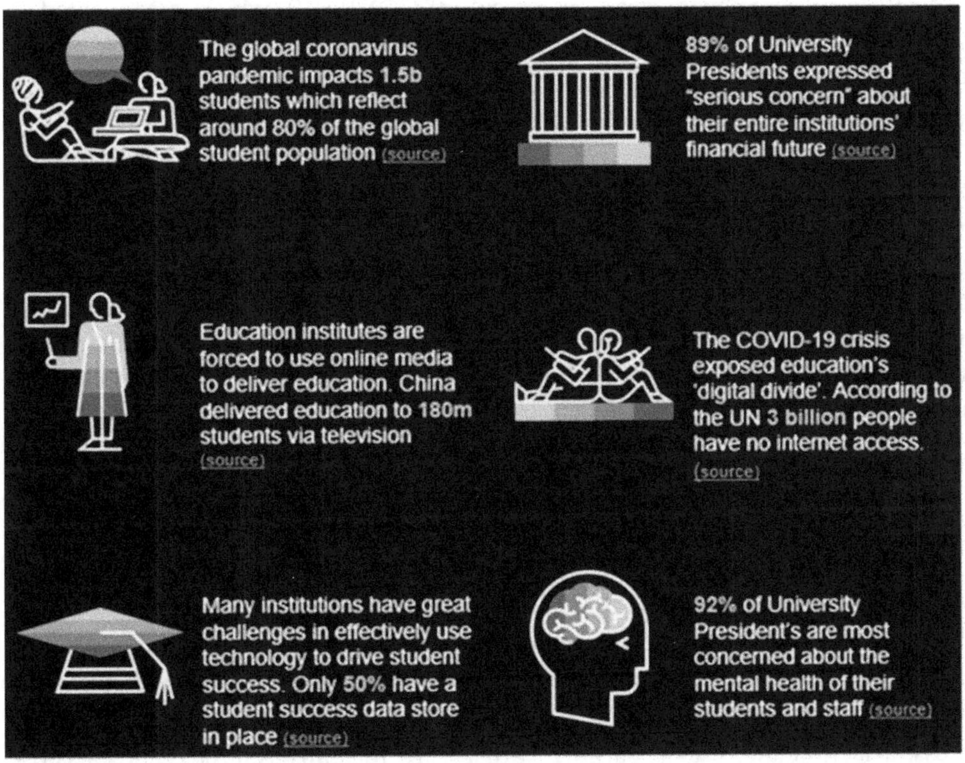

LITERATURE REVIEW

The COVID-19 pandemic had a substantial effect on more than 1.6 billion pupils' lives and educational experiences. In an effort to contain the pandemic, almost all the countries in the world began locking down schools and educational institutions in the middle of March 2020(Piper, 2020). The lockdown forced the institutions to quickly adopt and explore video conferencing-based remote learning(Hew et al., 2020). Numerous difficulties have been faced by the teachers, children, and their families, including an increase in stress and worry that has resulted in a decline in mental health(Barrot et al., 2021). The problems have been made worse by strict social isolation policies that have become necessary as a result of the scarcity of vaccines and the high mortality rates(Hager et al., 2020).

People, notably high school students, are feeling more stressed and anxious as a result of the COVID-19 pandemic-related circumstances. When compared to other pandemics, indicate a significantly larger fraction of young people experiencing psychiatric problems during the COVID-19 pandemic. According to the American Psychological Association (APA), approximately 81% of Gen Z youth ages between 13 to 17 face more severe stress as a result of COVID-19, which is connected to schooling (American Psychological Association (APA), 2020). The APA report, however, skips over the specifics of the stressors brought on by the changes in schooling brought on by the epidemic.

China was the first nation to experience COVID-19 pandemic effects(Li et al., 2020). As a result, numerous research looking at how the epidemic has affected students' mental health have been published (Viana *et al.*, 2020;Yuan *et al.*, 2020;Bakioğlu, Korkmaz and Ercan, 2020;Sharma and Vaish, 2020; Naser *et al.*, 2020). During the COVID-19 pandemic, Copeland *et al.*, 2021 spoke about the subject of mental health issues and suicidality among senior high school students. According to their findings, the percentages of depression, anxiety, PTSD, suicidal thoughts, and attempted suicide were, alarming. Academic pressure, pronged school closures, and societal stigma of COVID infection may be stresses, their study did not expressly focus on any stressors(Smit & Wandel, 2006). Resilience and well coping were preventative measures against the symptoms of stress, anxiety, and depression(Scheier & Carver, 1992). Most of the concern related to mental health in the COVID-19 population was associated with employment, educational attainment, and the use of unhealthy coping mechanisms(Naser et al., 2020).

Students are under more pressure to learn independently when there is disturbance in the academic process(Yasmin, 2020). Therefore, it makes sense to assume that stress, a lack of interest in learning, a disregard for daily routines, and possibly higher dropout rates may all be experienced by students as a direct result of public health initiatives. The pandemic aggravated pre-existing mental health disorders mostly because of the closure of academic institutions, the disruption of routine, and the loss of social ties(Larsen et al., 2022). In addition to students said they had a mental health issue that had been diagnosed in 2020, and one in four students said they were taking psychiatric medication(Engzell et al., 2021).

Anxiety among students is fueled by the disruption of their research projects and internships, which compromise their academic work and, in some cases, delay their completion of their degrees(Leal Filho et al., 2021). Other difficulties that college students experienced that had a negative impact on their mental health included financial difficulties brought on by the pandemic, health issues in their families, and deaths(Loayza, Norman and Pennings, 2020).

Furthermore, there are other notable unfavourable effects that require care, such as dependence on video games, emotional eating, and excessive social media use(Viana et al., 2020). Students found it difficult to create a lockdown habit despite the emphasis on doing so(Gonzalez et al., 2020). Additionally, COVID-19 introduced children to a tendency toward existential thinking and introspection, which at first did cause uneasiness(Khalil et al., 2020). Learning has been faced with a number of difficulties, and mental health vulnerabilities have grown. Some students experienced intensely negative emotions when they had to spend a lot of time away from the college, including dissatisfaction, worry, and betrayal(Rezapour et al., 2022). For many students studying abroad, homesickness was brought on by being away from home. Due to their lack of contact with friends, family and partners, some people experienced loneliness and isolation(Leal Filho et al., 2021). Numerous studies have shown that young people, notably college students, are experiencing higher levels of stress, worry, depressive thoughts, sleep disruptions, difficulties concentrating, feelings of denial, rage, and fear, as well as increasing worries about their academic success(Xiang et al., 2020).

Additionally, there is a propensity for the psychological symptoms of kids who already have a mental illness to worsen and raise certain students' risk for suicide(Tang et al., 2020). Another survey that looked at the impact of COVID-19 on students found that being a student was linked to a higher frequency of depressive symptoms, anxiety symptoms, perceived stress, and suicidal thoughts(Zhu et al., 2021). This confirms the same, an increasing trend of suicide among college students during the pandemic, warranting emergency services more than ever. Most of the students had negative mental health as a result of the epidemic, with social isolation, lack of attention, and anxiety being the three most prevalent of these symptoms, among many others(Kramer & Kramer, 2020). The main causes of mental health issues among students were concerns about reaching academic milestones, interpersonal connections, and financial security(Taylor et al., 2020).

The COVID-19 presents major and unanticipated obstacles to higher education institutions and their students. Numerous facets of the higher education experience have been examined by researchers in the COVID-19 period, both subjectively and quantitatively. In emergency scenarios like the novel COVID-19 pandemic, qualitative research is crucial in establishing newly explored factors or contexts that are not well understood(Carey, 2016). This can support and add to preliminary perceptions and insights that are currently developing in the investigation(Marshall, 1996).

METHODOLOGY

The study uses qualitative research design. Open ended question regarding worries about the COVID-19 pandemic were given and the responses were collected from google form and the results were compiled from textual analysis. The respondents forming part of this study is those who are at least 18 years old and be currently enrolled for a university degree such as undergraduate, post graduate or professional courses. The information and responses collected from the respondents were analyzed and presented as textual and content analysis.

RESULTS AND DISCUSSION

Many issues were found in the content analysis, spread across different themes. The identified themes as per the responses from university/higher education students are Academic and Education, Physical Safety concerns, mental health, job security and financial stability, social relationships, unforeseen future, concern about travel, politics, and economy etc. The thematic-wise details are as follows:

Academic and Education

The upcoming academic year's online or in-person format was the students' top concern regarding their education. Students were worried about maintaining engagement with peers and teachers, the caliber of online education, and their academic advancement. Prior studies shown that before the epidemic, pupils frequently expressed concerns of a similar nature. The stress of switching to online learning while lacking the necessary equipment or skills, as well as the unease caused by lecturers changing plans abruptly and without prior notice, were expressed by students. Some students were unsure of how the switch to online learning would affect their grades and thought that it had a detrimental impact on their performance. A student opined, "I have difficulty concentrating in my classes because they were never meant to take place online and I'm just not getting as much out of them in the virtual format."

Concerns about education also applied to study abroad and internship opportunities. Some students' degree programmes included substantial practical work related to internships or travel. The degree progress was undetermined when these opportunities ceased to exist. A student was concerned about the possible setback of graduation owing to internships not hiring, while another student was concerned about the opportunity to obtain education on practical skills if school is still online in the fall.

Physical Safety Concerns

Concerns concerning the safety of other COVID-19 groups, including parents, spouses, children, other family members, and the wider public, constituted the majority of the safety subcategories. Students studying away from their parents' homes were confused about whether they should go back since they were concerned about infecting others who were already at high risk. "I personally am in a scenario where I can't go home because my mother is immuno-compromised and I don't want to make her sick by travelling," a student stated. Those who had grandparents frequently expressed worry about unintentionally infecting others; worry about the safety of the elderly was a particular focus within the "safety of others" subcategory. During the lockdown, students also brought up rising domestic violence statistics and concerns for other people's safety that had nothing to do with the virus.

Another safety-related worry included other people's COVID-19 prevention actions, such as whether they used masks, maintained the proper distance, and kept their hands clean. Although there was a desire to reopen, most students understood that doing so required people to continue acting in ways that would reduce viral transmission in the community. Some students observed that "not everyone adopting the same measures to avoid the spread of the disease," and participants questioned if others would follow same protocols. Students looking for shared housing showed concern about how other people's actions may affect their health, since they are anxious to have to share a room with others.

Going to the doctor for non-COVID-19 health issues, going to school, going back to work, and regular travel all pose additional security risks. Participants' worries highlighted a conflict between wanting towns and schools to return and being concerned about the virus reemerging. Treatments for COVID-19 safety issues also addressed whether a prospective vaccination would be safe, how it would be disseminated, and when it would be accessible.

Mental Health

Many students who disclosed prior anxiety or depression issues mentioned that the pandemic had worsened their symptoms. Additionally, students started to worry more about their mental health. The majority of these psychological symptoms were brought on by worry about the future and worries about contracting an infection or spreading it to others. "General anxiety over not knowing I had it and constant dread of dying from it," opined by a student.

Anxiety was exacerbated by isolation and loneliness brought on by orders to stay at home. Negative feelings resulted from missing out on seeing loved ones. According to some students, "stressors related to contracting corona and giving it to an at-risk person in my home" and the accompanying duty or guilt were another issue that had an impact on students' mental health.

This study's findings showing women report greater rates of common mental health illnesses than men do are consistent with the proportion of female participants who answered questions about their mental health. Given that men are less likely to seek medical attention or practice preventative measures, the higher reported incidence may not accurately reflect real prevalence.

In proportionally higher numbers, students from the Indian higher education institutions voiced concerns about their mental health. This is consistent with the high overall rates of depression in the country. Although China has been found to have higher than average rates of depression globally, there have also been claims of widespread stigmatizing views. The students opined following major points related to mental health they experienced during the pandemic. The issues are presented in the order of intensity opined by the respondents.

- suicidal thoughts
- high level of anxiety
- severe distress
- high level of perceived stress
- severe depression

Job Security and Financial Stability

With regard to students' current financial situation and employment prospects, the pandemic caused volatility. Numerous students claimed to have worked to pay for their education, and the epidemic made finding or keeping a job difficult. Students must deal with job losses or a reduction in hours. "Since I was laid off, I'm worried about finding work. Because I am a full-time student, I am ineligible for any stimulus package and am unable to apply for unemployment benefits, said opined some students.

Future employment prospects were a further source of worry. "I am graduating and moving on to a postgraduate degree," one Irish woman student said. Concerns I have included jobs, relocating, the new course, and others. Students worried about "financial insecurity in the future, e.g., not finding a job" or "getting a job after graduating, especially in academia, due to budget cuts" as they were unsure if they would be able to find employment in their chosen area. Concerns about the volatility of safety net provisions were related to worries about employment stability. Concerns among students included childcare, unemployment insurance, and health insurance.

While the COVID-19 epidemic may make it easier for students to do online coursework from home, financial constraints may make it harder for them to continue to be students. Both male as well as female students expressed anxiety regarding employment security. In fact, COVID-19 has hindered women's ability to engage in paid work by widening the alarming gender gap in childcare and household duties. Contrarily, compared to mothers, non-fathers, and non-mothers, fathers have experienced greater employment stability and significantly fewer layoffs.

Social Relationships

Although important, keeping friendships and family ties proved difficult for students. Concern about "family members getting sick and dying while I am pursuing studies abroad" was expressed by a student. Students felt cut off from interpersonal ties, whether they were amorous or not: "I miss my pals and my lover". There was little interaction with their community's neighbors and other residents. A student opined "My life feels emptier now that the events I had been looking forward to have been postponed". Before the COVID-19 crisis abruptly put an end to everything, I had been arranging a very large event for already 8 months. I no longer feel a sense of connection to the college community that I once did. I miss interacting with the teachers and fellow students on a daily basis. Furthermore, I've experienced a lot of powerlessness, which has made me quite upset. I am now more conscious of how the world may be unfair and socioeconomic disparities.

Students questioned how these relationships could continue to develop and be built upon in the absence of face-to-face interaction.

Unforeseen Future

There was a pervasive sense of unease about the future for many pupils. One question frequently asked in general was "When would everything return to normal?" Along with this, there were concerns about the pandemic's duration and a desire for normalcy, but it was also understood that post-pandemic normalcy might not resemble pre-pandemic times. Comments from some students who asked "When will they find the cure and how long will we live like this" and "we are just worried about what the future holds, what the 'new normal' will look like, and all the uncertainties that come with that".

Travel Concerns

General travel worries to visit relatives, friends, or for the summer holidays fell under this group. There was a want to "go out," but not in the "open the stores, I need a haircut!" sense; rather, "I need to at least go window shopping every now and then to at least get my mind off of stuff and get out of my damn house" kind of attitude.

No matter where you were, "getting out" meant being allowed to go about without restriction. Concern over missing out on events was related to this: "family vacation because we have all been planning it for three years," said a student; "COVID-19 has merely made it even harder to organize for anything," someone who is stressed about getting married says. "I can't see my favorite singer's stage in person because COVID-19 made all concerts online or illegal."

Compared to domestic students, international students expressed higher worries about travel and staying in touch with loved ones. This is understandable given that overseas students typically face more difficulties getting in touch with family members back home due to factors including travel restrictions, safety concerns, and visa requirements. According to recent study, it is advisable to ask overseas students directly about their goals because they could differ from those of academic institutions. The first stage in creating an emergency/crisis response for this demographic is to identify these concerns.

Political Concern

Students voiced a lack of confidence in political officials, pointing out how politics affected choices made to contain the outbreak. Concerns ranged from "concern that the President is managing the issue poorly and that our country would be worse off as a result," expressed by a student studying abroad, to "insecurity in my own country and to the degradation of democracy". Concerns about "civil freedoms being disrespected and little to no concessions" were also raised.

Economic Concern

This theme covered a wide range of economic worries, such as the likelihood of an economic downturn, the state of the economy in the future, and the possibility of a recession. Among the comments on this subject were those from a student who said: "My concerns about COVID are less about getting the disease itself and more about how our nation's economy as a whole will be able to recover." Another student said: "I am concerned that businesses I used to frequent may go out of business".

Comparatively speaking, abroad studying students were more worried about the political and economic climate than their domestic counterparts. In fact, a student said, "I believe in the government and I'm not particularly scared about COVID-19." This is in line with the attention India has gotten from throughout the world due to its effective national responses to early cases and decline in COVID-19 positive rates. This variation in levels of worry between nations highlights the significance of open communication based on trustworthy information and scientific evidence, which should be represented in university emergency counselling even if local community policy differs in its approach. For instance, academic institutions might always demand safety precautions such as masks, social seclusion, and cleanliness regulations, regardless of what the local population thinks.

Misleading/Fake News About COVID-19

Conspiracy theories, media coverage, and questions about "how COVID-19 formed" were the main topics of student concerns over COVID-19 misinformation. Many students expressed skepticism about a potential vaccination due to their mistrust of information about treatments: "I would not be interested in the projected vaccines for the virus because everything looks to be a scam". Students were troubled by conflicting information concerning the virus. They feared that the conflicting messages would make people doubt the seriousness of the virus' threat or the value of safety precautions like wearing masks and avoiding close contact, which would have an adverse effect on the virus' ability to spread.

Practical Implications

Although the COVID-19 reaction may potentially be planned for in university contingency plans, the pandemic is distinct in the worldwide scope and duration of the response it has required. Universities had to quickly rethink and restructure how to educate students, with various degrees of success. In the future, colleges should create or revise emergency preparedness strategies while taking both immediate and long-term educational demands into account. Given that students' home realities differ, tailored approaches are necessary for some populations, such as those with unstable internet connectivity or dangerous home living situations. Students should be involved in the development of such plans because their welfare should be at the centre of any preparedness plans. Consideration needs to be given to vulnerable students, especially in the event that dormitories are closed for extended periods of time.

In the current study, students' primary worries related to their academic future and the general unpredictability of the future, both of which had an effect on their mental health. Communication issues between university administration and students regarding lockdowns, the start of classes, and feeling connected to classmates and teachers were frequently reported, and were occasionally exacerbated by the fact that students were distributed around the world. Student uncertainty and future worries may be reduced by open communication about university plans for post-pandemic and pandemic education. In situations of uncertainty, risk communication concepts including message consistency, process explanation, empathy and care, and genuine communication can offer predictability. Both boundary-spanning theory and the disaster-resistant university model require effective communication and information management systems.

Additionally, academics shouldn't be the exclusive focus of university readiness initiatives to ensure linkages between students and professors. Universities with vibrant student communities should look for online community development opportunities. This could involve expanding the services typically provided by campus support offices (such instructional design, information technology, and the library) through virtual excursions and non-academic workshops. Universities might also seek to broaden the idea of student life to include connecting with and taking care of loved ones in addition to mingling with classmates. Support for the family of the pupils may also be helpful. For instance, campus-sponsored student organisations may establish private or public Facebook Groups, which have been shown to suit students' demands for information and for making decisions. These actions may reduce students' worries about their loved ones. Educational institutions must be ready to help students who are returning to in-person instruction deal with the negative effects of loss and sadness brought on by COVID-19 on their mental health. To reach groups who feel unable to seek critical care, mental health initiatives must normalize treatment and fight stigma. The World Health Organization has created a Special Initiative for Mental Health to address requirements in twelve priority nations, including eradicating stigma. However, there is room for expansion in more anti-stigma projects.

CONCLUSION

The current study gathered qualitative data about the pandemic-related worries of college students from various part of the country. Education, personal and public safety, mental health, job and financial instability, future uncertainty, pandemic's effects on relationships, misinformation, politics, the economy, and travel were among the main topics of concern. Participatory research, enhanced communication, and the expansion of student services to include full virtual/online access could all be effective ways to solve these issues. The provision of mental health treatments, career planning and placement, social assistance, and technical help are among the key services. Overall, student feedback on issues can help higher education institutions support students more effectively during the COVID-19 epidemic and other events that call for a change in customary teaching strategies.

RECOMMENDATIONS

Programs for higher education should offer courses on environmental and public health issues. It is essential to adapt the curriculum as much as possible to the demands of the modern environment. All university students should be allowed to participate in the integration of essential environmental and health courses because everyone deals with environmental and health challenges. Learning resources connected to environmental literacy can be developed for use in classroom instruction and for educating a wider population in society.

Environmental science education programmes can create environmentally literate citizens who can serve as role models for environmental health issues in the community.

Environmental hygiene policies need to be strengthened across the board in school. The education of children in schools is the first step in making society more receptive. Teaching students about societal issues, in particular health issues, is difficult for universities. Students should also get information on infectious illness prevention, including behavioral recommendations and knowledge. The students can be given health management tools so they can practice the correct technique until it gets ingrained in the culture of the school. If the institution wants to achieve its goal, a policy to restrict the virus's source of transmission must be created. The sustainable environmental framework of a university should therefore serve as the foundation for the development of appropriate environmental and health policies.

The academic, career-counselling, and even medical services and programmes that should be provided to students both on-campus and online must take precedence in higher education due to the pandemic's global patterns. In fact, because mental problems are becoming more common among college students, there has been a lot of focus on the need for mental health services in colleges. Even when they are not in the centers, students should have easy access to free online health services from members of the medical staff and experts like psychologists and guidance counsellors, such as mental health teleconferencing and other relevant services.

Even while the need for online-driven competences in planning, carrying out, and evaluating student performance can be a hurdle for teachers, giving them access to sufficient training programmes can help them carry out the courses successfully. Teachers can access a selection of devices with cutting-edge features to support learning for children with a range of educational requirements.

REFERENCES

Acuti Martellucci, C., Flacco, M. E., Cappadona, R., Bravi, F., Mantovani, L., & Manzoli, L. (2020). SARS-CoV-2 pandemic: An overview. *Advances in Biological Regulation*, *77*, 100736. doi:10.1016/j.jbior.2020.100736 PMID:32773099

American Psychological Association (APA). (2020). *Stress in America, 2020: A National Mental Health Crisis*. APA. https://www.apa.org/news/press/releases/stress/2020/report-october

Bakioğlu, F., Korkmaz, O., & Ercan, H. (2020). Fear of COVID-19 and Positivity: Mediating Role of Intolerance of Uncertainty, Depression, Anxiety, and Stress. *International Journal of Mental Health and Addiction*, *1*. doi:10.100711469-020-00331-y PMID:32837421

Barrot, J. S., Llenares, I. I., & del Rosario, L. S. (2021). Students' online learning challenges during the pandemic and how they cope with them: The case of the Philippines. *Education and Information Technologies*, *26*(6), 7321–7338. doi:10.100710639-021-10589-x PMID:34075300

Carey, M. A. (2016). Comment: Concerns in the Analysis of Focus Group Data. *Sage*, *5*(4), 487–495. doi:10.1177/104973239500500409

Copeland, W. E., McGinnis, E., Bai, Y., Adams, Z., Nardone, H., Devadanam, V., Rettew, J., & Hudziak, J. J. (2021). Impact of COVID-19 pandemic on college student mental health and wellness. *Journal of the American Academy of Child and Adolescent Psychiatry*, *60*(1), 134–141. doi:10.1016/j.jaac.2020.08.466 PMID:33091568

De', R., Pandey, N., & Pal, A. (2020). Impact of digital surge during Covid-19 pandemic: A viewpoint on research and practice. *International Journal of Information Management*, *55*, 102171. doi:10.1016/j.ijinfomgt.2020.102171 PMID:32836633

Engzell, P., Frey, A., & Verhagen, M. D. (2021). Learning loss due to school closures during the COVID-19 pandemic. *Proceedings of the National Academy of Sciences of the United States of America*, *118*(17), e2022376118. Advance online publication. doi:10.1073/pnas.2022376118 PMID:33827987

Gonzalez, T., De la Rubia, M. A., Hincz, K. P., Comas-Lopez, M., Subirats, L., Fort, S., & Sacha, G. M. (2020). Influence of COVID-19 confinement on students' performance in higher education. *PLoS One*, *15*(10), e0239490. doi:10.1371/journal.pone.0239490 PMID:33035228

Hager, E., Odetokun, I. A., 2, I. D., Bolarinwa Id, O., Zainab, A., Okechukwu, O., & Al-Mustaphaid, A. I. (2020). *Knowledge, attitude, and perceptions towards the 2019 Coronavirus Pandemic: A bi-national survey in Africa*. PLOS Research. doi:10.1371/journal.pone.0236918

Hew, K. F., Jia, C., Gonda, D. E., & Bai, S. (2020). Transitioning to the "new normal" of learning in unpredictable times: Pedagogical practices and learning performance in fully online flipped classrooms. *International Journal of Educational Technology in Higher Education*, *17*(1), 1–22. doi:10.118641239-020-00234-x PMID:34778516

Khalil, R., Mansour, A. E., Fadda, W. A., Almisnid, K., Aldamegh, M., Al-Nafeesah, A., Alkhalifah, A., & Al-Wutayd, O. (2020). The sudden transition to synchronized online learning during the COVID-19 pandemic in Saudi Arabia: A qualitative study exploring medical students' perspectives. *BMC Medical Education*, *20*(1), 1–10. doi:10.118612909-020-02208-z PMID:32859188

Kramer, A., & Kramer, K. Z. (2020). The potential impact of the Covid-19 pandemic on occupational status, work from home, and occupational mobility. In *Journal of Vocational Behavior* (Vol. 119, p. 103442). Academic Press Inc. doi:10.1016/j.jvb.2020.103442

Larsen, L., Helland, M. S., & Holt, T. (2022). The impact of school closure and social isolation on children in vulnerable families during COVID-19: A focus on children's reactions. *European Child & Adolescent Psychiatry*, *31*(8), 1–11. doi:10.100700787-021-01758-x PMID:33770275

Leal Filho, W., Wall, T., Rayman-Bacchus, L., Mifsud, M., Pritchard, D. J., Lovren, V. O., Farinha, C., Petrovic, D. S., & Balogun, A. L. (2021). Impacts of COVID-19 and social isolation on academic staff and students at universities: A cross-sectional study. *BMC Public Health*, *21*(1), 1213. doi:10.118612889-021-11040-z PMID:34167494

Lekamwasam, R., & Lekamwasam, S. (2020). Effects of covid-19 pandemic on health and wellbeing of older people: A comprehensive review. *Annals of Geriatric Medicine and Research*, *24*(3), 166–172. doi:10.4235/agmr.20.0027 PMID:32752587

Li, M., Chen, J., & Deng, Y. (2020). *Scaling features in the spreading of COVID-19*. Ming Li.

Loayza, N. & Pennings, S. M. (2020). Macroeconomic Policy in the Time of COVID-19: A Primer for Developing Countries. *Our World in Data*. https://ourworldindata.org/coronavirus-source-data

Marshall, M. N. (1996). Sampling for qualitative research. *Family Practice © Oxford University Press, 13*(6). http://fampra.oxfordjournals.org/

Naser, A. Y., Dahmash, E. Z., Al-Rousan, R., Alwafi, H., Alrawashdeh, H. M., Ghoul, I., Abidine, A., Bokhary, M. A., AL-Hadithi, H. T., Ali, D., Abuthawabeh, R., Abdelwahab, G. M., Alhartani, Y. J., Al Muhaisen, H., Dagash, A., & Alyami, H. S. (2020). Mental health status of the general population, healthcare professionals, and university students during 2019 coronavirus disease outbreak in Jordan: A cross-sectional study. *Brain and Behavior*, *10*(8). doi:10.1002/brb3.1730 PMID:32578943

Nüchter, V., Abson, D. J., von Wehrden, H., & Engler, J. O. (2021). The concept of resilience in recent sustainability research. *Sustainability (Switzerland)*, *13*(5), 1–21. doi:10.3390u13052735

Piper, K. (2020). The devastating consequences of coronavirus lockdowns in poor countries. *VOX*. https://www.vox.com/future-perfect/2020/4/18/21212688/coronavirus-lockdowns-developing-world

Rezapour, M., Dehzangi, A., & Saadati, F. (2022). Students' negative emotions and their rational and irrational behaviors during COVID-19 outbreak. *PLoS One*, *17*(3), e0264985. doi:10.1371/journal.pone.0264985 PMID:35255106

Ronchi, A., Pagliuca, F., Zito Marino, F., Montella, M., Franco, R., & Cozzolino, I. (2020). Interventional cytopathology in the COVID-19 era. *Cytopathology*, *31*(6), 509–513. doi:10.1111/cyt.12886 PMID:32654199

Scheier, M. F., & Carver, C. S. (1992). Effects of optimism on psychological and physical well-being: Theoretical overview and empirical update. *Cognitive Therapy and Research*, *16*(2), 201–228. doi:10.1007/BF01173489

Schwartz, D. A., & Graham, A. L. (2020). Potential maternal and infant outcomes from coronavirus 2019-NCOV (SARS-CoV-2) infecting pregnant women: Lessons from SARS, MERS, and other human coronavirus infections. In Viruses, 12(2). MDPI AG. doi:10.3390/v12020194

Sharma, A., Tiwari, S., Deb, M. K., & Marty, J. L. (2020). Severe acute respiratory syndrome coronavirus-2 (SARS-CoV-2): A global pandemic and treatment strategies. *International Journal of Antimicrobial Agents*, *56*(2), 106054. doi:10.1016/j.ijantimicag.2020.106054 PMID:32534188

Sharma, N., & Vaish, H. (2020). Impact of COVID–19 on mental health and physical load on women professionals: An online cross-sectional survey. *Health Care for Women International*, *41*(11–12), 1255–1272. doi:10.1080/07399332.2020.1825441 PMID:33021925

Smit, B., & Wandel, J. (2006). Adaptation, adaptive capacity and vulnerability. *Global Environmental Change*, *16*(3), 282–292. doi:10.1016/j.gloenvcha.2006.03.008

Tang, W., Hu, T., Hu, B., Jin, C., Wang, G., Xie, C., Chen, S., & Xu, J. (2020). Prevalence and correlates of PTSD and depressive symptoms one month after the outbreak of the COVID-19 epidemic in a sample of home-quarantined Chinese university students. *Journal of Affective Disorders, 274*, 1–7. doi:10.1016/j.jad.2020.05.009 PMID:32405111

Taylor, S., Landry, C. A., Paluszek, M. M., Fergus, T. A., McKay, D., & Asmundson, G. J. G. (2020). Development and initial validation of the COVID Stress Scales. *Journal of Anxiety Disorders, 72*, 102232. Advance online publication. doi:10.1016/j.janxdis.2020.102232 PMID:32408047

Viana, R. B., Dankel, S. J., Loenneke, J. P., Gentil, P., Vieira, C. A., Andrade, M. dos S., Vancini, R. L., & de Lira, C. A. B. (2020). The effects of exergames on anxiety levels: A systematic review and meta-analysis. In Scandinavian Journal of Medicine and Science in Sports, 30(7), pp. 1100–1116. Blackwell Munksgaard. doi:10.1111ms.13654

Xiang, Y., Li, W., Zhang, Q., Jin, Y., Rao, W., Zeng, L., Lok, G. K. I., Chow, I. H. I., Cheung, T., & Hall, B. J. (2020). Correspondence Timely research papers about COVID-19 in. *Lancet, 6736*(20), 30375. doi:10.1016/S0140-6736(20)30375-5 PMID:32078803

Yasmin, H. (2020). Covid 19: Stress Management among Students and its Impact on Their Effective Learning. *International Technology and Education Journal, 4*(2).

Yuan, B., Li, W., Liu, H., Cai, X., Song, S., Zhao, J., Hu, X., Li, Z., Chen, Y., Zhang, K., Liu, Z., Peng, J., Wang, C., Wang, J., & An, Y. (2020). Correlation between immune response and self-reported depression during convalescence from COVID-19. *Brain, Behavior, and Immunity, 88*, 39–43. doi:10.1016/j.bbi.2020.05.062 PMID:32464158

Zhao, M., Wang, M., Zhang, J., Ye, J., Xu, Y., Wang, Z., Ye, D., Liu, J., & Wan, J. (2020). Advances in the relationship between coronavirus infection and cardiovascular diseases. In *Biomedicine and Pharmacotherapy* (Vol. 127). Elsevier Masson SAS., doi:10.1016/j.biopha.2020.110230

Zhu, Y., Zhang, L., Zhou, X., Li, C., & Yang, D. (2021). The impact of social distancing during COVID-19: A conditional process model of negative emotions, alienation, affective disorders, and post-traumatic stress disorder. *Journal of Affective Disorders, 281*, 131–137. doi:10.1016/j.jad.2020.12.004 PMID:33316718

Chapter 7
Psychological Impact of the COVID-19 Pandemic on Childless Couples:
A Review

Sri Raghavi Vasudevan
Vellore Institute of Technology, India

Bhuvaneswari Mohanraj
Vellore Institute of Technology, India

ABSTRACT

Infertility has been one of the most pressing challenges in recent years. Infertility services have been postponed and rescheduled globally due to the start of this deadly pandemic. The current study investigated the psychological distress and social consequences of infertile couples during the COVID-19 pandemic. This review study examined articles on infertility, psychosocial effects, and infertility-related stress and pandemic. From the reviewed data, it can be concluded that the pandemic has affected the mental health of childless couples. Increased anxiety, stress, feelings of hopelessness, and fear of uncertainty were common psychological distress experienced by infertile patients during the pandemic. The results of the investigations aid in identifying the psychological concerns of the COVID-19 pandemic on childless couples, knowledge gaps, contemporary patterns, and cutting-edge psychotherapeutic approaches to handling distress.

DOI: 10.4018/978-1-6684-7221-7.ch007

INTRODUCTION

The World Health Organization (WHO) designated the SARS-CoV-2-related coronavirus illness as Coronavirus Disease 19 (COVID-19), classifying it as a pandemic and a global public health emergency (Zhu et al., 2020). The first case of COVID-19 was discovered in Wuhan (China) in December 2019, and an outbreak quickly spread to Hubei Province and other regions of the nation (Huang et al., 2020). The virus spread rapidly across the population, which was spurred by its high virulence and long-lasting surface viability, posing possible harm to the community. India, the second-most populated nation on earth, is predicted to have the highest infection rate (Sarkar, Saha, & Arora, 2021). With an average of 36,000 new cases per day worldwide, India saw the most instances. The size of the epidemic has already put immense pressure on the nation's healthcare system because there were more patients than hospital beds available. One of the most severe issues in recent years has been infertility, or "the failure to naturally create a child after 12 months of sexual intercourse (Oquin & Lafontaine., 2010) without using birth control prophylactics" (WHO, 2018). In India, more than three million couples seek infertility treatment each year, with five lakhs having IUI and IVF procedures (Malhotra et al., 2020). Infertility services have decreased during this COVID-19 period. All around the world, infertility services have been rescheduled and postponed as a result of the outbreak of this fatal epidemic. Couples who wanted to establish a family never expected that the declaration of social lockdown in various provinces of the subcontinent starting in the middle of March would cause their next clinic visit to be delayed not just for days but several months (Sarkar, Saha, & Arora, 2021). Couples who were anxious to have children have experienced unspeakable mental and emotional costs owing to the delay of such treatments because of the high cost and complexity of IVF. Infecundity was shown to be the top stressor among the general public in a recent cross-sectional online study done in the USA, and it was nearly as common as the fear of the pandemic itself (66% vs. 63%) (Vaughan et al., 2020) (Sarkar, Saha & Arora, 2021). Many elective treatments, including reproductive services, have been suspended for 8 to 9 months as health systems throughout the world have worked to reduce the virulence of Covid-19. However, for infertile couples, "time" was the critical element (Gupta et al., 2021).

According to studies from several countries, women's stress levels were higher than those of COVID-19 infection due to infertility and forced treatment delays (Wiweko et al., 2021). This illustrates the widespread social stigmas and limitations associated with infertility, and the immediate need to start treatment for those who need it despite the pandemic might be the reason for the increase in stress levels (Gupta et al., 2021). Couples has suffered additional harm as a result of the COVID-19 epidemic, such as the loss of loved ones and unemployment, which has decreased their desire to have children. This attitude may lead to a decrease in birth rates in the near future. Although most couples had prolonged infertility, a minority (4.0%) of couples were able to conceive naturally on their own while the country was under lockdown. This may be due to increased closeness and spending more incredible time together (Cito et al., 2020).

While the biological approach has generated many pathophysiological data and suggestions for diagnostic and treatment modalities during the COVID-19 Pandemic, the aim of clinical and medical psychology was to evaluate how this physical condition impacts the mental health of infertile couples (Turabian, 2019). Even if there has been steady progress in medical and psychosocial therapy, there are still gaps in the study on the relationship between the COVID-19 epidemic and the psychological suffering endured by patients diagnosed with infertility.

Over the years, infertility has been studied using several approaches. The current study examines the psychological suffering of infertile couples and societal repercussions during the COVID-19 pandemic.

METHODOLOGY

Objective

To analyze studies on the psychological effects faced by infertile couples during Covid 19 Pandemic.

To understand whether the treatment suspension had an impact on the infertile patient.

Research Method

Literature Search

This review study examined articles on infertility, psychosocial factors, and infertility-related stress and pandemic among Indian populations. The search will be based on Pubmed, SCOPUS, MEDLINE, and Shodhganga databases and other relevant databases using the keywords "pandemic," "Infertility," "psychosocial consequences," "Treatment suspension," "Assisted reproductive technique," as well as "coping strategies." The aforementioned keywords turned up very few studies.

The titles of every manuscript that the search produced were read. Abstracts and publications that matched the interest area were examined. The bibliographies of the recovered texts were also reviewed for further reference. After reading the study abstracts, research that did not majorly focus on psychological consequences faced among childless couples during the pandemic was eliminated. Studies that satisfied the criteria for inclusion were collected as a result of these processes.

Inclusion Criteria

Studies with open access, full-text publications published during and post Covid 19 that primarily addressed the psychological challenges experienced by infertile couples were included. Only English-language publications and papers with English abstracts were included for review.

Exclusion Criteria

Studies that don't emphasize more on pandemic-related distress in infertile patients were excluded. Studies in the native language or other than the English language were eliminated.

Procedure

Following the core results being collected, each research was subjected to a qualitative analysis. The chosen articles were initially categorized by year of publication. Then, the selected study was arranged according to publishing year and given a content analysis.

As a result, the analyzed content was organized into six domains, a) Life on pause: effect of covid 19 on reproductive medicine, b) Psychosocial consequences faced by infertile couples during a lockdown, c) Covid-19 pandemic myths and their impact on infertile couples d) Treatment-seeking behavior among infertile couples e) Coping with the pandemic.

DISCUSSION

Life on Pause: Covid 19's Impact on Reproductive Medicine

Couples seeking infertility treatments in India and the entire world, doctors, and the medical community face enormous challenges due to the unprecedented COVID-19. According to medical experts, 30 lakh people seek fertility treatment in India each year, but during covid 19 pandemic, only 5 lakhs undergo IVF procedures. However, during the covid-19 pandemic, couples suffered greatly due to treatment suspension. Data analysis shows that from April to June 2021, there was a nearly 90% decrease in IVF cycles performed across the country. The annual number of IVF cycles has decreased since the epidemic began. In India, roughly 250,000 IVF rounds are carried out a year; by 2020, it was predicted that this number would have dropped from 150,000 to 180,000. This was concerning news because IVF treatment not only identifies any underlying illnesses that women may have but also assists them in becoming pregnant safely (Murdia K, 2021).

Covid 19 has an impact on fertility counselling in addition to assisted reproductive technology. Due to financial hardship, some of the participants abruptly stopped receiving counselling, and they weren't sure when or if they would start up again. More remote counselling has been shown to be beneficial and to be accessible. Concerns included exhaustion, practical and technological difficulties, and anonymity decreased therapeutic effectiveness (Pericleous et al., 2021).

Table 1 shows that few modifications were made to the IVF procedure following COVID-19. In the first wave, these protocol changes were complex for participants to adapt to, but by the second wave, they were well acclimated.

Table 1. IVF protocol modifications

BEFORE COVID 19	DURING AND POST-COVID 19
Physical examinations	Visits made through telemedicine
Visits with nurses and coordinators in person	Virtual conferences with coordinators and nurses.
Travel without restrictions or using a personal safety device	If they didn't already have one, all patients were given masks to wear while at the hospital, and all staff members were given masks to wear on their trips to and from the center.
Before stimulation, a test for hepatitis B, C, syphilis, HIV, and have performed.	Before the onset of stimulation, consider adding SARS-COV-2 tests.
Several visits during stimulation (usual consultations during stimulation should be spaced out as needed (3-4 trips before egg retrieval)	Patients checked in and went straight to their rooms. In the exam room, blood was drawn, and vital signs were taken.
Overcrowded waiting areas	Wherever practical, seating arrangements and personnel placement were adjusted to preserve a >6-foot distance.
The ultrasonography examination room has a high turnover rate.	Longer time between procedures, clean surfaces, and an empty waiting area.
Partner is recommended to accompany the patient to appointments	No spouses or visitors (promote using video-telephone services).
Consent sheets with signatures—regular pens	Clean pens are available if you need to sign any permission papers.

Source: Arya, J., & Mali, P. C. (2021). Influence of COVID-19 Pandemic on Assisted Reproductive Techniques Services in India: A Review. *J. Life Sci*, *7*(6S), 9S-16S

PSYCHOSOCIAL CONSEQUENCES FACED BY INFERTILE COUPLES DURING A LOCKDOWN

Despite the COVID-19 epidemic, infertility was a significant stressor (Vaughan et al., 2020). In a study, Respondents were asked to list their top three stressors in January 2020 (before the epidemic), early March 2020 (at the beginning of the COVID-19 pandemic), and in the midst of the pandemic (Vaughan et al., 2020). The study found that Infertility was the top stressor and most commonly reported at all three time periods.

According to research by Jaiswal et al. (2022), 72% of infertile women suffer from anxiety. According to this study, anxiety and stress among infertile women were predicted to be influenced by the length of infertility and any delays in treatment brought on by the suspension of services and concern over the covid-19 infection. The patients have had to deal with the ambiguity surrounding the possibility of achieving their long-term reproductive objectives in a general unpredictability regarding the length and degree of interruption of their treatment, as well as the worry of infection (Muhaidat et al., 2021). Similarly, case-control research examined the feelings of depression and stress experienced by infertile women whose treatment had been postponed because of COVID-19. According to the study's findings, infertile patients whose treatment was delayed felt more frustration and depression than those who were not receiving infertility treatment (Rasekh et al., 2022)

According to another study, increased distress was linked to a sense of helplessness, which reflected the difficulties in coping with unpredictable and uncontrolled unpleasant experiences like the Pandemic. The decision to abruptly discontinue the IVF treatment left them feeling abandoned and helpless, possibly making them even more vulnerable (Kimhy et al., 2020). Turocy et al., 2020 investigated the emotional impact of infertile participants whose treatment was suspended or halted. It was identified that 85% of respondents reported it was pretty painful to highly distressing, and 22% said it was comparable to losing a child. The emotional impact was the same regardless of the canceled cycle type. A study by Tokgoz, Kaya, & Tekin., (2022) found that anxiety levels were not only high in the women whose cycles were delayed as a result of the epidemic but also considerably increased when the ovarian reserve was depleted.

Similarly, it was believed that 25–60% of infertile couples experience psychological issues, and People may experience depression, shame, or even a sense of worthlessness due to this condition. Several variables, including gender, the length of infertility, and culture, might influence this occurrence (Lechner, Bolman, & van Dalen, 2007).

Despite experiencing such psychological discomfort, domestic violence—a more significant worldwide public health issue—is nevertheless perpetrated against women. Intimate partner abuse, the most prevalent type of violence against women, is estimated to affect 50% of infertile people during this pandemic (Bondade, et al., 2018). Women who are infertile were twice as likely to encounter domestic violence than persons who are fertile. Intimate partner violence was estimated to affect one in three women worldwide, and the current environment of exclusion, isolation, and associated social, emotional, and economic stressors was likely to increase the risk of this type of violence, making infertile women an easy target for domestic abuse during the pandemic (Dawson et al., 2022). The study also suggested that governments worldwide should keep women's health at the center of their policy changes and provide essential services to address violence against women during the pandemic as well as in preparation and response to long-term solutions post-pandemic (Hadler, 2002).

During the COVID-19 epidemic in China, It was found that age was also mentioned as a contributing factor to elevated anxiety levels (Huang, & Zhao, 2020). This study discovered that those under 35 were more prone to anxiety and depression symptoms. Although the risk of COVID-19 is higher in older persons, anxiety levels were elevated in young individuals, which can be explained by concerns about the future and the economic effects of the epidemic on the affected population (Tokgoz, Kaya, & Tekin., 2022).

Additionally, A study discovered that infertile women in the quarantine group paid more attention to the dynamics of the epidemic than infertile women in the non-quarantine group, and their mood, stress, and sleep were all in some way impacted. It suggested that the isolation could put more psychological strain on infertile women. The epidemic's second wave affects people differently than its first wave. People's anxiety during the second wave of the pandemic has decreased due to the first wave's quarantine experience. However, it was discovered that women's familial relationships are more stressful in the quarantine group of the second wave. The companionship and contact of family members and a range of entertainment options may assist in reducing anxiety. However, quarantine procedures have introduced numerous variables (isolation, illness, infection) that may exacerbate anxiety. The conflict between a husband and wife may be effectively reduced via intimacy, improved communication, and commitment. The COVID-19 epidemic not only significantly enhanced the anxiety of infertile women but also affected other negative feelings and family relations (Cao et al., 2021).

The internet became a sophisticated tool for women whose treatment had been postponed by the closure of reproductive clinics. Social media became a problematic means of a communication channel during the pandemic in the UK because patients felt emotionally upset by exposure to information about pregnancy or children, even though fertility forums were generally seen as positive Support Mechanisms (Tippett, 2022).

COVID-19 PANDEMIC MYTHS AND THEIR IMPACT ON INFERTILE COUPLES

The internet was empowering and disempowering for those contemplating or undergoing reproductive treatment. A woman's body will become resistant to this specific spike protein after receiving the COVID-19 vaccination, which will affect her fertility, claims a fake social media article. Due to exposure to these kinds of news, the patient's anxiety has increased. The two spike proteins are completely distinct from one another and have no impact on a woman's capacity to become pregnant, including through in vitro fertilization methods. 23 of the volunteer women who participated in the Pfizer immunization studies became pregnant, and the one woman who miscarried received a placebo rather than the actual vaccine (Hasan, Osborn, & Chauhan, 2022).

The doctor states that there was no evidence to support that the COVID-19 virus affects the ovarian reserves and hormones of expectant mothers receiving IVF treatment, and they must be checked before the treatment process begins (Veliscu et al., 2022). If the test is positive, the treatment will be stopped, was the myth around the general population. But due to this fear and misbelief among infertile women, treatment-seeking behavior had reduced during the pandemic (Murdia K, 2021).

During the pandemic, another widespread belief was that "Covid vaccinations aren't safe during IVF treatment." Medical bodies have affirmed the safety of the prescribed immunizations for patients. Because of this fallacy, women avoid vaccinations while receiving IVF treatment.

There was a pervasive myth among infertile couples that clinics have delayed IVF treatment due to the pandemic. Because of this, many would-be parents believe that delaying treatment is preferable to giving treatment in the pandemic situation. According to a survey, 5.0% of infertile couples decided to postpone fertility treatment because they were anxious about the virus's possible consequences on pregnancy and the risk of infection in the hospital. (Cito et al., 2020). However, most reputable IVF clinics adhere to strict safety protocols to guarantee a successful procedure.

Many misunderstandings regarding viruses, vaccines, and the treatment process led to higher anxiety among infertile couples. The population's fear may have been reduced if the government had adequately informed the public about the virus and its impact on reproductive medicine through various communication channels, including social media and newspapers, and so on.

TREATMENT-SEEKING BEHAVIOR AMONG INFERTILE COUPLES

The public health infrastructure in several of these underdeveloped nations has been stretched by the COVID-19 pandemic. Fertility services have been disproportionately impacted by limited healthcare resources and other issues like an economic downturn and job losses. Therefore, it is critical to comprehend infertile couples' viewpoints on the continuation of fertility treatment during the present COVID-19 epidemic, as they are the primary stakeholders in a shared decision-making process, especially for self-funded IVF cycles (Kamath et al., 2021).

The knowledge, anxiety levels, and attitudes of infertile couples concerning COVID-19 and its effect on self-funded reproductive treatment were examined by Kamath et al. (2021). The findings indicated that infertile couples visiting the infertility clinic had high levels of knowledge and awareness regarding COVID-19. Most participants were knowledgeable about the cause of the spread, typical symptoms (64.1-96.2%), and the significance of preventative actions (95.6-97.4%). The desire to continue fertility treatment was strongly impacted by the participants' educational levels. According to further analysis, those with lower levels of education (below graduate) were less inclined to continue fertility treatment. Despite the COVID-19 epidemic, 72% of respondents opted to continue fertility treatments. It was shown that increased age-related anxiety, emotional problems brought on by treatment delays, familial pressure, and domestic violence were the primary factors for resuming the treatment (Jaiswal et al., 2022).

Due to the epidemic, even the employment market suffered significantly, and individuals began expressing preferences for fertility in a broad socioeconomic context. Despite research indicating that treatment interruptions make infertile patients more anxious and distressed, one study found that more than 40% of women claimed to have altered their expectations for when and how many children to have. 34% of women said they would postpone having children or have fewer children. This may result from the couples' financial difficulties during the epidemic. Unexpectedly, and with considerable relevance to the field of infertility, these preferences changed more frequently among women who were childless (45%) than among those who were already mothers and suffering from secondary infertility (38%), indicating a significant degree of potential market contraction for fertility services, at least in the near- to medium-future (Gleicher, 2020).

Coping With the Pandemic

A study examines the association between intolerance of uncertainty (IU), situation appraisal, coping mechanisms, and overall discomfort among women who had a delayed IVF procedure. Situation appraisal refers to the perceived threat that COVID-19 poses to infertility treatment. The study used SEM (Structural Equation Modelling), and it was identified that avoidance coping has a role in mediating the relationship between situation appraisal and overall suffering. The amount of discomfort in this challenging situation for mental health was determined by situation appraisal and coping mechanisms, with IU serving as the primary predictor of the total reaction as a dispositional variable (Mitrović, Kostić, & Ristić, 2022).

In addition to directly impacting general distress, IU also has an effect via the avoidance strategy since it rises in response to highly unpredictable events (like a pandemic brought on by an unknown virus), which in turn triggers the avoidance strategy and raises general distress. This helps to explain how COVID-19's perceived danger to infertility treatment may have indirectly increased overall misery through coping mechanisms (Mitrovic, Kostic, & Ristic, 2022). As a result, people with a low threshold for uncertainty tend to overestimate their capacity to control a situation and their vulnerability to danger. In light of this, IU decides on situational appraisal. The emotion-focused coping strategy of avoidance, typically adopted in circumstances of elevated danger (Taha et al., 2014), was further determined by situational appraisal. This approach eventually contributes to an increase in overall distress, which was a negative effect (Mitrovic, Kostic, & Ristic, 2022)

Potential to lessen psychological stress and loneliness during the delay of ART treatment was increased communication between reproductive clinics and patients, and better use of internet platforms acted as a support system.

When Gordon and Balsom (2020) looked at the psychological effects of fertility treatment suspensions during the COVID-19 pandemic, they discovered that higher levels of acceptance and benefit-finding were linked to a lower mental health impact, while higher levels of helplessness were linked to a higher negative impact. Finding social support and expressing more optimism were linked to improved outcomes. On the other hand, avoidance of infertility reminders was linked to less favorable results. The study also revealed that defensive pessimism, a personality trait, was linked to a more significant decline in the quality of life and a more significant detrimental effect on mental health when reproductive treatments were halted. (Gordon., & Balsom, 2020).

FEW PROTECTIVE FACTORS AND THERAPIES AGAINST PSYCHOLOGICAL DISTRESS

The reviewed article observed that the Covid 19 pandemic has affected the mental health of infertile couples. Few studies have mentioned that hospitals and clinics provided counselling services to reduce stress and anxiety. Psychological therapies, like emotional focused therapy (Soltani et al., 2014), cognitive behavioral therapy, mind-body intervention (Frederiksen et al., 2015), and acceptance and commitment therapy (Hosseinpanahi et al., 2020), was efficacious in reducing emotional distress like anxiety, depression, and infertility-related stress among childless couples.

The journey of Fertility treatment during the Covid-19 Pandemic was considered less stressful when there was no pause in obtaining treatment, a clear understanding of the reason behind the halt in treatment, and involving them in the decision-making process (Seifer et al., 2021). Indulging in meaning-based coping techniques was an effective way of dealing with stress and anxiety (Gordon & Balsom,2020). Studies suggest that helping patients express their emotions, and providing them with simple relaxation techniques and self-emotional management skills was effective in relieving stress and anxiety among patients (Kong et al., 2020). Providing the proper knowledge and information about the COVID-19 virus, the vaccine, and its impact on reproductive treatment would have helped couples to lessen their fear of uncertainty and misconception about vaccination. Strategies like maintaining a healthy lifestyle and social connections, accepting anxiety and negative feelings, promoting self-efficacy, and knowing where to go for medical care if necessary were protective factors in combating the stress and anxiety about Covid-19 (Petzold et al., 2020).

LIMITATION

Due to limited accessibility, the researcher could not reach out to infertile couples to understand their subjective mental and emotional effects during the pandemic. Scopus, Pubmed, MEDLINE, Shodhganga, and Google Scholar were used to compile the research papers for this review report. However, due to journal accessibility, some documents may have been overlooked. Therefore, working papers, a few reports issued by the government and other organizations, eBooks, and Conference proceedings were excluded from the study.

CONCLUSION

Based on the literature review, most pertinent studies used cohort, cross-sectional, case-control, and self-controlled case series designs. From the reviewed data, it can be concluded that the pandemic has affected the mental health of childless couples. When there is a detrimental effect on mental health, it is essential to prepare and implement protective measures. Increased anxiety, stress, sense of hopelessness, and fear of uncertainty were common psychological distress among infertile patients during the pandemic. It was also found that treatment suspension has a significant negative effect on infertile patients. To minimize the adverse psychological effects that stress, anxiety, and depression have on individuals and interpersonal relationships, the current study set out to find more effective techniques for handling this critical circumstance.

IMPLICATIONS AND SUGGESTIONS

The study's findings help pinpoint information gaps, current trends, and current usage of psychotherapy techniques for handling distress, as well as the psychological consequences of the COVID-19 epidemic on childless couples. This study will also aid medical and mental health professionals in understanding the need for psychological support for infertile couples throughout their treatment. The biopsychosocial approach will help address the psychological and social repercussions infertile couples endure as a result of COVID-19, which may lessen the pandemic's aftereffects. Further research is required to determine the pandemic's long-term psychological effects on women receiving infertility treatments.

Regardless of the participants' background characteristics, this study offers information that may assist in building skills to enhance dealing with stressful external circumstances by strengthening and empowering personal resources and directly facing and addressing feelings of helplessness. These can include stress reduction methods like guided imagery and mindfulness that can help people feel more in control of their lives and less powerless (Stanisawski, 2019).

Competing Interests

All authors of this article declare there have no competing interests.

Funding

This research received no specific grant from any funding agency in the public, commercial, or not-for-profit sectors. The authors of the article covered funding for this research.

REFERENCES

Arya, J., & Mali, P. C. (2021). Influence of COVID-19 Pandemic on Assisted Reproductive Techniques Services in India: A Review. *Journal of Life Science*, *7*(6S), 9S–16S.

ASRM. (2020). *ASRM Patient Management and Clinical Recommendations During the Coronavirus (COVID-19) Pandemic*. ASRM. https://www.asrm.org/news-and-publications/news-and-research/announcements/update-1-released-to-the-asrm-patient-management-and-clinical-recommendations-during-the-coronavirus-covid-19-pandemic/

Ben-Kimhy, R., Youngster, M., Medina-Artom, T. R., Avraham, S., Gat, I., Marom Haham, L., Hourvitz, A., & Kedem, A. (2020). Fertility patients under COVID-19: Attitudes, perceptions, and psychological reactions. *Human Reproduction (Oxford, England)*, *2020*(12), 2774–2783. doi:10.1093/humrep/deaa248 PMID:32877507

Boivin, J., Harrison, C., Mathur, R., Burns, G., Pericleous-Smith, A., & Gameiro, S. (2020). Patient experiences of fertility clinic closure during the COVID-19 pandemic: Appraisals, coping and emotions. *Human Reproduction (Oxford, England)*, *35*(11), 2556–2566. doi:10.1093/humrep/deaa218 PMID:32761248

Bondade, S., Iyengar, R. S., Shivakumar, B. K., & Karthik, K. N. (2018). Intimate Partner Violence and Psychiatric Comorbidity in Infertile Women - A Cross-Sectional Hospital Based Study. *Indian Journal of Psychological Medicine*, *40*(6), 540–546. doi:10.4103/IJPSYM.IJPSYM_158_18 PMID:30533950

Cao, L. B., Hao, Q., Liu, Y., Sun, Q., Wu, B., Chen, L., & Yan, L. (2021). Anxiety Level During the Second Localized COVID-19 Pandemic Among Quarantined Infertile Women: A Cross-Sectional Survey in China. *Frontiers in Psychiatry*, *12*, 647483. doi:10.3389/fpsyt.2021.647483 PMID:34366908

Carp-Veliscu, A., Mehedintu, C., Frincu, F., Bratila, E., Rasu, S., Iordache, I., Bordea, A., et al. (2022). The Effects of SARS-CoV-2 Infection on Female Fertility: A Review of the Literature. *International Journal of Environmental Research and Public Health, 19*(2), 984. MDPI AG. doi:10.3390/ijerph19020984

Cito, G., Pizzarelli, C., Zurkirch, V., Basile, V., Ruggiero, M., & Coccia, M. E. (2022). Parenthood in Infertile Couples Attending Assisted Reproductive Technologies (ARTs) Centers: What Has Changed During the COVID-19 Pandemic? *Journal of Reproduction & Infertility*, *23*(2), 120–127. doi:10.18502/jri.v23i2.8997 PMID:36043127

Dawson, L., Einboden, R., McCloughen, A., & Buus, N. (2021). Beyond polyphony: Open Dialogue in a Women's Shelter in Australia as a possibility for supporting violence-informed practice. *Journal of Marital and Family Therapy*, *47*(1), 136–149. doi:10.1111/jmft.12457 PMID:32990992

Denis, A. V., Shah, J. S., Penzia, A. S., Domar, A. D., & Toth, T. L. (2020). Infertility remains a top stressor despite the COVID-19 pandemic. *Reproductive Biomedicine Online*, *41*(3), 425–427. doi:10.1016/j.rbmo.2020.05.015 PMID:32600945

Frederiksen, Y., Farver-Vestergaard, I., Skovgård, N. G., Ingerslev, H. J., & Zachariae, R. (2015). Efficacy of psychosocial interventions for psychological and pregnancy outcomes in infertile women and men: A systematic review and meta-analysis. *BMJ Open*, *5*(1), e006592. doi:10.1136/bmjopen-2014-006592 PMID:25631310

Gleicher, N. (2020). The COVID-19 pandemic through the eyes of an NYC fertility center: A unique learning experience with often unexpected results. *Reproductive Biology and Endocrinology*, *18*(1), 1–16. doi:10.118612958-020-00663-3 PMID:33148264

Gordon, J. L., & Balsom, A. A. (2020). The psychological impact of fertility treatment suspensions during the COVID-19 pandemic. *PLoS One*, *15*(9), e0239253. doi:10.1371/journal.pone.0239253 PMID:32946479

Gupta, M., Jaiswal, P., Bansiwal, R., Sethi, A., Vanamail, P., Kachhawa, G., Kumari, R., & Mahey, R. (2021). Anxieties and apprehensions among women waiting for fertility treatments during the COVID-19 pandemic. *International Journal of Gynaecology and Obstetrics: the Official Organ of the International Federation of Gynaecology and Obstetrics*, *152*(3), 441–443. doi:10.1002/ijgo.13468 PMID:33155288

Halder, A. (2021). Salient Yet Silent: A Need for Strategies to Cope with Violence against Infertile Women during COVID-19 Pandemic. *EC Gynaecology*, *10*, 29–31.

Hasan, S. D., Osborn, D. R., & Chauhan, A. (2022). Myths About COVID Vaccines. *KnowsWhy.com.* https://www.knowswhy.com/myths-about-covid-vaccines/

Hosseinpanahi, M., Mirghafourvand, M., Farshbaf-Khalili, A., Esmaeilpour, K., Rezaei, M., & Malakouti, J. (2020). The effect of counseling based on acceptance and commitment therapy on mental health and quality of life among infertile couples: A randomized controlled trial. *Journal of Education and Health Promotion*, *9*(1), 251. doi:10.4103/jehp.jehp_512_20 PMID:33224995

Huang, C., Wang, Y., Li, X., Ren, L., Zhao, J., Hu, Y., Zhang, L., Fan, G., Xu, J., Gu, X., Cheng, Z., Yu, T., Xia, J., Wei, Y., Wu, W., Xie, X., Yin, W., Li, H., Liu, M., & Cao, B. (2020). Clinical features of patients infected with 2019 novel coronavirus in Wuhan, China. *Lancet*, *395*(10223), 497–506. doi:10.1016/S0140-6736(20)30183-5 PMID:31986264

Huang, Y., & Zhao, N. (2020). Generalized anxiety disorder, depressive symptoms and sleep quality during COVID-19 outbreak in China: A web-based cross-sectional survey. *Psychiatry Research, 288*, 112954. doi:10.1016/j.psychres.2020.112954 PMID:32325383

Jaiswal, P., Mahey, R., Singh, S., Vanamail, P., Gupta, M., Cheluvaraju, R., Sharma, J. B., & Bhatla, N. (2022). *The psychological impact of suspension/postponement of fertility treatments on infertile women waiting during the COVID pandemic.* Psychological Impact of Suspension/Postponement of Fertility Treatments on Infertile Women Waiting During COVID Pandemic. doi:10.5468/ogs.21254

Kamath, M. S., Joseph, T., Karuppusami, R., Chinta, P., Pal, A., Nallamilli, S. R., Sarkar, S., Poobalan, A. & Kunjummen, A. T. (2021). Knowledge, anxiety levels and attitudes of infertile couples towards COVID-19 and its impact on self-funded fertility treatment: a cross-sectional questionnaire survey. *Human reproduction open*, *2021*(4).

Kong, X., Kong, F., Zheng, K., Tang, M., Chen, Y., Zhou, J., Li, Y., Diao, L., Wu, S., Jiao, P., Su, T., & Dong, Y. (2020). Effect of psychological–behavioral intervention on the depression and anxiety of COVID-19 patients. *Frontiers in Psychiatry, 11*, 586355. doi:10.3389/fpsyt.2020.586355 PMID:33329130

La Rosa, V. L., Barra, F., Chiofalo, B., Platania, A., Di Guardo, F., & Conway, F. (2019). An overview on the relationship between endometriosis and infertility: The impact on sexuality and psychological well-being. *Journal of Psychosomatic Obstetrics and Gynaecology*, 1–5. PMID:31466493

Lechner, L., Bolman, C., & van Dalen, A. (2007). Definite involuntary childlessness: Associations between coping, social support, and psychological distress. *Human Reproduction (Oxford, England)*, *22*(1), 288–294. doi:10.1093/humrep/del327 PMID:16920722

Mahey, R., Sharma, A., Kumari, A., Kachhawa, G., Gupta, M., Meena, J., & Bhatla, N. (2020). The impact of a segregated team roster on obstetrics and gynecology services in response to the COVID-19 pandemic in a tertiary care center in India. *International Journal of Gynaecology and Obstetrics: the Official Organ of the International Federation of Gynaecology and Obstetrics*, *151*(3), 341–346. doi:10.1002/ijgo.13408 PMID:33011974

Malhotra, N., Shah, D., & Pai, R. (2013). Assisted reproductive technology in India: A 3-year retrospective data analysis. *Journal of Human Reproductive Sciences*, *6*(4), 235–240. doi:10.4103/0974-1208.126286 PMID:24672161

Mitrović, M., Kostić, J. O., & Ristić, M. (2022). Intolerance of uncertainty and distress in women with delayed IVF treatment due to the COVID-19 pandemic: The mediating role of situation appraisal and coping strategies. *Journal of Health Psychology*, *27*(11), 2515–2528. doi:10.1177/13591053211049950 PMID:34670414

Muhaidat, N., Alshrouf, M. A., Karam, A. M., & Elfalah, M. Jnr. (2021). Infertility Management Disruption During the COVID-19 Outbreak in a Middle-Income Country: Patients' Choices, Attitudes, and Concerns. *Patient Preference and Adherence*, *15*, 2279–2288. doi:10.2147/PPA.S327055 PMID:34675492

Murdia K, (2021) Covid-19 and IVF: Long wait for women trying to be mothers through Assisted Reproductive Technology. NEWS 18.COM.Last update, 2021; 16:14 IST

Peoquin, K., & Lafontaine, M. F. (2010). What are the correlates of infertility-related clinical anxiety? A literature review and the presentation of a conceptual model. *Marriage & family review, 46*(8), 580-620.

Pericleous-Smith, A., Dark, S., McCluskey, G., Mizen, L., & Crawshaw, M. (2021). Survey of fertility counseling provision in UK licensed treatment centers during the first phase of the COVID-19 pandemic. *Human Fertility*, 1–11. doi:10.1080/14647273.2021.1898053 PMID:33749479

Petzold, M. B., Bendau, A., Plag, J., Pyrkosch, L., Mascarell Maricic, L., Betzler, F., Rogoll, J., Große, J., & Ströhle, A. (2020). Risk, resilience, psychological distress, and anxiety at the beginning of the COVID-19 pandemic in Germany. *Brain and Behavior*, *10*(9), e01745. doi:10.1002/brb3.1745 PMID:32633464

Rasekh Jahromi, A., Daroneh, E., Jamali, S., Ranjbar, A., & Rahmanian, V. (2022). Impact of COVID-19 pandemic on depression and hopelessness in infertile women. *Journal of Psychosomatic Obstetrics & Gynecology*, 1-7.

Rooney, K. L., & Domar, A. D. (2018). The relationship between stress and infertility. *Dialogues in Clinical Neuroscience*, *20*(1), 41–47. doi:10.31887/DCNS.2018.20.1/klrooney PMID:29946210

Sarkar, A., Saha, P. K., & Arora, A. (2021). COVID-19 Pandemic and infertility: Gynecological Dilemma from an Indian perspective. *Reproductive Sciences (Thousand Oaks, Calif.)*, *28*(4), 1020–1022. doi:10.100743032-021-00474-w PMID:33544338

Seifer, D. B., Petok, W. D., Agrawal, A., Glenn, T. L., Bayer, A. H., Witt, B. R., Burgin, B. D., & Lieman, H. J. (2021). Psychological experience and coping strategies of patients in the Northeast US delaying care for infertility during the COVID-19 pandemic. *Reproductive Biology and Endocrinology*, *19*(1), 1–16. PMID:33397418

Soltani, M., Shairi, M. R., Roshan, R., & Rahimi, C. R. (2014). The impact of emotionally focused therapy on emotional distress in infertile couples. *International Journal of Fertility & Sterility*, *7*(4), 337. PMID:24520504

Stanisławski, K. (2019). The coping circumplex model: An integrative model of the structure of coping with stress. *Frontiers in Psychology*, *10*, 694. doi:10.3389/fpsyg.2019.00694 PMID:31040802

Tippett, A. (2022). Life on pause: An analysis of UK fertility patients' coping mechanisms after the cancellation of fertility treatment due to COVID-19. *Journal of Health Psychology*, *27*(7), 1583–1600. doi:10.1177/1359105321999711 PMID:33685265

Tokgoz, V. Y., Kaya, Y., & Tekin, A. B. (2022). The level of anxiety in infertile women whose ART cycles are postponed due to the COVID-19 outbreak. *Journal of Psychosomatic Obstetrics and Gynaecology*, *43*(2), 114–121. doi:10.1080/0167482X.2020.1806819 PMID:32812477

Torales, J., O'Higgins, M., Castaldelli-Maia, J. M., & Ventriglio, A. (2020). The outbreak of COVID-19 coronavirus and its impact on global mental health. *The International Journal of Social Psychiatry*, *66*(4), 317–320. doi:10.1177/0020764020915212 PMID:32233719

Turabian, J. L. (2019). Doctor-Patient Relationship in the Case of Infertility: A Vision from General Medicine. [CrossRef]. *Adv. Reprod. Sci. Reprod. Health Infertil*, *1*, 104.

Turocy, J. M., Robles, A., Hercz, D., D'Alton, M., Forman, E. J., & Williams, Z. (2020). THE EMOTIONAL IMPACT OF THE ASRM GUIDELINES ON FERTILITY PATIENTS DURING THE COVID-19 PANDEMIC. *Fertility and Sterility*, *114*(3), e63. doi:10.1016/j.fertnstert.2020.08.194

Varvogli, L., & Darviri, C. (2011). Stress management techniques: Evidence-based procedures that reduce stress and promote health. *Health Science Journal*, *5*, 74–89.

Vaughan, D. A., Shah, J. S., Penzias, A. S., Domar, A. D., & Toth, T. L. (2020). Infertility remains a top stressor despite the COVID-19 pandemic. *Reproductive Biomedicine Online*, *41*(3), 425–427. doi:10.1016/j.rbmo.2020.05.015 PMID:32600945

Vitale, S. G., La Rosa, V. L., Rapisarda, A. M., & Lagana, A. S. (2017). Psychology of infertility and assisted reproductive treatment: The Italian situation. *Journal of Psychosomatic Obstetrics and Gynaecology*, *38*(1), 1–3. doi:10.1080/0167482X.2016.1244184 PMID:27750491

Vitale, S. G., La Rosa, V. L., Rapisarda, A. M. C., & Laganà, A. S. (2017). Endometriosis and Infertility: The Impact on Quality of Life and Mental Health. *Journal of Endometriosis and Pelvic Pain Disorders*, *9*(2), 112–115. doi:10.5301/je.5000274

WHO. (2020). *Coronavirus disease (COVID-19), Situation Report*. WHO. https://apps.who.int/iris/handle/10665/332151

Wiweko, B., Ho, T. M., Tanaka, A., Raggio, V., Lee, J. R., Patil, M., Chan, C. C. W., Wutayavanich, T., Diao, F., Nair, S., & Mendiola, R. F. (2021). COVID-19 Pandemic Impacts Decision-Making and Psychosocial Behavior in Women Seeking Fertility Treatment in APAC—An ASPIRE Patient Experience Report. *Fertility & Reproduction*, *3*(03), 58–77. doi:10.1142/S2661318221500080

World Health Organization. (2018). *Infertility*. International Classification of Diseases, 11th Revision (ICD-11)

Zhu, N., Zhang, D., & Wang, W. (2019). A novel coronavirus from patients with pneumonia in China. *The New England Journal of Medicine*, *2020*(382), 727–733. PMID:31978945

Chapter 8
Family Carers During the COVID-19 Pandemic:
A Paradigm Shift in Caregiving

Krishna Priya Balachandran
Vellore Institute of Technology, India

Bhuvaneswari Mohanraj
Vellore Institute of Technology, India

ABSTRACT

Ultimately, every individual will find themselves in a caregiving or care-receiving situation at some point in life. As a family caregiver, an individual's effort to support their loved one during difficult times leaves them in a laborious situation. A remarkable number of caregivers caring for a loved one suffering from an acute illness experience a sense of meaning, fulfillment, and profound emotional and psychological rewards. However, lifelong caregiving for a significant one diagnosed with a chronic illness or disability could be onerous. The current book chapter elucidates to the readers the lived experiences of family caregivers of children with neurodevelopmental disorders. The caregivers of children with neurodevelopmental disorders go through a life-long caregiving process. Thus, this book chapter will attempt to illustrate narratives of primary caregivers of children with neurodevelopmental disorders and the paradigm shift they experienced during COVID-19. This research is a determined effort to ensure that the stories of these unsung heroes reach a wider audience.

DOI: 10.4018/978-1-6684-7221-7.ch008

INTRODUCTION

It is indisputable that a substantial section of the community takes up the role of an informal caregiver at a particular time in their life. Every individual at a given point in life would have become a caregiver for their significant one for at least a brief period. The role of an informal caregiver takes work. It requires an indispensable amount of time, energy, and resources that an individual invests in their daily life during caregiving. An individual is least prepared and holds limited capacity and skill set. At the same time, they are inevitably obligated to assume the role of an informal caregiver as their significant one is diagnosed with some form of illness, disorder, or condition. The lack of preparedness and a critical diagnosis that may appear as a bolt out of the blue will stick around the family caregivers for a significant time.

The challenges faced by a family caregiver are multifaceted. It is non-viable to restrict the challenges they face as financial, physical, and psychological concerns. It surpasses these customary challenges, and it is imperative to integrate the impact of caregiving on an individual's normative life events, namely career, marriage, parenthood, families, and several other domains of life. The family caregivers experience many negative emotions, such as guilt, remorse, helplessness, anger, and denial, as they navigate through several stages of caregiving. Caregiving is associated with numerous burdens and stress for family caregivers.

The COVID-19 pandemic has amplified the challenges faced by family caregivers due to several pandemic-related restrictions, work from home, and the closure of healthcare services and educational institutions. During the pre-covid period, the primary caregiver looking after the primary needs of the person with a disability experienced utmost stress and burnout. However, during the pandemic individualistic responsibility of a caregiver shifted to a shared familial duty that would ensue as relationship strain, familial conflict, and complex crisis. In the Indian context, family caregivers are not officially recognized and lack the provision to seek physical and psychological support to ameliorate their well-being.

The outbreak of COVID-19 affected people from all walks of life, including children, adolescents, older adults, employees, women, the minority section of the community, and innumerable humankind. The challenges faced by different sections of the community are diverse. An enthralling observation during the COVID-19 scenario is that the informal caregivers providing care for any form of illness, disability, or diagnosis of COVID-19 itself would represent and constitute one or more of the sections of the community as mentioned above of the community. For instance, an informal caregiver could be a youth, an older adult, an employee, a woman, or anyone belonging to the minority sections of the community. It indicates that informal caregivers experience additional strain during the pandemic exacerbating their challenges and the pressure to carry through the other existing roles.

Primary caregivers of children with neurodevelopmental disorders likely experience higher stress levels and disruptions to their quality of life and well-being. (Khan,2018; Ganjiwale et al., 2016; Hooda,2020). Neurodevelopmental disorders (NDDs) are behavioral and cognitive conditions that appear throughout the developmental phase and are characterized by significant difficulties in the development and performance of a particular set of intellectual, motor, and social functions (World Health Organization, 2019). Children with chronic medical disorders are more likely to acquire comorbid neurodevelopmental issues that interfere with their daily activities (King-Dowling et al., 2019).

The COVID-19 restrictions, such as complete lockdown leading to home quarantine, work from home, and closure of health-care services, educational institutions, and recreational services added to the already experiencing stress among family caregivers. The limited form of recreation or opportunity that the caregivers' received while the child was away at special schools or rehabilitative centers had come to stand still during the COVID-19 pandemic. Although the initial days of lockdown were seen as an ideal opportunity for self-growth and family bonding, over time, feelings of detachment, uncertainty, lack of control, and loss of time and security increased the likelihood of adverse mental health problems, violence, and trauma among parents and children (Fontanesi et al., 2020). Parents of children with neurodevelopmental disorders already undergo high levels of stress and burden compared to parents of children with typical development or children with other chronic diseases. (Hoffman et al., 2009).

There is an exponential rise in mental health problems, familial conflict, violence, disruption in physical and psychological well-being, and trauma experienced by parents of children with neurodevelopmental disorders during the COVID-19 pandemic. (Masi et al., 2021; Wang et al.,2021). Home quarantine and full-time caregiving for a child with a neurodevelopmental disorder become burdensome and back-breaking for parents (Fontanesi et al., 2020). Lack of expertise and skills possessed by the parents to manage children with behavioral problems and inability to seek social support from extended family members, especially the elderly in the caregiving process due to lockdown regulations and fear of contracting the virus have amounted to increased parental stress and disruption of both parents and children's psychological well-being (Zhang et al., 2020). Low levels of parental stress, depression, anxiety, and milder maladaptive behaviors in children were associated with the pre-covid period (Ueda et al., 2021). Symptomatic changes in children with neurodevelopmental disorders during COVID-19 were also associated with parental distress (Burnett et al., 2021; Kong, 2020).

Caregivers of children with neurodevelopmental disorders reported lowered level of quality of life compared to caregivers of children with typical development (Pecor et al., 2021). Alterations in daily routine, functional limitations in carrying out activities of daily life, and termination of regular support present abundant threats to the family of children with neurodevelopmental disorders(Shorey et al., 2021). Mental health professionals and other relevant stakeholders have advocated for mental health issues experienced during this unfortunate pandemic. Efforts in imparting psychosocial intervention to individuals to effectively deal with the pandemic have been carried out constructively. A parenting recommendation issued by the World Health Organization (WHO) and United Nations International Children's Emergency Fund (UNICEF) in the form of a parental guide as an attempt to promote family well-being during the pandemic (World Health Organization,2020; United Nations International Children's Emergency Fund,2021).

There need to be more such guidelines, support, and recommendations rendered to parents or caregivers of children with neurodevelopmental disorders. Therefore, it is paramount to illuminate the shift in caregiving challenges faced by family caregivers before and during the pandemic. This current book chapter aims to provide insights into the shift in caregiving challenges faced by family members and caregivers to adapt to the new normal.

AIM AND OBJECTIVE OF THE RESEARCH

The primary aim of the current book chapter is to throw light on the paradigm shift experienced by family or primary caregivers in caregiving in the new normal situation of COVID-19. The current chapter will address the challenges faced by caregivers before the pandemic and the extent to which these challenges are similar or contrasting in the given state of the "new normal" where every individual is learning and adapting to live with the COVID-19 pandemic. The chapter will attempt to explicate the lived experience of family caregivers during the pandemic through narrative case illustrations of family caregivers rendering primary care for children with neurodevelopmental disorders. A section of the chapter would enfold the narrative case study of a few primary caregivers of children with neurodevelopmental disorders sharing their lived experiences and chronicles during the pandemic.

A section of the chapter will illustrate the lived experience of primary caregivers of children with neurodevelopmental disorders. Every story narrated by the caregivers would be unique and different, yet it would establish a sense of similarity as they share a common caregiving experience. The COVID-19 pandemic situation is changing, but it is still ongoing. Therefore, the current study will help us understand their challenges and the coping strategies to navigate effectively to enhance the caregiver's and their children's physical, mental, and social well-being.

METHODOLOGY

Research Design

A case narrative research method was adopted to conduct the current research study. It is a qualitative study in which the researcher collects in-depth information or data from a person or a group of persons about a particular life event or events that occurred in a specific order to share and retell the narratives told by the person.

Sampling Design

A non-probability sampling design and snowball sampling technique were employed to identify and recruit primary caregivers of children with neurodevelopmental disorders fulfilling the inclusion criteria and willingness to participate in the study. Six participants were recruited for the narrative case analysis.

Inclusion Criteria

1. Primary caregivers between the age group of 25-60 years.
2. Caregivers (Mother, Father, Grandparents, or significant others) involved in the child's primary care.
3. Caregivers who can comprehend and converse in English and/or Tamil.
4. Primary caregivers of children with a neurodevelopmental disorder (ASD, Cerebral Palsy, Learning Disability, and Intellectual Disability) and its comorbidities were included in the study.
5. Primary caregiver who has lived with the child for at least four years and takes care of their essential needs.

Exclusion Criteria

1. Primary caregivers of children or persons with other physical or mental health conditions apart from NDDs chosen for the current study (ASD, Cerebral Palsy, Learning Disability, and Intellectual Disability) and their associated comorbidities.
2. Caregivers having other significant persons with psychiatric or medical illness for whom they are caregiving.

Sample Description

Primary caregivers (Parents or other significant family members) have been involved in the primary care of the child with neurodevelopmental disorders for at least four years or more and, for the most part, have provided care during the COVID-19 pandemic. Neurodevelopmental disorders are a group of disorders that affects individuals functioning in multiple domains of life such as physical, psychological, social, cognitive, and vocational. Individuals diagnosed with neurodevelopmental disorders unlike other chronic or acute ailments require constant attention and care from parents or primary caregivers to carry out their activities of daily living based on the severity levels.

Neurodevelopmental disorders do not have a complete cure. Hence, the caregiving process is lifelong. The complexities of providing care for children with neurodevelopmental disorders could pose physical and psychological turmoil as caregivers need to provide care for an extended period. Therefore, primary caregivers of children with neurodevelopmental disorders were chosen to understand the paradigm shift in caregiving by identifying the opportunities and challenges faced by caregivers of children with neurodevelopmental disorders is imperative.

The rationale of having at least four years of caregiving experience to be a part of the case study is to determine the change in caregiving experience before and during the pandemic. The current study included case narratives of six primary caregivers of children diagnosed with neurodevelopmental disorders. Two of the primary caregivers were mothers of children diagnosed with autism spectrum disorder, one of the primary caregivers was a mother of a child with an Intellectual disability, another primary caregiver was a grandmother of a child with cerebral palsy, and two more caregivers who were mothers of children diagnosed with cerebral palsy and learning disability.

Procedure

The present study was conducted as a telephonic interview in which the primary caregivers of children with neurodevelopmental disorders who agreed to participate in the study were asked to narrate their lived experience of providing primary care for their child before and during the COVID-19 pandemic. In addition, the researchers asked relevant leading questions to understand the challenges experienced, positive experiences (if any), and the needs and requirements of these caregivers. During the narration, the researcher noted down the key concepts and themes that emerged during the caregivers' narration of their lived experiences.

The following instructions were given to the participants

"I hope we all have come out of this covid 19 pandemic. We all have experienced some changes and adapted to the new normal due to the pandemic's impact. So, I would like you to recollect memories of nursing or care provided to your children before and during the pandemic. What was the new normal that each of you had adopted in treating your children, and what concerns did you experience during the covid-19 period regarding looking after your child? I would like you to narrate your experiences continuously. I would ideally not interrupt in between your narration. However, if necessary, I'll ask you questions in-between to probe into specific events or instances. I assure you that your response will be kept confidential with complete anonymity, and the collected data will be used only for research purposes."

ANALYSIS

Each caregiver's story was carefully heard, interpreted, and analyzed qualitatively to identify themes and contents. Qualitative content and thematic analysis procedures were carried out to analyze the collected data. The researcher conducted content analysis to identify themes, and classify, summarize, and tabulate the data. The researcher interpreted the qualitative data through word and phrase repetitions and primary and secondary data comparisons. In the word and phrase repetition method, the researcher compared the words and phrases most commonly used by respondents. Through primary and secondary data comparison, data collected through focus group discussion was compared with literature review findings.

SUMMARY OF THE CASE NARRATIVES

Following is the summary of the narratives provided by each of the six primary caregivers of children with neurodevelopmental disorders. Each narrative was carefully listened, interpreted, and analyzed to produce a summary of each participant's narratives.

Case Narrative 1

Caregiver MK is a 54-year-old female providing care for her 7-year-old grandchild diagnosed with cerebral palsy. She reported being the primary caregiver for her grandchild soon after his birth and continues to take care of his activities of daily living, such as bathing, dressing, feeding, and assisting with other essential needs. She expressed her caregiving strain as an ongoing experience that she cannot differentiate between the 'before' and 'after' pandemic scenarios. A noteworthy change in caregiving during the covid-19 pandemic that she pointed out is the share of roles and duties by family members. The child's parents were at home due to the Lockdown, which enabled the respondent (MK) to receive some time off from her duties of looking after the grandchild. Before the pandemic, she reported a stressful experience of having to do most household chores by herself and engage her grandchild in his activities of daily living as both his parents were working full-time. She reported having less time for herself during the weekdays as her workload would exceed the usual limit. As a result, she felt tired and exhausted by the end of the day. She also reported experiencing severe irritability, anger, and physical signs of aches and pains. The respondent also reported that accompanying her grandchild thrice a week to a neurodevelopmental center 15 kilometers away from their home for treatment added to her strain and exhaustion. In addition, her constant assistance for her grandchild with motor movements has substantially strained her physical health. During the pandemic, the family members shared the caregiving responsibility, reducing her stress and burden.

Case Narrative 2

Caregiver SL is a 32-year-old female providing care for her 8-year-old son diagnosed with an autism spectrum disorder. She is a homemaker and accompanies her son daily to a special school. She reported her experience of providing care and looking after her son during the covid-19 Lockdown as overwhelming and highly stressful. She emphasized the statement that before the pandemic, for 6 hours every day, she stitched dresses at home for women in the neighboring households while her son was away at school. During the pandemic, as the nation collectively experienced a lockdown, institutions were also closed, hindering the small work she did at home. She stated that her son required her constant attention during the Lockdown as he began to engage himself in self-harming behavior (head banging). He also began to exhibit increased anger and irritability towards family members. These actions of his required constant attention from the caregiver SL that hindered her everyday household chores. She also informed about having relationship strain and verbal arguments with her partner as he often complained about their sons' actions but did not share the duty of providing care. She also reported experiencing crying spells several times during the Lockdown, which was rare before the Lockdown. There were instances in which the child's maladaptive behavior was beyond control, which led caregiver SL to hit her child, after which she had an intense feeling of remorse and guilt.

Case Narrative 3

Caregiver RK is a 42-year-old female providing care for her 15-year-old daughter diagnosed with a learning disability. RK works as a corporate lawyer and often finds herself busy. She described her experience of Lockdown during the covid-19 pandemic as an opportunity to bond with her family and transition from offline academic interaction to online academic interaction with her daughter. She stated that the special school in which her daughter studies took considerable time to comprehend and work out the transition of all the learners to an online medium to continue their education. As a parent with special needs, she felt equally part of this transitioning process. However, she described the entire process as learning, acquiring knowledge, and orientation to novel technological skills. She also stated that the period of Lockdown was an occasion to spend quality time with the family members enabling positive family interaction and warmth. Although a few instances were stressful, she felt it was possible to sail through the tides with determination.

Case Narrative 4

Caregiver LS is a 29-year-old-female providing care for her 5-year-old son diagnosed with cerebral palsy with co-morbid conditions such as occasional seizures. She described her experience of providing care during the Lockdown as highly stressful and overwhelming. There were several instances during which her son fell sick and also experienced multiple seizures, due to which he had to get hospitalized. LS reported that this made her always look out for her son's health condition and feel apprehensive. She stated that before covid-19 Lockdown, she had the opportunity to ask the healthcare professionals' opinions and seek medical advice as she visited the neurodevelopmental center for her son's treatment. In the neurodevelopmental center, the occupational and speech therapists assisted and guided her on the seating posture and ways to feed food to enable chewing and digestion. However, during the Lockdown, she found it challenging to carry out these practices at home. She reported constantly calling the healthcare professionals at the neurodevelopmental center during the Lockdown to receive assistance and guidance on providing care. She reported experiencing an emotional meltdown and questioned her capability to provide care for her son, and she felt guilty. She also conveyed that her husband was understanding of her feelings and emotions during such an uncertain situation and reassured her frequently, leading to better understanding and positive interaction between them. The caregiver also reported enrolling herself in a support group for parents of children with special needs.

Case Narrative 5

Caregiver TR is a 30-year-old female providing care to her 7-year-old son diagnosed with autism. Her experience providing care for her son during the Lockdown was highly stressful as she had to do everything herself. Her husband had gone on a business trip to Australia, and due to covid-19 Lockdown, he was stranded there, figuring out alternative options to return. Meanwhile, TR had a difficult time with her son alone at home as her house help also did not turn up due to Lockdown. Amidst such a nerve-wracking situation, TR tested positive for covid-19 and could not quarantine herself in her son's presence. Unusual to the scenario before the Lockdown, her son began throwing temper tantrums and exhibiting extreme irritability. She also described that her son began to regress into maladaptive behaviors such as repetitive actions which were observed to be decreased through intervention provided at the neurodevelopmental center. She felt that caregiving for children with special needs during the covid-19 pandemic poses many challenges. One of the main contributing factors is the inability to get in touch with other people to seek help and social support.

Case Narrative 6

Caregiver SK is a 34-year-old female providing care to her 8-year-old girl child diagnosed with an intellectual disability. She described her experience of caring for her daughter during the Lockdown as exhausting and stressful. She complained about feeling low in energy and lacked interest in pursuing activities that she found pleasurable before the covid-19 pandemic. In addition, she reported experiencing a change in sleep and appetite, where she found herself excessively eating and sleeping throughout the day. As her mastery over tasks such as dressing, feeding, and toilet training is limited, this led to an indispensable strain on the caregiver to be present with her to fulfil these essential needs. These had to be fulfilled even before the Lockdown; however, during the Lockdown adapting to the changes of uncertainty and working from home, and taking care of her daughter around the clock made it more challenging. These challenging times made her realize the importance of taking care of her physical and mental health to provide care for her daughter. She enrolled herself in therapy and found the process of counselling rewarding.

RESULTS AND DISCUSSIONS

Based on the case narrative analysis, eight themes emerged from the thematic analysis with related key concepts for each derived theme.

Table 1. Themes derived from caregivers' narratives

Themes	Key concepts
Physical and Psychological distress	Physical health concerns and psychological disturbances
Multifold Strains	Physical, psychological, emotional, and financial strains.
Lack of awareness	Lack of knowledge about the disorder, lack of caregiving skills
Need for Social and familial support	Lack of social support, lack of assistance
Caregiver burden	Change in appetite, experience negative emotions, loss of control, poor treatment or caregiving.
Coping	Quality time with family, taking time for oneself, seeking help from the mental health professional
Fear of contracting covid-19	Difficulty in quarantine, inability to follow social distancing rules and prevention measures
Positive outcomes	Quality time with family, positive family interaction

From table 1, it can be inferred that the eight emerging themes and their related key concepts related to the caregivers' shift in the process of caregiving during the covid 19 pandemic. The uncertainties and shift in adapting to the new normal of the pandemic had both positive and negative impacts on the primary caregivers of children with neurodevelopmental disorders. The eight themes that emerged from the six case narratives include psychological and physical distress, multifold strain, lack of awareness, need for social and familial support, caregiver burden, coping, fear of contracting covid-19, and positive outcomes. Each of these themes with their related key concepts is discussed below with the description of the case narratives and existing literature review of studies conducted on primary caregivers or parents of children with neurodevelopmental disorders.

Physical and Psychological Distress

During the pandemic, families of children with neurodevelopmental disorders experienced increased physical and psychological distress as they were required to be around the child round the clock. The caregivers reported experiencing tiredness, aches, and body pain throughout the lockdown. Few mothers also reported experiencing psychological concerns such as a lack of interest in activities they initially found pleasurable, loss of appetite and sleep, and feelings of hopelessness and helplessness. Similar findings, such as behavioral issues and health concerns, extreme stress, symptoms of anxiety and depression, were noted in numerous research studies conducted on families and caregivers of children with neurodevelopmental disorders (Shorey et al., 2021; Lee et al.,2021; Grumi et al., 2021)

Multifold Strain

A disability cannot be viewed through an individualistic lens; focusing on the impact of an individual with a disability at a community level is imperative. The community level includes the family and the primary caregivers and the influence of caregiving on a multidimensional level. A family caregiver involved in caregiving for their loved one faces challenges from multiple domains, such as deterioration of physical and psychological health, financial crisis, strain and conflict in social and familial interaction, and occupational stress. Caregivers experienced strain in multiple dimensions of their life, which has exaggerated to a greater extent with the occurrence of the pandemic. The financial crisis, shortage of food and other essential resources, unpaid leave from work by mothers, and reporting of domestic and familial violence were on the rise during the pandemic (Christie et al., 2022). Parents or informal caregivers also reported increased family conflicts and family-life interference during the covid 19 pandemic (Nylen-Eriksen et al., 2022).

Lack of Awareness

Primary caregivers reported having limited knowledge about their child's disability leading to challenges in providing care for them. Caregiver LS, the mother of a 5-year-old boy diagnosed with cerebral palsy and occasional seizures, reported feeling guilty about not knowing the effective way to bring her child to ease when he felt some form of uncomfortableness. This reflected the lack of guidance and education received from healthcare professionals during the pandemic due to the lockdown and closure of institutions. Most caregivers sensed a feeling of pressured responsibility to take up their children's complex educational, medical, and other treatment needs. Lack of specialist services, lack of guidance from professionals and teachers, and lack of face-to-face medical support or contact from neurodevelopmental clinics and special schools from which they sought rehabilitation led to increased worry among parents (Gillespie-Smith, 2021). Caregivers also reported worsening symptoms among their children over the course of the pandemic. Children diagnosed with neurodevelopmental disorders regressed to their maladaptive behavior of headbanging and self-harming. The caregivers' narrative is consistent with a cross-sectional study in which out of 149 primary caregivers, almost one-third of them reported that the neurodevelopmental disorder symptoms of their child worsened over time (Nisha & Bakul, 2022).

Need for Social and Familial Support

The pandemic came along with stringent restrictions and protocols on social distancing, hindering close human interaction, even among family members. This led to difficulties among parents and primary caregivers in caring for their children with disability. However, before the pandemic presence of another individual at home, like a household or grandparents, made it possible for parents to seek assistance while providing care for their children. Lack of social support during the pandemic crisis was found to be a contributing factor to parental stress (Burnett et al.,2021). The disruption of family support during the lockdown also had an immense impact on the caregivers' mental health (Currie et al., 2022). Apart from familial and social support, caregivers also felt that they were receiving inadequate support from healthcare professionals during the pandemic to clarify their queries regarding the disorder and its appropriate caregiving procedure (Nisha & Bakul, 2022).

Caregiver Burden

Caregivers during the interview reported extreme changes in appetite, excessive sleep or reduced sleep, tiredness, and the experience of negative emotions like irritability, anger outbursts, throwing temper tantrums, feeling a sense of loss of control over their daily routine and planned life events, feeling of providing poor treatment or caregiving to their child altogether aggravating caregiver burden (Gillespie-Smith, 2021; Lee et al., 2021; Paulauskeite et al., 2021). Parents or primary caregivers of children with neurodevelopmental disorders also reported experiencing an overwhelming feeling of anxiety, depression, worry, increased exhaustion, and loneliness (Currie et al., 2022).

Coping

Most caregivers reported adopting a problem-focused coping style to resolve the challenges faced during the COVID-19 pandemic. The primary caregivers began to have a positive outlook toward the situation and their caregiving duties through cost-benefit analysis. It is noteworthy to point out that during the narration, caregiver MK reported that her duty as a caregiver continues; however, other sources are been received. Few caregivers also pointed out seeking help from mental health professionals and enrolling in support groups for parents of children with special needs to alleviate their stress and improve their well-being and provide effective care for their children (Martinsone & Tzivian., 2021). Few caregivers also began to spend quality time with other family members and also began to take out time for themselves from the hectic schedule of caregiving and amidst the uncertain daily routine during the covid-19 pandemic.

Fear of Contracting Covid-19

Caregivers reported experiencing extreme stress and exhaustion while providing care for their children while being tested covid positive. The inability of their child to comprehend and understand the current situation and how covid19 is contracted. This situation made it difficult for caregivers to maintain social distancing and quarantine themselves when they tested positive for covid as their children required constant attention from the caregivers. The difficulty following social distancing, isolation rules, and the child's activity constantly had the parents and other family members worry and fear about the child contracting covid-19 (Paulauskeite et al., 2021; Suzuki & Hiratani, 2021). Most caregivers felt that their children were facing the issue of not being able to follow the covid-19 protocols and rules of social distancing (Nisha & Bakul, 2022). A cross-sectional study on 150 primary caregivers pointed out that 84.1% of children with neurodevelopmental disorders exhibited challenges in the implementation of social distancing and covid-19 prevention measures (Yamamoto et al., 2022).

Positive Outcomes

Amidst all the challenges and concerns experienced by the parents or primary caregivers during the pandemic, few of them did not miss out on the opportunity to describe how the covid-19 crisis brought positive outcomes within the family. The pandemic empowered the family of children to overcome this stressful situation by allowing shared responsibilities of caregiving, spending quality time with members of the family, and holding positive interaction that strengthens familial and couple relationships through the expression of love and assurance. These positive outcomes cannot be overlooked as it indicates that family can act as a positive resource to overcome the negative impact of a crisis such as the covid-19 pandemic.

CONCLUSION

The case narrative analysis enabled us to understand the multidimensional challenges faced by the family members, especially the primary caregivers. It comprehensively elucidates the concerns faced by caregivers in physical, psychological, social, emotional, and occupational domains of life. The case narrative analysis illustrates the paradigm shift in caregiving during the covid 19 pandemic increasing the stress and burden among caregivers as they strive to adapt to the new normal.

IMPLICATIONS

An in-depth understanding of the lived experience of the caregivers of children with neurodevelopmental disorders will enable mental health professionals and other predominant stakeholders in the relevant discipline to formulate guidelines and recommendations. The caregivers' guide would improve the caregivers' family's well-being during the new normal of the COVID-19 pandemic. Providing caregiver-centric services and interventions to improve well-being and enable providing effective care for children with special needs during such stressful life events.

The coping skills adopted to face the COVID-19 crisis will determine positive outcomes for the child and their primary caregivers. Training caregivers to adopt effective coping strategies and ensuring accessibility to counselling services and providing Tele-mental health services to family members of children with special needs will enable the caregivers to seek benefits and insights from credible professionals regarding their child's condition and one's physical and mental health. The current study would benefit in understanding the magnitude, costs, and impact of caregiving for the policymakers to view caregivers' concerns as a public health concern.

Conflict of Interest

All authors of the current book chapter declare that they have no conflict of interest.

Funding

The research study was not funded by any government or private body.

ACKNOWLEDGMENT

The authors of the research study would like to thank the parents and primary caregivers of children with neurodevelopmental disorders for their participation and cooperation in conducting the research.

REFERENCES

Bjørnnes, A. K. (2022). *Fighting the waves; COVID-19 family life interference in a neurodevelopmental disorder-caregiver.*

Burnett, D., Masi, A., Diaz, A. M., Rizzo, R., Lin, P. I., & Eapen, V. (2021). Distress levels of parents of children with neurodevelopmental disorders during the COVID-19 pandemic: A comparison between Italy and Australia. *International Journal of Environmental Research and Public Health, 18*(21), 11066. doi:10.3390/ijerph182111066 PMID:34769585

Christie, H., Hiscox, L. V., Halligan, S. L., & Creswell, C. (2022). Examining harmful impacts of the COVID-19 pandemic and school closures on parents and carers in the United Kingdom: A rapid review. *JCPP Advances, 2*(3). doi:10.1002/jcv2.12095 PMID:36247724

Currie, G., Finlay, B., Seth, A., Roth, C., Elsabbagh, M., Hudon, A., Hunt, M., Jodoin, S., Lach, L., Lencucha, R., Nicholas, D. B., Shakako, K., & Zwicker, J. (2022). Mental health challenges during COVID-19: Perspectives from parents with children with neurodevelopmental disabilities. *International Journal of Qualitative Studies on Health and Well-being, 17*(1), 2136090. doi:10.1080/17482631.2022.2136090 PMID:36309898

Fontanesi, L., Marchetti, D., Mazza, C., Di Giandomenico, S., Roma, P., & Verrocchio, M. C. (2020). The effect of the COVID-19 lockdown on parents: A call to adopt urgent measures. *Psychological Trauma: Theory, Research, Practice, and Policy, 12*(S1), S79–S81. doi:10.1037/tra0000672 PMID:32525382

Ganjiwale, D., Ganjiwale, J., Sharma, B., & Mishra, B. (2016). Quality of life and coping strategies of caregivers of children with physical and mental disabilities. *Journal of Family Medicine and Primary Care, 5*(2), 343. doi:10.4103/2249-4863.192360 PMID:27843839

Gillespie-Smith, K., McConachie, D., Ballantyne, C., Auyeung, B., & Goodall, K. (2021). The impact of COVID-19 restrictions on psychological distress in family caregivers of children with neurodevelopmental disability in the UK. *Journal of Autism and Developmental Disorders*. doi:10.100710803-021-05132-3 PMID:34286392

Grumi, S., Provenzi, L., Gardani, A., Aramini, V., Dargenio, E., Naboni, C., Vacchini, V., & Borgatti, R. (2020). Rehabilitation services lockdown during the COVID-19 emergency: The mental health response of caregivers of children with neurodevelopmental disabilities. *Disability and Rehabilitation, 43*(1), 27–32. doi:10.1080/09638288.2020.1842520 PMID:33167738

Hoffman, C. D., Sweeney, D. P., Hodge, D., Lopez-Wagner, M. C., & Looney, L. (2009). Parenting Stress and Closeness: Mothers of Typically Developing Children and Mothers of Children With Autism. *Sage, 24*(3), 178–187. doi:10.1177/1088357609338715

Hooda, S. (2020). *Stress and coping strategies in Primary caregivers of children with intellectual disability* [Doctoral dissertation]. Shodhganga: a reservoir of Indian theses.

Khan, F. M. (2018). *A Study of Perceived Stress Quality of Life and Coping Strategies of Parents of Children with Special Needs* [Master's thesis]. Shodhganga: a reservoir of Indian theses.

King-Dowling, S., Proudfoot, N. A., & Obeid, J. (2019). Comorbidity Among Chronic Physical Health Conditions and Neurodevelopmental Disorders in Childhood. *Current Developmental Disorders Reports*, *6*(4), 248–258. doi:10.100740474-019-00173-x

Kong, M. (2020). What COVID-19 means for non-neurotypical children and their families. *Pediatric Research, 89*(3), 396–397. doi:10.1038/s41390-020-0913-7

Lee, V., Albaum, C., Tablon Modica, P., Ahmad, F., Gorter, J. W., Khanlou, N., McMorris, C., Lai, J., Harrison, C., Hedley, T., Johnston, P., Putterman, C., Spoelstra, M., & Weiss, J. A. (2021). The impact of <scp>COVID</scp> -19 on the mental health and wellbeing of caregivers of autistic children and youth: A scoping review. *Autism Research, 14*(12), 2477–2494. doi:10.1002/aur.2616 PMID:34591373

Martinsone, B., & Tzivian, L. (2021). Differences in stress and coping during the COVID-19 pandemic in families with and without children with developmental disorders or chronic conditions. *Frontiers in Public Health*, *9*, 704577. doi:10.3389/fpubh.2021.704577 PMID:34490186

Masi, A., Mendoza Diaz, A., Tully, L., Azim, S. I., Woolfenden, S., Efron, D., & Eapen, V. (2021). Impact of the COVID-19 pandemic on the well-being of children with neurodevelopmental disabilities and their parents. *Journal of Paediatrics and Child Health, 57*(5), 631–636. doi:10.1111/jpc.15285 PMID:33426739

Nisha, S. I., & Bakul, F. (2022). Parents/primary caregivers' perspectives on the well-being, and home-based learning of children with neurodevelopmental disorders during COVID-19 in Bangladesh. *International Journal of Developmental Disabilities*, 1–10. doi:10.1080/20473869.2022.2121140

Nylén-Eriksen, M., Lara-Cabrera, M. L., Grov, E. K., Skarsvaag, H., Lie, I., Dahl-Michelsen, T., Sæterstrand, T. M., Mandahl, A., Hafstad, H., Lersveen, M. B., & United Nations Children's Fund (2020). *6 ways parents can support their kids through the COVID-19 outbreak*. UNICEF. https://www.unicef.org/coronavirus/6-ways-parents-can-support-their-kids-through-coronavirus-covid-19

Paulauskaite, L., Farris, O., Spencer, H. M., & Hassiotis, A.EPICC-ID group. (2021). My son can't socially distance or wear a mask: How families of preschool children with severe developmental delays and challenging behavior experienced the COVID-19 pandemic. *Journal of Mental Health Research in Intellectual Disabilities*, *14*(2), 225–236. doi:10.1080/19315864.2021.1874578

Pecor, K. W., Barbayannis, G., Yang, M., Johnson, J., Materasso, S., Borda, M., Garcia, D., Garla, V., & Ming, X. (2021). Quality of Life Changes during the COVID-19 Pandemic for Caregivers of Children with ADHD and/or ASD. *International Journal of Environmental Research and Public Health 2021, 18*(7), 3667. doi:10.3390/ijerph18073667

Shorey, S., Lau, L. S. T., Tan, J. X., Ng, E. D., & Aishworiya, R. (2021). Families With Children With Neurodevelopmental Disorders During COVID-19: A Scoping Review. *Journal of Pediatric Psychology*, *46*(5), 514–525. doi:10.1093/jpepsy/jsab029 PMID:33758930

Suzuki, K., & Hiratani, M. (2021). The association of mental health problems with preventive behavior and caregivers' anxiety about COVID-19 in children with neurodevelopmental disorders. *Frontiers in Psychiatry*, *12*, 713834. doi:10.3389/fpsyt.2021.713834 PMID:34335341

Ueda, R., Okada, T., Kita, Y., Ozawa, Y., Inoue, H., Shioda, M., Kono, Y., Kono, C., Nakamura, Y., Amemiya, K., Ito, A., Sugiura, N., Matsuoka, Y., Kaiga, C., Kubota, M., & Ozawa, H. (2021). The quality of life of children with neurodevelopmental disorders and their parents during the Coronavirus disease 19 emergency in Japan. *Scientific Reports, 11*(1), 1–8. doi:10.1038/s41598-021-82743-x

Wang, L., Li, D., Pan, S., Zhai, J., Xia, W., Sun, C., & Zou, M. (2021). The relationship between 2019-nCoV and psychological distress among parents of children with autism spectrum disorder. *Globalization and Health*, *17*(1), 1–14. doi:10.118612992-021-00674-8 PMID:33632259

World Health Organization. (2019). *International statistical classification of diseases and related health problems* (11th ed.). WHO. https://icd.who.int/

World Health Organization. (2020). *Coronavirus disease (COVID-19) advice for the public: Advocacy*. WHO. https://www.who.int/emergencies/diseases/novel-coronavirus-2019/advice-for-public/healthy-parenting

Yamamoto, T., Tanaka, S., Yoshizaki, A., Yoshimura, Y., Fauzi, A. A., Syarinaz, A., Adlan, A., Jayanath, S., Hamzah, N., Fujino, H., & Tachibana, M. (2022). *Relationship between children with neurodevelopmental disorders and their caregivers and friends during early phase of COVID-19 school closure in Japan: Association with difficulty in implementing infection prevention.*

Zhang, J., Shuai, L., Yu, H., Wang, Z., Qiu, M., Lu, L., Cao, X., Xia, W., Wang, Y., & Chen, R. (2020). Acute stress, behavioural symptoms and mood states among school-age children with attention-deficit/hyperactive disorder during the COVID-19 outbreak. *Asian Journal of Psychiatry*, *51*, 102077. doi:10.1016/j.ajp.2020.102077 PMID:32315967

Chapter 9
Mental Health and Well-Being Products/Apps and Their Challenges

Saubhagya Sooradas
Vellore Institute of Technology, India

Harman Singh
Vellore Institute of Technology, India

Amisha Vatsa
Vellore Institute of Technology, India

Aditya Mantri
Vellore Institute of Technology, India

Annanya Negi
Vellore Institute of Technology, India

Sanchit Khedkar
Vellore Institute of Technology, India

Rohan Varshney
Vellore Institute of Technology, India

ABSTRACT

Over recent times, multitudinous internal health apps (MHapps) have been developed and made available to smartphone druggies. The pandemic, of course, has put employees under a kind of mental strain few have likely experienced before, so it's no wonder more businesses are looking for ways to help workers who are struggling with anxiety, depression, and sleeplessness. In recent years, apps aiming to address all of those issues have proliferated. The boon of mental health application downloads during Covid-19 soared, and while interest will remain, there are bound to be some digital health apps that disappear. During those strange times, people couldn't go and see a doctor face to face about their mental ill-health or go to therapy appointments. Just as with most areas of healthcare impacted by the pandemic, mental health had to go digital. Digital mental health products and digital and virtual therapy have been shown to be comparable to real-life therapy for many patients.

DOI: 10.4018/978-1-6684-7221-7.ch009

INTRODUCTION

Several in-house health apps (MHapps) have recently been developed to make medicine available on smartphones. These apps aim to improve inner health and well-being, from guiding recovery from internal ailments to encouraging healthy habits that enhance emotional health (Donker et al., 2013c). Demand for MHapps is strong, with a recent poll showing that 76 out of 525 respondents said they would use their mobile phones for proper operation and internal sound surveillance if the service were free, (Donker et al., 2013c).

A 2018 study showed that internal health apps could improve both the monitoring and operation of internal health, (Wang et al., 2018b). It is also suggested that the app works because it is easy to use, increases participation in treatment plans, and facilitates symptom monitoring. These types of apps have been trending since the outbreak of the epidemic. The incidence of internal diseases is a global problem. However, there are high barriers to entry into formal psychotherapy, resulting in the exclusion of large segments of the population from home care. Mobile internal health operations (mMHealth) (app) appear to be a promising new development to address this care gap and build on the success of mHealth (mobile health) apps in general. Unfortunately, the overall quality of similar apps does not match their numbers. The end of this manuscript is to propose a standard for building internal health-related mM Health apps, including a process for evaluating and evaluating usability and impact, (Grist et al., 2017c).

Improving mental health and well-being using digital technologies such as mobile applications, online programs, and wearable devices has received widespread attention recently. These products and apps can increase accessibility, convenience, anonymity, and personalization. Digital mental health and well-being products and apps can improve access to mental health services and reduce the stigma of seeking treatment. They provide users with evidence-based resources, interventions, and tools to manage and improve their mental health. In addition, lifestyle factors such as poor diet, Lack of exercise, chronic stress, and substance abuse can contribute to poor mental health and increase the chances of mental health problems such as depression, panic attacks, and anxiety. There is nature. Ensuring that digital mental health products and apps are developed with user input and evidence is essential. Lifestyle factors are considered for maximum effectiveness and user trust.

However, it also faces some challenges related to development, implementation, and effectiveness (Baumel et al., 2019). This proposal aims to explore these challenges and suggest possible research directions. Several studies have examined the benefits of products and apps for mental health wellness. For example, a systematic review of mobile health interventions in mental health found that such interventions can improve symptoms of depression, anxiety, and stress (Firth et al., 2017). Another review suggested that online cognitive-behavioral therapy programs may be more effective and comfortable than face-to-face therapy for some mental illnesses (Andrews et al., 2018). However, these studies also highlight some challenges and limitations of these techniques.

Mental health is a huge concern worldwide, and India is no exception. Unfortunately, mental health disorders are highly stigmatized in India, resulting in a lack of awareness and resources to address this issue. As a result, the country faces multiple challenges, including a shortage of mental health professionals, Lack of funding, Lack of access to mental health care in rural areas, and high treatment dropout rates. Traditional beliefs and cultural stigma surrounding mental health have also given rise to these. In recent years, the mental health space has become a focus for innovation and investment, with many startups and businesses developing new products and services to address mental health challenges. However, scaling these solutions can be challenging due to several factors, such as regulatory barriers, a fragmented market, a lack of interoperability between different solutions, and limited access to capital. Furthermore, mental health is a complex and sensitive issue that requires a deep understanding of the cultural, social, and psychological factors that influence mental well-being. Startups and businesses need to address these challenges by developing robust business models, establishing partnerships with key stakeholders, investing in user research and co-creation, and developing solutions tailored to the needs and preferences of different user groups (Mohr et al., 2017b).

Although digital platforms provide a venue for self-management of depression and anxiety, despite the vast offerings in the market, only a handful are widely used, and the momentum gain for digital mental well-being platforms is relatively slow (Torous et al., 2021). Digital platforms like mental health apps offered on app stores can be beneficial in monitoring mental health status across the broad spectrum of mental health issues, including mood disorders like bipolar disorder and the various range of depressive disorders, psychotic disorders like schizophrenia, anxiety disorders, and much more. For example, smartphone-based monitoring can help collect data on mood instability in patients diagnosed with bipolar disorder. The collected data can facilitate the management of the same (Stanislaus et al., 2020; Anstosik-Wójcińska et al., 2020). Passive data collected from other intelligent devices, such as smartphones and smartwatches, indicate psychotic relapse in patients diagnosed with schizophrenia (Ben-Zeev et al., 2017). The collected data can be used for timely intervention and provided (Gumley et al.,2007,202). Of course, this epidemic has put workers under the kind of internal tension that many would have endured before. So it is no wonder that more companies are looking for ways to help workers who struggle with anxiety, depression, and wakefulness. I am here. The benefits of downloading medical surgeries during Covid-19 have skyrocketed, and while interest remains, some digital health apps may disappear. People will find more differences in the apps they use when evaluating utility. March 11 marked his second year of WHO protests against the Covid-19 epidemic, leading to global and public lockdowns and strict stay-at-home measures—government guidelines. Covid-19 is an indivisible problem of being locked down, quarantined, and losing loved ones, and the impact on internal health is enormous. Some people suffering from internal health problems are experiencing worsening symptoms.

In contrast, those who had not reported problems before the epidemic began to show symptoms of poor sleep, stress, anxiety, depression, and debilitating fatigue. Numerous studies in the UK have documented a pattern of declining internal health and wellness from March to May 2020 during the initial lockdown. This was followed by a period of improvement in July, August, and September 2020, according to many reports, when lockdowns lifted conditions similar to those before the outbreak began. From October 2020 to February 2021, he said, people's internal health alternated between bad and good.

OVERVIEW OF MENTAL HEALTH AND WELL-BEING PRODUCTS/APPS

Importance of Mental Health and Well-Being Products/Apps

In recent years, many mental health apps (MHapps) have been developed by many developers and made available to smartphone users, which comes in handy. These apps aim to improve mental health and well-being, from guiding recovery from mental illness to encouraging beneficial habits to enhance emotional health (Donker et al., 2013e). As a result, MHapps are in high demand, with a recent public survey showing that 76% of 525 respondents would use their mobile phones for mental health self-management and self-monitoring if the service were free. As a result, interest has emerged (Proudfoot et al., 2010).

There is a growing number of mobile apps for monitoring and treating mental health symptoms and disorders. However, clinically validated evidence for most of them is unknown. Therefore, its benefits for patients with long-term use are controversial. Mental health apps can potentially improve the monitoring and treatment of mental health symptoms, difficulties, and disorders. However, most currently available apps lack clinically validated evidence of their effectiveness. Given the number and pace of mobile health (mHealth) apps being released, more robust research is needed to develop and test evidence-based programs (Grist et al., 2017b).

MHapps and other technology-based solutions may play an essential role in the future of mental health care by making mental health support more accessible and reducing barriers to seeking help (Watts & Andrews, 2014b). However, innovative solutions for managing mental health problems are precious, given that many people suffering from mood and anxiety problems seek professional help (Mojtabai et al., 2002b). Moreover, even when people are aware of their problems and willing to seek help, service is not always readily available geographically, economically, or socially.

Types of Mental Health and Well-Being Products/Apps

Databases such as PsycInfo, Scopus, and ProQuest were searched for peer-reviewed sources. Search terms include (but are not limited to) 'health,' 'anxiety,' 'depression,' 'seek help,' 'self-help,' 'self-help,' 'smartphone,' and 'gamification.' not). Articles published between March 1975 and March 2015 were considered for inclusion, and meta-analyses and systematic reviews were requested for each relevant study area. In addition, some overview texts were referenced to explain the theoretical concepts related to the mobile app and recommended products. DESIGN (Becker et al., 2014b), (Luxton et al., 2011b). Sources not directly related to mental health or computer-based health interventions were excluded from the review. This was not a systematic review based on a single literature search, so the number of found and excluded articles was not recorded. In addition, we used multiple searches to explore concepts and formulate the recommendations presented. The lead author (DB) conducted this research and made basic recommendations. Secondary authors provided individual feedback on the review, suggested sources, and directed further research conducted by the primary author.

Current Market Offerings

The recommendations explored in this review should be considered in the context of the current range of MHapps available. The suggested recommendations are as follows: (1) cognitive behavioral therapy based; (2) address both anxiety and low mood; (3) designed for use by nonclinical populations; (4) automated tailoring; (5) reporting of thoughts, feelings, or behaviors; (6) recommend activities; (7) mental health information; (8) real-time engagement; (9) activities explicitly linked to specific reported mood problems; (10) encourage nontechnology-based activities; (11) gamification and intrinsic motivation to engage; (12) log of past app use; (13) reminders to engage; (14) simple and intuitive interface and interactions; (15) links to crisis support services; (16) experimental trials to establish efficacy. This is a recommended direction for future research. To demonstrate the necessity of such a future review or some form of an accreditation system to ensure the quality of healthcare apps (Jorm et al., 2004b), the lead author conducted a brief overview of the range of currently available MHapps via a series of preliminary searches of the iTunes App Store. The search terms used included "anxiety," "depression," "low mood," "mental health," "therapy," "relaxation," and "self-help." Inspection and use of the apps found in these searches revealed some significant gaps in their capabilities when compared with the recommendations

Lifestyle Factors Causing a Mass Decline in Mental Health

Poor Diet

Studies show that undernourishment is associated with poorer mental health. A deficiency of certain nutrients can affect mood, behavior, and cognitive function, as the brain needs these nutrients to function correctly. For example, studies have linked diets high in sugar and saturated fats to increased risk of depression and anxiety. These foods often lack essential mental and cognitive health nutrients, such as vitamins, minerals, and antioxidants. A diet containing it has also been associated with an increased risk of depression (1,2).

On the other hand, a healthy diet rich in essential vitamins, proteins, and minerals such as vitamin B12, folic acid, and omega-3 fatty acids is associated with a lower risk of depression and other diseases and similar mental conditions. In addition, a diet rich in fruits, vegetables, fish, and whole grains is beneficial for mental health (3). Conversely, a low-fiber diet, including whole grains, fruits, and vegetables, has increased the risk of depression. In addition, low vitamin D levels in dairy products have also been associated with depression (4,5).

Lack of physical exercise: Disruption of neurobiological brain function is one of the main reasons inactivity leads to poor mental health. Studies suggest that physical activity stimulates the production of neurotrophic factors, proteins that support the growth, maintenance, and survival of neurons in the brain (6). Regular exercise increases the production of neurotrophic factors and improves overall brain health, especially cognitive function (7). However, a sedentary lifestyle has the opposite effect, decreasing the body's production of neurotrophic factors and increasing the risk of cognitive decline and neurodegenerative diseases (8). This can lead to many mental health issues, including depression, anxiety, and cognitive impairment (9). Has been shown to decrease HPA axis activity and reduce levels of the stress hormone cortisol (10). A sedentary lifestyle causes chronic activation of the HPA axis and may contribute to developing mood disorders such as depression and anxiety (11). In summary, regular physical activity increases the brain's production of endorphins, chemicals that increase well-being and reduce symptoms of depression and anxiety. Not only does it make you feel better, but it also positively impacts your mental health.

Chronic Stress

Chronic stress is long-lasting and often triggered by challenging or traumatic events (12). Chronic stress can alter brain chemistry and function, disrupt the regulation of the stress response system, and cause other physiological and psychological changes, which can significantly negatively impact mental health. Chronic stress increases activity in the body's central stress response system, the hypothalamic-pituitary-adrenal (HPA) axis, leading to mental health problems. Cortisol, a stress-related hormone, is released upon activation of the HPA axis (13). Long-term activation of the HPA axis can lead to dysregulation of cortisol levels, which may contribute to developing mood disorders such as depression and anxiety (14). Chronic stress can also affect how the brain looks and functions, especially in areas of the brain associated with controlling emotions and processing thoughts. Long-term stress shrinks the hippocampus, a part of the brain important for learning and memory (15). This can lead to memory and cognition problems and an increased risk of depression, panic attacks, and anxiety. Prolonged stress increases the production of neurotransmitters, chemicals in the brain that control mood, behavior, and cognitive function. It can affect your level. Prolonged stress has been shown to lower serotonin levels, a neurotransmitter associated with happiness and happiness (16). This can facilitate the development of depression and other emotional disorders.

Substance abuse: Using drugs or alcohol to damage or disrupt someone's life is called substance abuse. Substance abuse can alter how the brain works and structures, leading to mental health problems such as depression and anxiety (17). Moreover, substance abuse can exacerbate current mental health problems and contribute to the emergence of new ones. Substance abuse can lead to severe mental health problems because it disrupts the balance of neurotransmitters in the brain. The brain uses chemicals called neurotransmitters to communicate between neurons. Drug or alcohol abuse can lead to neurotransmitter imbalances that alter mood, behavior, and cognition (18). For example, regular alcohol consumption can decrease serotonin levels, a neurotransmitter that regulates mood, increasing the risk of depression (19). Structural and functional (fundamental)changes in the brain can also result from substance abuse. Chronic drug use, such as cocaine, methamphetamine, and marijuana, is associated with changes in brain structure, such as decreased amounts of gray matter in specific brain regions (20). These changes can lead to memory and attention problems and an increased risk of mental health problems such as anxiety and psychosis. In addition, substance abuse may increase the risk of stress and trauma, which are known to increase the chances of developing mental health problems. Alternatively, they are more likely to be exposed to other traumatic events that can lead to mental health issues such as PTSD (21). Substance abuse can impair mental health through various mechanisms, including altered neurotransmitter levels, altered brain structure and function, and increased risk of stress and trauma. Mental illness, such as psychosis, can develop or worsen due to these factors.

Social isolation: Loneliness, a personal experience brought about by a Lack of social connections and support, can result from social isolation (22). Long-term loneliness is associated with various detrimental effects, including depression, anxiety, and cognitive decline (23, 24). In addition, loneliness is associated with brain changes that may facilitate the development of mental health problems (25). Lack of social support, an essential tool for reducing stress, may result from another risk factor, social isolation (26). Social support can provide emotional, practical, and educational resources to help people cope with stressors and reduce their risk of developing mental health problems (27). Lack of social support is associated with an increased risk of anxiety and depression (28). Social isolation can lead to a lack of opportunities for meaningful social interactions and activities necessary for maintaining cognitive function and overall well-being (29). Evidence shows that social engagement reduces the risk of dementia and cognitive decline (30). Fulfilling activities such as volunteerism and hobbies gives people purpose and fulfillment and help prevent depression and other mental health problems (31).

Benefits of Mental Health and Well-Being Products/Apps

Mobile applications for mental health and well-being offer users a range of benefits. These apps can provide access to mental health care to people who might otherwise not have the resources, such as in remote and rural areas. It also provides flexibility by allowing users to access services anytime, anywhere, making it more convenient than traditional forms of treatment that require in-person appointments, ultimately allowing individuals to access mental health care. In addition, these apps offer a sense of privacy not found in traditional therapies. Some people feel more comfortable and open to sharing personal information or discussing sensitive topics through apps than in person.

Additionally, these apps offer personalized treatment options tailored to each user's specific needs. For example, some apps provide guided meditations and cognitive-behavioral therapy exercises that address a user's symptoms and goals. It also helps reduce the stigma of seeking mental health care by providing easily accessible and discreet services., helps people better understand their mental health status and give them a sense of control over their symptoms. This encourages people to seek help with their mental health issues. In addition, these apps also help increase self-efficacy and enable individuals to manage their mental health better.

Other benefits of these applications are mentioned below:

Improved Mental Health and Well-Being

Mental health and well-being applications have proven effective in enhancing mental health and well-being through various interventions, including self-help strategies, psychoeducation, cognitive-behavioral therapy, mindfulness practices, and positive psychology techniques. In addition, they have improved access to mental health care, particularly for individuals who may not seek conventional mental health services for various reasons.

A systematic review conducted by Bucci et al. (2019) found that digital mental health interventions can provide access to care for individuals with mild to moderate mental health issues who might not seek face-to-face therapy. In addition, mental health apps have improved the convenience of mental health care delivery, as individuals can access mental health support anytime and anywhere, eliminating the need to travel to appointments. Sucala et al. (2017) also found that mental health apps provide a more convenient and accessible alternative to traditional face-to-face therapies. Additionally, mental health apps offer increased privacy and confidentiality for individuals who can receive care without fear of stigmatization or judgment by others. While privacy policies are often in place to protect personal information, mental health apps should prioritize transparency and trust to ensure that individuals feel safe and secure while using the app, as highlighted by Torous and Roberts (2017).

These apps often use algorithms and machine learning techniques to identify patterns in user data and provide recommendations for personalized treatment plans, as Schueller et al. (2017) noted. Personalization is a critical factor in the effectiveness of mental health apps, as it enables individuals to receive interventions tailored to their unique needs. In addition, Firth et al. (2017) found that mental health apps can reduce anxiety symptoms and potentially reduce the stigma associated with seeking help for mental health issues.

In addition, these apps have been found to increase self-efficacy and empower individuals to manage their mental health more effectively, as Mohr et al. (2018) suggested. By providing users with tools and strategies to manage their mental health, individuals can develop a sense of mastery over their mental health. Mental health apps have been found to improve mental health outcomes. Andrews et al. (2018) found that computer-based therapy was effective, acceptable, and practical for mental health care, just as effective as traditional face-to-face therapy, and with the added benefits of convenience and accessibility.

Increased Access to Mental Health Services

Mental health and well-being applications offer a promising solution to increase access to mental health services by overcoming common barriers that hinder individuals from seeking traditional mental health services. These apps cater to the needs of individuals facing challenges such as stigma, cost, or geographical location, providing remote access to mental healthcare. Teletherapy and online mental health support groups are examples of remote mental health care that have proved to be effective in improving mental health outcomes.

A systematic review of teletherapy found that it is as effective as in-person therapy, thereby improving access to mental health care for individuals who face geographical barriers to care. Similarly, online mental health support groups provide social support, reduce social isolation, and improve mental health outcomes. By providing a cost-effective and accessible solution, mental health and well-being apps have reduced the cost of mental health care, with some available for free or charge a nominal fee. Additionally, smartphone apps for mental health are cost-effective and can offer an alternative to traditional mental health services.

Moreover, mental health and well-being apps offer increased privacy and convenience, which can encourage individuals to seek help for mental health concerns. These apps' anonymity can reduce stigma and increase comfort with seeking help. The flexibility offered by these apps to access mental health care at any time and in any location allows individuals to seek help when and where they need it. Therefore, mental health and well-being apps can significantly improve access to mental health care and address mental health concerns.

To conclude, the emergence of mental health and well-being apps presents a hopeful prospect of revolutionizing mental healthcare delivery. These apps offer a range of advantages, including enhanced access to care, greater convenience, more privacy, customized treatment, diminished stigma, heightened self-efficacy, and better outcomes, making them a convenient, accessible, and effective intervention for those dealing with mental health issues. However, it is essential to underscore the significance of utilizing only evidence-based apps subjected to rigorous research, as not all apps are equal. Despite facing some obstacles, such as efficacy and quality control, the potential gains of mental health and well-being apps cannot be overlooked. It is, therefore, vital to continuing exploring and enhancing these apps to fully realize their potential in transforming mental health care delivery.

A Spectrum of Mental Health Issues

Mental, behavioral, and neurodevelopmental disorders are syndromes characterized by clinically significant disturbances in an individual's cognition, emotional regulation, or behavior, reflecting dysfunction in the underlying psychological, biological, or developmental processes. The distress or impairment caused by these abnormalities affects the essential personal, familial, social, educational, occupational, or other domains of functioning. These disorders are vast and encompass various conditions. Concerning digital mental well-being, the most common issues people seek to treat are one of two categories:

Mood disorders are a category of mental health illnesses characterized by persistent fluctuations in an individual's emotional state, significantly affecting their everyday functioning. These disorders influence how individuals feel, think, and act. The primary disorders discussed in this area are manic-depressive and bipolar disorders.

Anxiety or fear-related disorders are characterized by excessive fear and anxiety, accompanied by behavioral abnormalities that significantly impair an individual's functioning. Fear and anxiety are closely related phenomena; fear is a reaction to a perceived impending threat in the present, while anxiety refers to a perceived anticipated threat in the future. The fundamental differences between Anxiety and Fear-Related Disorders are the stimuli or events that induce fear or anxiety. Typically, this category includes Generalized Anxiety Disorder, Panic Disorder, Particular Phobia, Agoraphobia, Social Anxiety Disorder, Separation Anxiety Disorder, and Selective Mutism.

Preventive Mental Health Care

Preventative mental health treatment aims to prevent the emergence or worsening of mental health disorders by promoting mental health and well-being, lowering the risk of developing mental illnesses, and improving the overall quality of life. This type of care can be provided in various ways, including through electronic interventions, community-based programs, and individual interventions. In recent years, digital preventive mental health care treatments have become popular due to their accessibility, affordability, and scalability. Apps and other digital platforms for mental health provide a method for monitoring the mental health status of various conditions, including mood disorders such as bipolar disorder, various depressive disorders, psychotic disorders such as schizophrenia, and anxiety disorders, among others. Digital phenotyping, also known as the data acquired by smartphones and mental health apps regarding a patient's condition, vitals, mood, etc., assists mental health practitioners and digital mental health services in treating clients successfully (Insel, 2017b). Smartphone apps for mental health give users access to resources and tools for managing their mental health, which is beneficial in reducing depression and anxiety symptoms and enhancing the quality of life. (Depp et al., 2019b). For example, passive data acquired by smartphones and other intelligent devices, such as smartwatches, can signal psychotic relapse in schizophrenia patients, allowing for prompt intervention based on the obtained data, (Gumley et al., 2020c).

Therapy and Counseling

Therapy and counseling are helpful methods for improving mental health and enabling individuals to manage mental health difficulties effectively. In recent years, the introduction of digital mental health services has enhanced access to care and decreased stigma, despite several constraints, such as restricted technological access in specific locations, trust concerns with digital mental health services, and usability issues (Torous et al., 2021c). However, despite the availability and exposure to many digital platforms for mental health, only a few are extensively adopted, and the adoption rate is slow. Cognitive Behavioural Therapy (CBT) and Psychodynamic Therapy (PDT) are the most often used treatments for mental health issues, with Interpersonal Therapy (IPT) and positive psychology being valuable procedures in the context of digital mental health services. CBT is more successful than IPT in reducing depression symptoms. However, IPT is more effective in reducing anxiety symptoms as CBT focuses on cognitive and behavioral aspects linked with depression. In contrast, IPT focuses on interpersonal interactions and communication patterns associated with anxiety (Etzelmueller et al., 2020c).

Cognitive Behavioral Therapy

CBT is a well-established psychological intervention based on the assumption that thoughts, emotions, and behaviors are interdependent and mutually influential. CBT has successfully treated various mental disorders, such as anxiety, depression, PTSD, and OCD (Etzelmueller et al., 2020b). It is supported by the theoretical frameworks of cognitive and behavioral psychology, which propose that an individual's thoughts and beliefs can influence their behavior and emotions. CBT holds that bad ideas can drive negative behaviors and emotions, reinforcing the negative thinking pattern and sustaining the negative reinforcement cycle (Sachetta, 2021). When offered via the Internet, CBT is referred to as Internet-based CBT (iCBT) or Internet-based CBT. CBT is as successful as face-to-face CBT, with no apparent differences in efficacy across illnesses or intervention modalities (guided vs. unguided). However, the quality of evidence for iCBT tends to be poorer than that for face-to-face therapy (Andersson et al., 2012b). iCBT has potential where there is a shortage of trained professionals (Etzelmueller et al., 2020c).and where face-to-face therapy presents a challenge, with one example being the COVID-19 pandemic, and can prove just as effective.

CHALLENGES OF MENTAL HEALTH AND WELL-BEING PRODUCTS/APPS

Mental health and well-being products/apps have gained popularity recently as a cost-effective and accessible way to address mental health issues. However, several challenges are associated with these products/apps, including ethical concerns with data privacy and security, Lack of regulation and oversight, inadequate user support, limited access for disadvantaged populations, little evidence of effectiveness, and the potential unintended consequences.

Ethical Concerns with Data Privacy and Security

Mental health and well-being products/apps collect sensitive personal data, including mental health diagnoses, mood patterns, and other personal information. This data collection, storage, and use raise critical ethical concerns around privacy and security. Several studies have highlighted the need for robust privacy policies and security measures to protect users' sensitive information (Firth, Torous, Nicholas, Carney, Rosenbaum, et al., 2017b). In addition, it is necessary to check that user data is protected and secure and that users have control over their data and how it is used (Firth, Torous, Nicholas, Carney, Rosenbaum, et al., 2017b).

Lack of Regulation and Oversight

Mental health and well-being products/apps are not regulated by a central authority, which raises concerns about their safety and efficacy (Berry et al., 2016b). This Lack of oversight also contributes to inadequate user support, as there are few guidelines or requirements for supporting users struggling with mental health issues. Therefore, there is a need for more robust regulation and oversight of these products/apps to ensure that they are safe, secure, and effective for users (Berry et al., 2016b).

Inadequate User Support

Mental health and well-being products/apps often rely on automated support systems that may not adequately address users' needs. There is a need for more personalized support systems that can provide tailored support to users who may be struggling or dealing with mental health issues or problems (Resources, 2021). Additionally, there is a need for more comprehensive user support systems that can address a wide range of mental health issues, including severe mental health disorders (Resources, 2021).

Limited Access for Disadvantaged Populations

Mental health and well-being products/apps may not be accessible to all people and populations, particularly those disadvantaged. For example, underprivileged populations may have limited access to smartphones or the internet, making using mental health and well-being products/apps difficult. Furthermore, cultural barriers may prevent these populations from seeking mental health care (Wainberg et al., 2017). There is a need for more accessible mental health and well-being products/apps that can address the needs of disadvantaged populations (Wainberg et al., 2017), (Murthy, 2017d).

Limited Evidence of Effectiveness

There is limited evidence of the effectiveness of mental health and well-being products/apps in improving mental health outcomes. Many studies are small-scale and lack rigorous scientific evaluation (Murthy, 2017d). This Lack of evidence raises concerns about the potential unintended consequences of these products/apps, such as overreliance on technology and neglect of other important aspects of mental health care (Firth, Torous, Nicholas, Carney, Pratap, et al., 2017b). There is an urge for a more robust scientific evaluation of these products/apps to determine their effectiveness and potential unintended consequences (Murthy, 2017d),

The Potential Unintended Consequences

Mental health and well-being products/apps can potentially cause unintended consequences, such as overreliance on technology and neglect of other important aspects of mental health care (Firth, Torous, Nicholas, Carney, Pratap, et al., 2017c). Additionally, these products/apps may exacerbate mental health issues if not used correctly or fail to provide adequate support to users (Firth, Torous, Nicholas, Carney, Pratap, et al., 2017c). Therefore, there is a need for more research to understand the potential unintended consequences of mental health and well-being products/apps and how they can be mitigated.

Challenges to Solving Mental Health, Especially in India

India is one of the countries facing significant challenges in addressing mental health issues. The stigmatization of mental health problems in India is a significant barrier to providing adequate care to those in need (Wainberg et al., 2017b). Moreover, mental health care is underfunded, and the country lacks trained mental health professionals (Wainberg et al., 2017b). The Indian government's National Mental

Health Survey found that almost 14% of the Indian population requires active and sudden intervention for one or more mental health conditions. However, only a tiny fraction of those people receive adequate care (Murthy, 2017e).In addition, cultural norms and beliefs surrounding mental health also play a crucial role in mental health stigma and treatment. These issues pose significant challenges to developing practical solutions that are accessible and acceptable to the Indian population (Wainberg et al., 2017b). Therefore, product startups/businesses operating in this space must understand the cultural nuances and the unique challenges faced by the Indian population to create successful and practical solutions.

Challenges for a Product Startup/Business to Disrupt this Space With Scale

While mental health and well-being products/apps have the potential to address and deal with some of the challenges facing traditional mental health care, they also face several challenges of their own. One significant challenge is the Lack of regulation and oversight in the mental health technology space, which can lead to untested, ineffective, or potentially harmful products being available to consumers (Torous & Roberts, 2017b). In addition, there are concerns about the ethical implications of data privacy and security in collecting and using user data by mental health apps (Murthy, 2017f).

Moreover, many mental health apps lack adequate user support, including access to trained professionals who can provide personalized care (Vaidyam et al., 2019b). Limited evidence of the effectiveness of mental health and well-being apps is another challenge, as many of these products have not undergone rigorous scientific evaluation [50]. This limited evidence of effectiveness can lead to a lack of trust in these products and lower user engagement.

Furthermore, another challenge is limited access to mental health and well-being products for disadvantaged populations, such as those in low-income areas or rural communities (Henson et al., 2019). These populations often lack access to the technology required to use these products, and language or cultural barriers may further limit their ability to benefit.

Finally, there is also a potential for unintended consequences of these products, such as over-reliance on technology for mental health care, which may not be appropriate or effective for all users (Bakker et al., 2016c).

In conclusion, while mental health and well-being products/apps can improve access to mental health care and support, they face several challenges. These include ethical concerns with data privacy and security, Lack of regulation and oversight, inadequate user support, limited access for disadvantaged populations, little evidence of effectiveness, and potential unintended consequences. Additionally, startups/businesses operating in this space must be aware of the unique challenges or problems faced by different populations, particularly in countries like India, where mental health stigma, limited access to care, and cultural differences pose significant obstacles to developing practical solutions.

DISCUSSION OF CASE STUDIES

People of various ages, genders, and origins are affected by mental health concerns, which are becoming a global concern. By providing a variety of interventions, such as cognitive-behavioral therapy, mood tracking, and mindfulness-based stress reduction, among others, mental health apps have emerged as a potential alternative to assist in addressing these difficulties. This essay aims to summarize the efficacy of the three mental health applications, Headspace, Calm, and Moodfit, and the challenges mental health companies and startups face in a building in this space concerning the Indian market.

Figure 1. Mental health as a spectrum

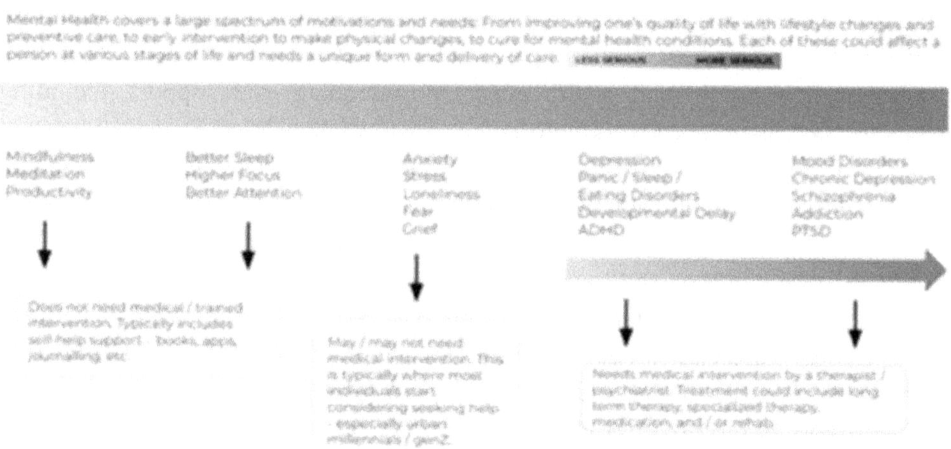

The focus on mental health has increased in India over the past few years as more millennials openly discuss their therapy experiences, more employers offer mental health benefits, more managers are encouraged to receive coaching, and more celebrities openly discuss their struggles with mental health issues. In addition, the delivery of these services is becoming increasingly online as the need grows, taking the form of teleconsults, AI-driven apps, and online support groups.

The phrase "mental health" is broad, just like people's various demands and problems. We consider it a continuum of requirements, from actively seeking aid to preserving a healthy mind.

Figure 2. Market size and opportunity

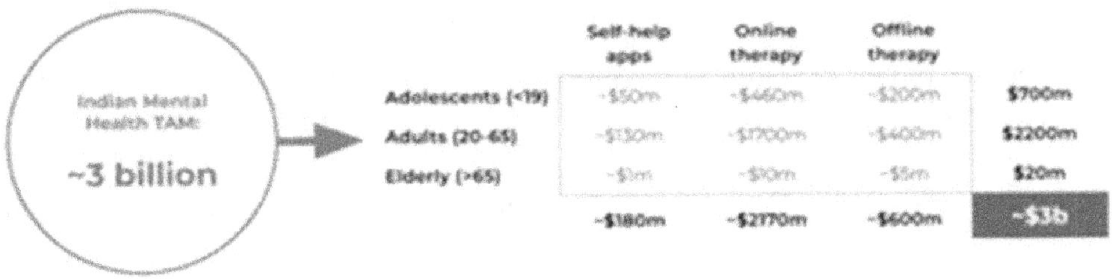

Figure 3. Differences in theraputical need and suppy

Therapist	Supply needed (per global standard)	India's actual supply*	Deficit
Psychiatrist	13k	3.5k	9.5k
Clinical Psychologists	20k	1k	19k
Psychiatric Social Workers	35k	1k	34k
Psychiatric Nurses	30k	1.5k	28.5k

Nevertheless, there are striking obstacles to building products in this domain.

1. India's population cannot be adequately served by its current supply: To administer a population of our size, India should have 20 000 clinical psychologists and 35 000 psychiatric social workers, according to WHO criteria. However, unfortunately, our actual supply of qualified professionals is significantly less than that.

2. The cost of therapy is high. A typical one-hour session of traditional therapy costs between 1-2k INR and clients are advised to attend at least one session per week for several months, if not years. Also, the most excellent counselors and therapists are frequently found in Tier 1 cities, which limits the availability of traditional offline therapy for users in other locations.
3. Scaling up high-quality services is challenging. Due to its reliance on individualized attention and highly skilled experts, traditional treatment is complicated to scale. You frequently sacrifice quality as you try to scale this service (by incorporating group sessions, AI, and self-help). Scalability, quality, and affordability are in intrinsic conflict with one other in mental health.

It is like a trilemma. For example, in mental health products, you can choose 2 out of 3: scalability, quality, and affordability.

Case Study 1: Headspace

Headspace is a popular meditation app that provides users with guided meditation sessions ranging from three minutes to an hour. The app has been evaluated in several studies, with the results indicating that it is an effective intervention for reducing symptoms of anxiety and depression.

In one study, Flett et al. (2021) evaluated how well Headspace worked to lessen sadness and anxiety symptoms in college students. One hundred seventy-four individuals in the study were randomly assigned to the Headspace or the control group. The Headspace group's participants were told to use the app for ten straight days at a rate of 10 minutes per day. According to the findings, participants in the Headspace group had much fewer symptoms of anxiety and depression than those in the control group. According to the study, Headspace can be a practical intervention for lessening sadness and anxiety symptoms among college students.

Another study by Wuthrich et al. (2020) assessed Headspace's efficiency in lowering depressive and anxiety symptoms in a clinical population. Ninety-six people with mild to moderate symptoms of anxiety and depression were enrolled in the study. Randomization was used to assign participants to the Headspace or control groups. For 30 days straight, participants in the Headspace group were instructed to use the app for 10 minutes each day. According to the findings, participants in the Headspace group had much fewer symptoms of anxiety and depression than those in the control group. According to the study's findings, Headspace can be a practical intervention for lessening sadness and anxiety symptoms in a clinical population.

Case Study 2: Calm

Calm is another popular mental health app that offers a range of interventions, including meditation, sleep stories, and breathing exercises, among others. The app has been evaluated in several studies, indicating that it is an effective intervention for managing stress, anxiety, and depression. Huberty et al. (2019) . 's randomized controlled experiment assessed Calm's efficiency in easing adult stress and anxiety symptoms. The study randomly assigned two hundred twenty-two individuals to the Calm or control groups. The Calm group's participants were told to use the app daily for 10 minutes for 30 days. According to the findings, participants in the Calm group had significantly fewer signs of stress and anxiety than those in the control group. According to the study, Calm can be a valuable strategy for treating adult pressure and anxiety.

A different study by Mani et al. (2020) assessed the efficiency of Calm in enhancing university students' sleep quality. 26 people were involved in the trial and randomly assigned to the Calm or the control group. For 14 days straight, participants in the Calm group were instructed to use the app for 10 minutes before bed. According to the findings, participants in the Calm group had significantly better sleep than those in the control group. According to the study's findings, Calm can be a helpful intervention for raising university students' sleep quality.

Case Study 3: Moodfit

Moodfit is a mood-tracking app that allows users to monitor their moods, set goals, and track progress. The app uses cognitive-behavioral therapy techniques to help users develop positive habits and behaviors.

Mohr et al. (2017) conducted a randomized controlled experiment to assess the efficacy of Moodfit in lowering adult depressive symptoms. Five hundred people participated in the trial and were randomly assigned to the control or Moodfit groups. The Moodfit group's participants were told to use the app daily for 10 minutes for 30 days. According to the findings, the Moodfit group had significantly fewer depressive symptoms than the control group. According to the study's findings, Moodfit may be a helpful intervention for easing the symptoms of depression in adults.

Another study by Wang et al. (2021) assessed the efficiency of Moodfit in enhancing cancer survivors' moods and quality of life. Fifty people participated in the trial and were randomly assigned to the control or Moodfit groups. The Moodfit group was instructed to use the app daily for 10 minutes for 30 days. Comparing the Moodfit group to the control group, the results revealed that participants in the Moodfit group significantly improved their mood and quality of life. According to the study's findings, Moodfit can be a practical intervention for raising cancer survivors' moods and quality of life.

In a nutshell, mental health applications like Headspace, Calm, and Moodfit have demonstrated promising benefits in lowering symptoms of anxiety, depression, and stress and enhancing mood and quality of life among various demographics. However, more investigation is required to ascertain the applications' long-term efficacy and explore the possibility of incorporating them into standard mental healthcare. By giving users simple and accessible tools for self-management and intervention, mental health apps can be a helpful complement to conventional mental healthcare.

CONCLUSION

Summary of Mental Health and Well-being Products/Apps

In recent years, the development of mental health and well-being products and apps has increased significantly. These products and apps are designed to provide individuals with resources to help manage their mental health and well-being. While these products and apps can be valuable tools, it is essential to remember that they should not be taken as a substitute for professional mental health treatment.

Many mental health and well-being products and apps offer features such as mood tracking, guided meditation, and stress reduction techniques. These tools can be helpful for individuals looking to improve their mental health and well-being. Additionally, some products and apps offer access to mental health professionals, which can be a valuable resource for those seeking professional support.

However, it is essential to note that not all mental health and well-being products and apps are created equal. Some may make unrealistic promises or lack scientific evidence to support their effectiveness. Therefore, it is crucial to do research and consult with a mental health professional before using any mental health and well-being products or apps.

In conclusion, mental health and well-being products and apps can be helpful resources for individuals looking to manage their mental health and well-being. However, they should not be used as a professional mental health treatment substitute. Therefore, it is essential to carefully evaluate their effectiveness and consult a mental health professional before using them.

Benefits and Challenges of Mental Health and Well-Being Products/Apps

In conclusion, mental health and well-being products/apps have benefits and challenges. The benefits of these products include increased access to mental health resources, greater convenience and flexibility, cost-effectiveness, and reduced stigma surrounding mental health. However, these products also pose challenges, such as concerns about privacy and data security, the potential for over-reliance on technology, Lack of regulation, and the potential for ineffective or even harmful products.

It is essential for individuals to evaluate mental health products/apps carefully and to seek professional help when needed. However, mental health products/apps should not be viewed as a substitute for professional care but as a supplement. Additionally, policymakers and regulators should work to ensure that these products meet standards for safety and effectiveness while protecting users' privacy and data security. Overall, mental health products/apps have the potential to play a positive role in improving mental health and well-being. Still, they must be used responsibly and in conjunction with professional care.

Future Directions for Mental Health and Well-Being Products/Apps

The future of mental health and well-being products/apps looks promising. Advancements in technology and data analytics have opened up new opportunities for personalized and effective interventions. The increasing popularity of these products/apps indicates a growing demand for accessible mental health resources. However, several challenges must be addressed, such as ensuring privacy and security, minimizing biases, and increasing access to underrepresented populations.

To overcome these challenges and further improve mental health and well-being products/apps, future directions could include a greater focus on evidence-based interventions, integration with healthcare systems, and collaboration with mental health professionals. In addition, further research and development of these products/apps can help ensure they remain relevant and effective in meeting users' needs.

Overall, mental health and well-being products/apps have the potential to play a significant and vital role in improving the mental health of individuals and communities. By addressing the challenges and continuing to innovate, these products/apps can help make mental health resources more accessible, convenient, and effective.

Call to action for increased regulation and oversight of mental health and well-being products/apps

As the use of mental health and well-being products/apps continues to grow, it is essential to recognize the potential risks associated with their service. While these products and apps can offer valuable support and resources, they can also be ineffective or harmful if not adequately regulated or overseen.

Therefore, a clear call to action is needed for increased regulation and oversight of mental health and well-being products/apps. This includes mandatory safety testing, transparent and accurate marketing, and regular user feedback and complaints monitoring. In addition, mental health professionals should be involved in developing and testing these products/apps to ensure they are evidence-based and effective.

By taking these steps, we can help ensure that mental health and well-being products/apps are safe and adequate resources for those seeking support and help manage their mental health. It is the responsibility of regulators and developers to prioritize users' well-being and take steps to ensure that these products/apps are serving their intended purpose without causing harm.

REFERENCES

Andersson, G., Carlbring, P., & Furmark, T.SOFIE Research Group. (2012). Therapist experience and knowledge acquisition in internet-delivered CBT for social anxiety disorder: A randomized controlled trial. *PLoS One*, *7*(5), e37411. doi:10.1371/journal.pone.0037411 PMID:22649526

Andersson, G., Carlbring, P., & Hadjistavropoulos, H. D. (2017). Internet-based cognitive behavior therapy. In S. G. Hofmann & G. J. G. Asmundson (Eds.), *The science of cognitive behavioral therapy* (pp. 531–549). Academic Press. doi:10.1016/B978-0-12-803457-6.00021-0

Bakker, D., Kazantzis, N., Rickwood, D., & Rickard, N. (2016). Mental Health Smartphone Apps: Review and Evidence-Based Recommendations for Future Developments. *JMIR Mental Health*, *3*(1), e7. doi:10.2196/mental.4984 PMID:26932350

Baumel, A., Muench, F., Edan, S., & Kane, J. M. (2019). Objective User Engagement With Mental Health Apps: Systematic Search and Panel-Based Usage Analysis. *Journal of Medical Internet Research*, *21*(9), e14567. doi:10.2196/14567 PMID:31573916

Beck, J. S., & Beck, A. (2011). *Cognitive behavior therapy*. Guilford Publication.

Becker, S., Miron-Shatz, T., Schumacher, N., Krocza, J., Diamantidis, C., & Albrecht, U. V. (2014). mHealth 2.0: Experiences, Possibilities, and Perspectives. *JMIR mHealth and uHealth*, *2*(2), e24. doi:10.2196/mhealth.3328 PMID:25099752

Ben-Zeev, D. (2017). CrossCheck: Integrating self-report, behavioral sensing, and smartphone use to identify digital indicators of psychotic relapse. *Psychiatric rehabilitation journal, 40*(3) 266.

Berry, N., Lobban, F., Emsley, R., & Bucci, S. (2016). Acceptability of Interventions Delivered Online and Through Mobile Phones for People Who Experience Severe Mental Health Problems: A Systematic Review. *Journal of Medical Internet Research*, *18*(5), e121. doi:10.2196/jmir.5250 PMID:27245693

Coyle, D., Doherty, G., & Sharry, J. (2012). An evaluation of a solution focused computer game in adolescent interventions. *Clinical Child Psychology and Psychiatry*, *17*(2), 225–242. doi:10.1177/1359104511417264 PMID:19515752

Depp, C. A., Perivoliotis, D., Holden, J., Dorr, J., & Granholm, E. L. (2019). Single-Session Mobile-Augmented Intervention in Serious Mental Illness: A Three-Arm Randomized Controlled Trial. *Schizophrenia Bulletin*, *45*(4), 752–762. doi:10.1093chbulby135 PMID:30281086

Dominiak, M., Kaczmarek-Majer, K., Antosik-Wójcińska, A. Z., Opara, K. R., Olwert, A., Radziszewska, W., Hryniewicz, O., Święcicki, Ł., Wojnar, M., & Mierzejewski, P. (2022). Behavioral and Self-reported Data Collected From Smartphones for the Assessment of Depressive and Manic Symptoms in Patients With Bipolar Disorder: Prospective Observational Study. *Journal of Medical Internet Research*, *24*(1), e28647. doi:10.2196/28647 PMID:34874015

Donker, T., Petrie, K., Proudfoot, J., Clarke, J., Birch, M. R., & Christensen, H. (2013). Smartphones for smarter delivery of mental health programs: A systematic review. *Journal of Medical Internet Research*, *15*(11), e247. doi:10.2196/jmir.2791 PMID:24240579

Donker, T., Petrie, K., Proudfoot, J., Clarke, J., Birch, M. R., & Christensen, H. (2013). Smartphones for smarter delivery of mental health programs: A systematic review. *Journal of Medical Internet Research*, *15*(11), e247. doi:10.2196/jmir.2791 PMID:24240579

Elkholy, H., Tawfik, F., Ibrahim, I., Salah El-din, W., Sabry, M., Mohammed, S., Hamza, M., Alaa, M., Fawzy, A. Z., Ashmawy, R., Sayed, M., & Omar, A. N. (2021). Mental health of frontline healthcare workers exposed to COVID-19 in Egypt: A call for action. *The International Journal of Social Psychiatry*, *67*(5), 522–531. doi:10.1177/0020764020960192 PMID:32972298

Etzelmueller, A., Vis, C., Karyotaki, E., Baumeister, H., Titov, N., Berking, M., Cuijpers, P., Riper, H., & Ebert, D. D. (2020). Effects of Internet-Based Cognitive Behavioral Therapy in Routine Care for Adults in Treatment for Depression and Anxiety: Systematic Review and Meta-Analysis. *Journal of Medical Internet Research, 22*(8), e18100. doi:10.2196/18100 PMID:32865497

Firth, J., Cotter, J., Torous, J., Bucci, S., Firth, J. A., & Yung, A. R. (2016). Mobile Phone Ownership and Endorsement of "mHealth" AmongPeople With Psychosis: A Meta-analysis of Cross-sectional Studies. *Schizophrenia Bulletin, 42*(2), 448–455. doi:10.1093chbulbv132 PMID:26400871

Firth, J., Torous, J., Nicholas, J., Carney, R., Pratap, A., Rosenbaum, S., & Sarris, J. (2017). The efficacy of smartphone-based mental health interventions for depressive symptoms: A meta-analysis of randomized controlled trials. *World Psychiatry; Official Journal of the World Psychiatric Association (WPA), 16*(3), 287–298. doi:10.1002/wps.20472 PMID:28941113

Firth, J., Torous, J., Nicholas, J., Carney, R., Rosenbaum, S., & Sarris, J. (2017). Can smartphone mental health interventions reduce symptoms of anxiety? A meta-analysis of randomized controlled trials. *Journal of Affective Disorders, 218*, 15–22. doi:10.1016/j.jad.2017.04.046 PMID:28456072

Giota, K., & Kleftaras, G. (2014). Mental Health Apps: Innovations, Risks and Ethical Considerations. *E-Health Telecommunication Systems and Networks, 3*(03), 19–23. doi:10.4236/etsn.2014.33003

Grist, R., Porter, J., & Stallard, P. (2017). Mental Health Mobile Apps for Preadolescents and Adolescents: A Systematic Review. *Journal of Medical Internet Research, 19*(5), e176. doi:10.2196/jmir.7332 PMID:28546138

Gualano, M. R., Bert, F., Martorana, M., Voglino, G., Andriolo, V., Thomas, R., & Siliquini, R. (2020). How digital health technologies facilitate the implementation of the principles of person-centered healthcare. *Health Policy and Technology, 9*(4), 361–367.

Gumley, A., Bradstreet, S., Ainsworth, J., Allan, S., Alvarez-Jimenez, M., Beattie, L., Bell, I., Birchwood, M., Briggs, A., Bucci, S., Castagnini, E., Clark, A., Cotton, S. M., Engel, L., French, P., Lederman, R., Lewis, S., Machin, M., MacLennan, G., ... Gleeson, J. (2020). Early Signs Monitoring to Prevent Relapse in Psychosis and Promote Well-Being, Engagement, and Recovery: Protocol for a Feasibility Cluster Randomized Controlled Trial Harnessing Mobile Phone Technology Blended With Peer Support. *JMIR Research Protocols, 9*(1), e15058. doi:10.2196/15058 PMID:31917372

Gumley, A., Bradstreet, S., Ainsworth, J., Allan, S., Alvarez-Jimenez, M., Beattie, L., Bell, I., Birchwood, M., Briggs, A., Bucci, S., Castagnini, E., Clark, A., Cotton, S. M., Engel, L., French, P., Lederman, R., Lewis, S., Machin, M., MacLennan, G., ... Gleeson, J. (2020). Early Signs Monitoring to Prevent Relapse in Psychosis and Promote Well-Being, Engagement, and Recovery: Protocol for a Feasibility Cluster Randomized Controlled Trial Harnessing Mobile Phone Technology Blended With Peer Support. *JMIR Research Protocols*, *9*(1), e15058. doi:10.2196/15058 PMID:31917372

Harari, G. M., Lane, N. D., Wang, R., Crosier, B. S., Campbell, A. T., & Gosling, S. D.(2016, November). Using Smartphones to Collect Behavioral Data in Psychological Science: Opportunities, Practical Considerations, and Challenges. *Perspectives on Psychological Science*, *11*(6), 838–854. doi:10.1177/1745691616650285 PMID:27899727

Henson, P., Wisniewski, H., Hollis, C., Keshavan, M., & Torous, J. (2019). Digital mental health apps and the therapeutic alliance: Initial review. *BJPsych Open*, *5*(1), e15. doi:10.1192/bjo.2018.86 PMID:30762511

Hofmann, S. G., & Smits, J. A. (2008). Cognitive-behavioral therapy for adult anxiety disorders: A meta-analysis of randomized placebo-controlled trials. *The Journal of Clinical Psychiatry*, *69*(4), 621–632. doi:10.4088/JCP.v69n0415 PMID:18363421

Insel, T. R. (2017). Digital Phenotyping: Technology for a New Science of Behavior. *Journal of the American Medical Association*, *318*(13), 1215–1216. doi:10.1001/jama.2017.11295 PMID:28973224

Jorm, A. F., Griffiths, K. M., Christensen, H., Parslow, R. A., & Rogers, B. (2004). Actions taken to cope with depression at different levels of severity: A community survey. *Psychological Medicine*, *34*(2), 293–299. doi:10.1017/S003329170300895X PMID:14982135

Kessing, L. V., Hansen, H. V., Christensen, E. M., Dam, H., Gluud, C., & Wetterslev, J. (2014). Do young adults with bipolar disorder benefit from early intervention? *Journal of Affective Disorders*, *152–154*, 403–408. doi:10.1016/j.jad.2013.10.001 PMID:24268595

Lattie, E. G., Adkins, E. C., Winquist, N., Stiles-Shields, C., Wafford, Q. E., & Graham, A. K. (2019). Digital Mental Health Interventions for Depression, Anxiety, and Enhancement of Psychological Well-Being Among College Students: Systematic Review. *Journal of Medical Internet Research*, *21*(7), e12869. doi:10.2196/12869 PMID:31333198

Luxton, D. D., McCann, R. A., Bush, N. E., Mishkind, M. C., & Reger, G. M. (2011). mHealth for Mental Health: Integrating Smartphone Technology in Behavioral Healthcare. *Professional Psychology, Research and Practice*, *42*(6), 505–512. doi:10.1037/a0024485

Mohr, D. C., Lyon, A. R., Lattie, E. G., Reddy, M., & Schueller, S. M. (2017). Accelerating Digital Mental Health Research From Early Design and Creation to Successful Implementation and Sustainment. *Journal of Medical Internet Research*, *19*(5), e153. doi:10.2196/jmir.7725 PMID:28490417

Mojtabai, R., Olfson, M., & Mechanic, D. (2002). Perceived need and help-seeking in adults with mood, anxiety, or substance use disorders. *Archives of General Psychiatry*, *59*(1), 77–84. doi:10.1001/archpsyc.59.1.77 PMID:11779286

Murthy, R. S. (2017). National Mental Health Survey of India 2015-2016. *Indian Journal of Psychiatry*, *59*(1), 21–26. doi:10.4103/psychiatry.IndianJPsychiatry_102_17 PMID:28529357

Proudfoot, J., Parker, G., Hadzi Pavlovic, D., Manicavasagar, V., Adler, E., & Whitton, A. (2010). Community attitudes to the appropriation of mobile phones for monitoring and managing depression, anxiety, and stress. *Journal of Medical Internet Research*, *12*(5), e64. doi:10.2196/jmir.1475 PMID:21169174

Romate, J., & Rajkumar, E. (2022). Exploring the experiences, psychological well-being and needs of frontline healthcare workers of government hos-pitals in India: A qualitative study. *Humanit Soc Sci Commun.*, *9*(1), 89. doi:10.105741599-022-01093-9

Schellong, J., Lorenz, P., & Weidner, K. (2019). Proposing a standardized, step-by-step model for creating post-traumatic stress disorder (PTSD) related mobile mental health apps in a framework based on technical and medical norms. *European Journal of Psychotraumatology*, *10*(1), 1611090. doi:10.1080/20008198.2019.1611090 PMID:31143412

Simon, G. E., & Ludman, E. J. (2009). It's time for disruptive innovation in psychotherapy. *Lancet*, *374*(9690), 594–595. doi:10.1016/S0140-6736(09)61415-X PMID:19699995

Torous, J., Bucci, S., Bell, I. H., Kessing, L. V., Faurholt-Jepsen, M., Whelan, P., Carvalho, A. F., Keshavan, M., Linardon, J., & Firth, J. (2021). The growing field of digital psychiatry: Current evidence and the future of apps, social media, chatbots, and virtual reality. *World Psychiatry; Official Journal of the World Psychiatric Association (WPA)*, *20*(3), 318–335. doi:10.1002/wps.20883 PMID:34505369

Torous, J., Bucci, S., Bell, I. H., Kessing, L. V., Faurholt-Jepsen, M., Whelan, P., Carvalho, A. F., Keshavan, M., Linardon, J., & Firth, J. (2021). The growing field of digital psychiatry: Current evidence and the future of apps, social media, chatbots, and virtual reality. *World Psychiatry; Official Journal of the World Psychiatric Association (WPA)*, *20*(3), 318–335. doi:10.1002/wps.20883 PMID:34505369

Torous, J., & Roberts, L. W. (2017). Needed Innovation in Digital Health and Smartphone Applications for Mental Health: Transparency and Trust. *JAMA Psychiatry*, *74*(5), 437–438. doi:10.1001/jamapsychiatry.2017.0262 PMID:28384700

Vaidyam, A. N., Wisniewski, H., Halamka, J. D., Kashavan, M. S., & Torous, J. B. (2019). Chatbots and Conversational Agents in Mental Health: A Review of the Psychiatric Landscape. *Canadian Journal of Psychiatry*, *64*(7), 456–464. doi:10.1177/0706743719828977 PMID:30897957

Wainberg, M. L., Scorza, P., Shultz, J. M., Helpman, L., Mootz, J. J., Johnson, K. A., Neria, Y., Bradford, J. E., Oquendo, M. A., & Arbuckle, M. R. (2017). Challenges and Opportunities in Global Mental Health: A Research-to-Practice Perspective. *Current Psychiatry Reports*, *19*(5), 28. doi:10.100711920-017-0780-z PMID:28425023

Wang, K., Varma, D. S., & Prosperi, M. (2018). A systematic review of the effectiveness of mobile apps for monitoring and management of mental health symptoms or disorders. *Journal of Psychiatric Research*, *107*, 73–78. doi:10.1016/j.jpsychires.2018.10.006 PMID:30347316

Watts, S. E., & Andrews, G. (2014). Internet access is NOT restricted globally to high income countries: So why are evidenced based prevention and treatment programs for mental disorders so rare? *Asian Journal of Psychiatry*, *10*, 71–74. doi:10.1016/j.ajp.2014.06.007 PMID:25042956

World Health Organization. (2004). *International Statistical Classification of Diseases and related health problems: Alphabetical index* (Vol. 3). World Health Organization.

Chapter 10
Workplace Well-Being During and Post Pandemic

Ayush Gupta
Indian Institute of Management, Bodh Gaya, India

ABSTRACT

The chapter will give a broad overview of the changes in the well-being of individuals in the workplace during and post-pandemic. The chapter focuses on the problems faced by the people in the pandemic era, which has affected their physical and mental well-being, and some recommendations to be taken by them post-pandemic. The well-being term is complicated as the authors define it in many other ways. In simple words, well-being means dealing with how well a person's mind works and how happy a person is. The whole chapter consists of two major parts: First, based on the role, and second based on demographic factors. Based on role, there are two categories: employees, and employers and business owners. There are three demographic factors: Age, gender and sexuality, race and religion. In the end, two case studies of reputed organizations are given, which came up with innovative measures to improve employees' well-being.

INTRODUCTION

Before moving on to know how a workplace impacts the well-being of a person, let us understand what well-being means. Well-being means dealing with how well a person's mind works and how happy a person is. Let us now dive into understanding the changes in the well-being of a workplace, where people work in factories and offices during the pandemic and post-pandemic period; in order to boost their well-being, some suggestions are given. During the Covid-19 pandemic, new and

DOI: 10.4018/978-1-6684-7221-7.ch010

innovative ways to perform work-related activities like WFH (Work From Home) rather than doing the same traditional office work methods have emerged. This can be seen in today's workplaces with video conferencing, flexible timing, more opportunities like internships, and less cost incurred by organizations to maintain a physical workplace. However, these innovations significantly impact an individual's well-being, irrespective of role and gender. The chapter is divided into two major sections on well-being differences, first based on the role played by a person and second based on demographic factors of the employee. In the end, two cases: Google and PayU are given, which highlights certain well-being measures taken by them.

WELL-BEING DIFFERENCES: BASED ON ROLE

According to the role played by a person in the workplace, he/ she experiences different perceived well-being. Here, we will focus on the two distinct roles: employees, employers, and business owners.

Employee

Every employee is different from the others. Each has its own needs and wants, and they have certain expectations from the organizations. The main problem lies with the organizations finding the root cause behind the employees' changing behavior which affects their well-being. Some of the causes are:

Social Isolation

Social isolation is considered to be one of the factors affecting the well-being of an employee during a pandemic period. Social isolation means an objective lack of social connectedness with friends and family, and lonely people may be very well connected yet feel lonely regardless. Over the past four decades, research studies have found an inverse relationship between social isolation and its impact on our health and well-being in various ways. Social isolation can be seen as a lack of non-verbal and verbal communication among colleagues, as no tea breaks lead to a need for socialization. In its practical form, this can lead to alienation from work, which means the person is not motivated to work.

Consequently, he/she will reduce his performance affecting the organizational effectiveness. This phenomenon is prevalent in countries with a collectivist culture because people embrace personality traits and attributes like cohesion and harmony.

Post-Pandemic measures:

- Increasing employees' participation in non-work related activities such as playing games, making teams for fun events, and celebrating on occasions. Such actions will foster relationships among employees and create a cooperative environment.
- Employees should have informal groups where they can openly chat with anyone and use memes and emojis in their conversation, making it informal communication and nurturing relationships beyond work. A research survey found that 95 percent of people are likely to send an emoticon to a co-worker, and 62 percent feel closer to their co-workers when using emoticons in their chat conversations.

Disruption in Work-Life Balance

Work-life balance means the time employees dedicate to balancing their personal and professional lives. It is crucial as it improves the efficiency of employees as they divide their time based on priorities. With the WFH model, there has been an imbalance in the work-life balance of employees. Employees become lazy working remotely, and during office hours, they watch web series and movies, trying to avoid work and enjoy as much as possible between working hours. This ultimately decreases the work output and impacts organizational effectiveness on an individual level; the person becomes uninterested in work, and therefore their performance declines, eventually affecting their physical and mental well-being. Sometimes, late-night calls and shifts increase the working hours. Employees get less time for enjoyment, thereby overburdening a person and ultimately impacting their mental well-being.

(Mann, 2021) Emotional exhaustion is a significant factor behind employees working from home and maintaining a work-life balance. The home environment for doing work is terrible for a work environment. Therefore, this emotional exhaustion became a challenge for the employees to maintain the work-life balance during the covid pandemic. This emotional exhaustion positively impacts an employee's health, disturbing his/her well-being.

"McKinsey" research warns that companies must adequately address the WFH model to positively impact productivity, employee engagement, and well-being and eventually increase turnover. In December 2021, after analyzing the productivity trends of millions of Microsoft users around the globe, it was discovered that since the advent of remote work, the average person has sent 42% more emails outside of business hours, and the time spent in Teams meetings has more than doubled. From April to November of 2020, satisfaction with work-life balance decreased by 13%. Overworked employees were unable to experience uninterrupted periods of concentration, which was a significant factor in their diminished work-life satisfaction. The more individuals collaborated, whether by attending meetings or sending emails, the lower their work-life satisfaction compared to coworkers who collaborated less. In addition, individuals were foregoing vacations. The study discovered that the average vacation time for Microsoft's U.S. employees by an astounding 83%, and that when people work remotely, they are more likely to forgo lunch breaks and work late. The Microsoft data revealed that employees who were able to take time off in March or April 2020 were 8% more satisfied with their work-life balance in May than thoplummeted se who had no time off. According to a survey conducted, it is observed that 28.64% of Indians have reported that due to an increase in workload pressure, their overall work-life balance has also been disturbed. Additionally, 32.9% of the country's population has reported that due to the changed working style, which is the WFH model, they are uncomfortable and unsatisfied with the changed mode of working.

Post-Pandemic measures:

- Employers can provide technology support such as remote access to work systems, collaboration tools, and mobile devices that allow employees to work more efficiently and flexibly.
- Monitoring the performance of the employees in order to remove any unnecessary rest intervals by taking daily updates. Employees should use technology mindfully to avoid burnout and maintain a healthy work-life balance. They should set boundaries around checking emails and taking breaks from screens throughout the day.
- Employees should assume that it is their responsibility to have a separate room with a desk and chair and finish quality work as soon as possible to have enough time to spend with their family.
- Employees should also make time for self-care activities, like spending time in nature, exercise, meditation, or. One should take care of oneself as it helps to reduce stress and improve one's overall well-being.
- Late-night calls and night shifts are infrequent; if there are, employees are/should be informed beforehand about such meetings, so they should plan out their schedules accordingly.

Employers and Business Owners

Employers and business owners hire people to carry out organizational activities. These business owners mean entrepreneurs with not only startups and large businesses but also small-scale vendors who carry out the activities. So, during this phase of the pandemic, there are several difficulties that employers and business owners have faced. Some are listed below:

Minimal Knowledge of the Use of Technology

Technology has played an essential role during the pandemic era. During COVID-19, all businesses came onto laptops and computers. The importance of technology has increased multifold in the HR process, from pre-hire planning to post-retirement planning. Employers and big businesses need to integrate the processes of HR with technology; for this, the employers should be able to use Big Data and HR analytics and strategic HR tools such as the digital dashboard. MSMEs yet to integrate technology into their processes and make their workforce accustomed to it have faced problems as many older people are unaware of Google meet, Zoom, and Microsoft Teams. The business owners were coping with this changing environment so on their hands, so it was difficult for them to train their staff. According to an interview conducted by the author on an MSME, the author learned that around 60% of the employees were taking time to get updated with the new technology. Among those, 26% of employees suffered from anxiety and mental distress; their mental well-being was disturbed.

Post-Pandemic measures:

- The employers should be trained to use new methods by conducting video lectures or giving them a simulated situation for some time and assessing their performance. This will help smoothly carry out the processes, and the organization works in a structured manner.
- Small-scale vendors and suppliers should use technology because such events are uncertain and can affect their business, and they may suffer losses. They should maintain customer relationships through WhatsApp or Facebook and contact repeat customers weekly to know whether they want some items and offer them a discount.
- Executives and business owners, especially small and medium-sized businesses (MSMEs), should switch to e-commerce areas or online stores to advertise their products and use social media to attract new customers. The presence of social media is valuable, and companies have started doing this to prepare for such events and gain a competitive edge over others post COVID-19.

Employee Cheating

As domestic demand and exports have plummeted, almost all sectors have been severely impacted, with notable exceptions including the IT, Outsourcing, Technology, E-commerce, Pharma, and Health Care sectors, which have experienced significant growth. During the pandemic, the world was beset by uncertainty in all directions, the economy was disintegrating, and all industries, including recruitment, were negatively affected. The pandemic imposed a considerable hurdle for employers to hire the right people for vacant positions. The problem is cheating in order to get selected for the interview done by the candidates.

The other problem is that even the existing employees commit fraud so that their positions are reserved, and they do not have any risk of job loss. One factor behind employees doing fraud is employee anxiety which impacts their well-being. According to research (Hillebrandt, 2022), people may feel anxious when perceiving danger and unsure about what may happen. They claim that worry centers people on self-interest and leads to behavior aligning with this focus (i.e., self-interested behavior). Anxiety may lead to workplace stealing, immoral behavior meant to promote one's interests while breaking widely held norms or rules (e.g., misrepresenting work activity to appear more productive). Such acts harm business owners as they will not be able to see the real value hidden due to malpractices.

Post-Pandemic measures:

- For the applicants, employers should make sure that the questions asked should be innovative and application based as the applicants will find it difficult to answer them.
- For the applicants, the employers should conduct a rapid-fire question interview to assess an individual's mental aptitude and ensure that their cameras are on, and no one is sitting beside them telling them answers. This will make the interview process fair and just.
- Employers should assure their employees about job security and list guidelines for when they will be removed from the organization. This will reduce the activity of fraud committed by the existing employees.
- Setting up a grievance redress mechanism allows the organization to manage employees facing any grievances/perceived danger. It is said that if all the steps of the grievance mechanism are followed, any grievance can be handled.

B-Problems (Business Problems)

B-Problems refer to an accumulation of operating problems faced by business owners, primarily SMEs, in managing a business: Money Management and Disruption in the Supply Chain. Following a cash flow guideline that balances the outflow with the inflow during the pandemic is a tremendous challenge. The credit period has increased and made business operations a bumpy road. The suppliers favored big businesses instead of SMEs, and this affected the operations of SMEs. According to a study (Lathabhavan, 2022), small business entrepreneurs in India faced difficulties during the pandemic with reduced or nil financial support as a resource. Significant positive relationships between economic distress and depression, anxiety, and tension were among the findings. This suggests a lack of financial resources can contribute to depression and increase anxiety.

Additionally, this causes elevated levels of tension among entrepreneurs. This study contributed to the literature on financial threat by demonstrating its positive associations with various mental health outcomes, including depression, anxiety, and stress. This suggests that business proprietors are more prone to depression, anxiety, and stress when their financial security is uncertain. This strengthened the relationships observed in various employment categories and among the unemployed. The study also discovered a substantial negative correlation between financial well-being and stress, anxiety, and depression among Indian entrepreneurs. This suggests that financial confidence can reduce mental health problems. When these business problems accumulate and become overburdening for the owner, then his/her well-being gets affected, and faces mental health issues.

Post-Pandemic measures:

- For Money Management, business owners can go to the Small Business Administration (SBA) for assistance. Moreover, they can also reach the federal government, which recently implemented the Paycheck Program Act to obtain small loans to keep up with payroll and operational expenses.
- For Supply Chain Management, the owners should give the suppliers a reasonable discount on bulk orders to build strategic relationships. Due to impositions on trade, the owners should have a plan B ready if such events happen again so that time is well-spent in executing the plan.

WELL-BEING DIFFERENCES: BASED ON DEMOGRAPHIC FACTORS

Demographic factors are a population or group's characteristics used to describe or analyze its composition. According to the age, gender, race, and religion of an employee, he/ she experiences different perceived well-being. Here, we will focus on how these factors affect an employee and recommendations for the same.

Age

An employee's well-being in the organization varies depending on his or her age. According to studies, younger employees, particularly those in their 20s and early 30s, were more likely to experience adverse mental health and well-being effects during the pandemic. This may result from factors such as increased job insecurity, financial instability, and disruptions to social connections and career advancement. Older employees may have encountered various challenges, including caregiving responsibilities, health and mortality concerns, and difficulties adapting to remote work technologies. Some are:

WFH Model: Boon or Bane

Providing the WFH Model to the employees is perceived differently by different age groups. This model might act as an opportunity for some, and for some, it might be a challenge. The author conducted a survey and found that people of different age groups that people in the age group of 30-50 and primarily those who have a family at that time, are happy with the WFH facility, which gives them time to handle the household chores simultaneously, however people of age group under 30 were initially delighted. Still, they soon realized the need for an office environment and socialization. The WFH model thereby impacted the psychological well-being of employees, primarily those under 30.

Job Loss (Bellotti, 2021)

According to research, unemployment increased across all age categories, though in varying patterns. Younger employees exhibited a more significant proportion of job loss at the onset of the pandemic. However, they appeared to rapidly recover with a more stable job loss rate in the final months of the pandemic. However, older workers' job loss rates were generally lower than younger workers. However, they did not stabilize, and it is believed that they will have more difficulty finding a new occupation once they lose their jobs. A study of "Bangladeshi youth" (15–29 years old) revealed that approximately nearly 10% lost one of their current positions, 5% of individuals lost their current job, and roughly 9% had their job offers delayed.

Intention To Leave (Bellotti, 2021)

Several researchers hypothesized that job insecurity, caused by COVID-19 and exacerbated by the unpredictability of the crisis's scope and intensity, can influence people's intentions to quit. In this situation, younger employees were more inclined to leave their jobs than their older counterparts. Multiple studies supported this observation. According to the results of a "cross-sectional study" of "Serbian employees", increased levels of job insecurity during COVID-19 led to greater intentions to leave the workforce. In addition, the authors discovered that older participants (40+) had a lower intention to abandon their organization and a higher job motivation than younger employees. Similar results were observed in various countries (e.g., Bolivia, South Korea, and Peru): workers' age was negatively associated with attrition intentions, so older employees were more likely to remain than younger ones.

Post-pandemic measures:

- Employees under the age of 30 should conduct social and team-building activities, and the organizations should shift to the Hybrid Work Model, which is defined as one that provides support for both in-office and remote employees.
- Instead of engaging in layoffs and creating job loss for many employees, which will significantly reduce a company's brand image, it is advised that the organizations should go for layoffs only when the company is suffering losses.
- In order to make sure that there is low attrition among younger employees, they should be provided certain perquisites and benefits as the youth are full of energy and bring a new approach to doing activities; thereby, they are required for the success of the organization.

Gender and LGBTQ+

COVID-19 has impacted the well-being of all genders and LGBTQ+ in various ways. There are two categories in gender - male, and female, and in addition to that, the focus is also given to LGBTQ+ community.

Male

During this pandemic, men faced several challenges while working from home; however, there is less research on them. Some are:

Family Responsibility

Since most countries have a patriarchal society where it is expected that men should work and women take care of the household, this ideology persists, which overburdens men as he must fulfill various responsibilities as father, son, brother, and husband in a family. Men also took on increased caregiving responsibilities during the pandemic, as schools and childcare centers closed, and family members became ill. This has put pressure on male employees to balance work and family responsibilities. During this pandemic, when people were at risk of job loss as many organizations were doing layoffs. Then, the financial pressure on a man affects his mental well-being, and he suffers from anxiety and psychological distress.

Post-pandemic measures:

- The family should support men and encourage them during this phase of COVID-19. For this, the family must create a happy environment because, in the WFH model, the home environment becomes the work environment. This will boost their morale and productivity.
- The company should conduct motivational sessions by collaborating with various speakers so that their motivation to work is maintained.

Increase Risk of Exposure

During the pandemic, men who worked in essential industries, such as healthcare, grocery stores, and public transportation, faced an increased risk of exposure to the virus. They are considered to bear the family's responsibility and fulfill all their needs. This pressurizes them to go and look for a job if they have lost their job in this pandemic and satisfy their family's needs, or else if they have a job, then they are obliged to work for the company in whatever way the company is treating them.

Post-pandemic measures:

- A family must give emotional support whenever men suffer from this fear, as men are told not to express their emotions. As a result, they suffer deep within and tolerate pain by staying quiet.
- The company should ensure that the policies being adopted are for the betterment of the employees' health.

Female

Research shows that women are disadvantaged relative to men in the workplace. Glass ceiling is one of the most prevalent invisible barriers in organizations that restricts them from climbing higher positions. According to McKinsey, women are 1.2% more likely than men to report acute difficulties with burden increases, workplace connectivity, and belonging, a healthy and secure workplace, performance reviews, and physical health. In the UK and the United States, women are 2,9 and 2,6 times more likely than men to disclose acute mental health issues. In emerging economies, conditions for women are far worse. Severe or moderate difficulties afflict more than sixty percent of women in emerging economies, often twice the rate of their counterparts in developed nations. Women in India, China, and Brazil are two to three times more likely than their counterparts in the United States and Europe to report facing severe mental health challenges. The WFH model has impacted women in three ways:

Lack of Work Visibility

Per the prevailing stereotypes concerning women, they are generally assumed to be less committed to their work than men. In addition, working remotely increases their risk of being less committed than their in-office colleagues since their hard work away from the office is less visible. This results in stress, anxiety, and other mental disorders which impact their well-being. According to McKinsey & Company, compared to one in five males, one in four women is contemplating abandoning the workforce or switching professions. While all women have been affected, women in higher level positions, working mothers, and Black women have faced the most significant obstacles. This disparity was most pronounced among parents of children under ten, where ten percentage points more women than males contemplated abandoning their jobs. Women whose husbands are also working and having children reported a more significant increase in time spent on domestic duties since the beginning of the pandemic.

Post-pandemic measures:

- Employers/ Raters should have a proper plan for how they will rate individually to all the employees. A proper plan will guide both parties in appraising the performance of women.
- Companies can facilitate networking opportunities that allow women employees to connect with other professionals in their field. This can include hosting networking events or sponsoring professional organizations that focus on women in the workplace.

Speaking Up

Women generally find it harder to have a say in the meetings than men and live continuously, fearing that they would be heard carefully and thoughtfully. The WFH model has increased this fear as women do not know when to raise a point. According to a Harvard Business Review, a survey was done on U.S. working adults, which observed that 45% of women leaders find it challenging to speak up in virtual meetings, and 20% of women said their colleagues ignored them during meetings.

Post-pandemic measures:

- Women should be encouraged to speak up by giving recognition because, from the organization's view, having a perspective from both genders encourages the innovation cycle of ideas. From the women's perspective, they will be more confident and feel pride in their suggestions.

- Talk shows like stand-up comedy, debate, and other related activities can be organized twice/thrice a month, where women are encouraged to speak about a topic. This will help women to express their emotions and will enable them to have the courage to speak in front of their peers.

Juggling Between Household and Work

With the WFH model, women with families cannot distinguish between their professional and personal lives. Women cannot concentrate on their work as previously they worked far away from home, which helps them to focus on their work and have proper time management. Thus, the model has made women's lives difficult instead of relaxing their lives. They are in a dilemma that results in mental health issues and impacts their mental well-being. Studies show that women with children are less productive than their in-office counterparts.

Post-pandemic measures:

- Women should maintain their daily schedules in consultation with their employers so that they can efficiently work from home at their convenience. However, that does not mean that the employers would need to keep meetings scheduled because they should not discriminate against other genders. This will also help the organizations in a way that their employees will be motivated.

LGBTQ+

While many straight and cisgender people also feel isolated during the COVID-19 crisis, the negative impact is felt more acutely by LGBTQ+ people, who may find themselves even more isolated in the absence of interactions with LGBTQ+ colleagues, their employee resource group, or other support structures.

In a pandemic, the data demonstrated unequivocally that LGBTQ+ employees across all geographies struggle with their jobs. Compared to heterosexual and cisgender employees, LGBTQ+ respondents are 1.4 times more likely to report acute difficulties with fair performance evaluations and burden increases. They face similar difficulties with a loss of workplace connectivity and belonging. It is perhaps not remarkable that two out of three LGBTQ+ employees report acute or moderate mental health issues.

Geographically, the differences between LGBTQ+ and heterosexual and cisgender employees are most pronounced in Asia. Nearly twice as many LGBTQ+ respondents as straight and cisgender ones cited severe difficulties with equitable performance reviews and burden increases.

According to a study, 9% of LGBT employees experienced discrimination in 2020, and 11% of LGBT employees of color reported being fired or hired in 2020.

Post-pandemic measures:

- The "Hire Transgender" (Contratá Trans) training program, which Manuel is implementing within the "Impacto Digital" non-profit organization, aims to assist companies in Argentina in instituting inclusive policies and providing more transgender people with respectable employment.
- Organizations should allocate resources to support LGBTQ+ individuals and communities, particularly those disproportionately affected by the pandemic. This can include funding for healthcare, mental health services, and social support programs.
- Organizations can create safe spaces for LGBTQ+ individuals to connect and access resources. This can include LGBTQ+ community centers, virtual support groups, and peer-to-peer mentorship programs.
- Organizations should ensure that their workplaces are inclusive and welcoming for LGBTQ+ employees. This can include training employees on LGBTQ+ issues, creating policies that protect against discrimination, and offering benefits that support LGBTQ+ employees and their families.
- Organizations can use their influence to advocate for LGBTQ+ rights locally, nationally, and internationally. This can include lobbying for policy changes, engaging in public education campaigns, and supporting LGBTQ+ organizations and initiatives.
- Organizations should make a conscious effort to promote diversity and inclusion in all aspects of their operations. This can include diversifying their leadership and staff, creating opportunities for marginalized groups, and promoting LGBTQ+ representation in their marketing and communications.

Race and Religion

Race and religion are the two discriminating factors still prevalent today in global companies and have become more relevant during the COVID-19 pandemic. It is seen that organizations are trying to prevent racial and religious discrimination in the workplace but face obstacles in doing so because of a certain number of people having an orthodox mindset.

Asian American (Kantamneni, 2020)

Since the spread of the COVID-19 pandemic, Asians and Asian Americans have been held responsible for the spread of the virus. This can be seen in Donald Trump's tweet, which referred to the virus as the "Chinese virus," As a result, Asian Americans have been subjected to increased discrimination and are frequently portrayed as disease carriers. During COVID-19, for instance, the Asian Pacific Policy and Planning Council launched a website for Asian Americans to report discrimination. In its first eight weeks, it received 1497 reports of workplace discrimination, of which 57% occurred in California and New York, two of the states hardest impacted by discrimination. Similarly, a recent survey of over 1,000 adults conducted by IPSOS on behalf of the Center for Public Integrity found that 30% of Americans accuse China or Chinese people of COVID-19, and 32% of respondents have witnessed someone blaming Asians for the pandemic. These findings indicate that Asians and Asian Americans are currently experiencing heightened discrimination in the United States. Human Rights Watch was informed by senior members of several Asian-American and other non-governmental organizations that many members of the Asian-American community with whom they work have experienced abuse or harassment or know someone who has. The Federal Bureau of Investigation (FBI) and other federal agencies have not taken any specific actions to address the rise in racist attacks and discrimination, although several state and local governments have set up hotlines and directed authorities to investigate cases of attacks or discrimination.

African American Women

Black women are disproportionately impacted by the challenging events of 2020. During the COVID-19 pandemic, they are more than twice as likely as women overall to identify the loss of a loved one as one of their most significant obstacles. Moreover, incidents of ethnic violence throughout the United States exact a significant emotional toll.

Work would ideally be a supportive environment for Black women during these national and global crises. Unfortunately, this is not the situation for many. Black women are less likely than other women to report that their manager has inquired about their burden or taken measures to accommodate their work-life requirements. Less than one-third of Black women report their manager has checked in on them or nurtured an inclusive culture on their team in the wake of recent racial violence. In addition, Black women are significantly less likely than White women to report having influential allies at work.

All of this affects African American women, and they are more prone than employees of other races to feel awkward discussing the impact of recent events on their community and their sorrow and loss with co-workers. They are also more hesitant to express their views on ethnic inequality. Comparatively, Black women feel more excluded at work. Also, they are less likely to say they can bring their whole selves to work than other employees.

Muslim Community

Compared to their non-Muslim counterparts, more Indian Muslims are unemployed and encounter discrimination in accessing salaried positions and income through self-employment. During the first quarter of the COVID-19 pandemic, unemployment among Muslims in rural areas increased by 17% relative to non-Muslims, bringing the rural Muslim unemployment rate to 31.4%. In 2019-20, only 15.6% of the urban Muslim population aged 15 and older had regular salaried employment, compared to roughly 23.3% of non-Muslims. In 2019-20, discrimination against Muslims in the labor market increased to 68.3%, contributing to their low employment rate. The report reveals that Muslims faced 59.3% discrimination in 2004-2005, indicating a 9% increase in discrimination over the past sixteen years. Non-Muslims in urban regions with a regular salary earn an average of 20,346 Indian rupees (approximately $255), 49% more than Muslims, who earn 13,672 Indian rupees (approximately $160). Self-employed non-Muslims earn an average of 15,878 Indian rupees (approximately $199), whereas self-employed Muslims earn an average of 11,423 Indian rupees (approximately $143) despite being overrepresented in urban self-employment. This implies that non-Muslims earn one-third more in self-employment than Muslims. The majority of urban India's Muslim population is self-employed compared to other communities, according to a report, primarily due to low-quality family professions and related difficulties in locating other employment opportunities. During COVID-19, Muslim employees may have faced challenges in observing religious practices, such as praying five times a day, during work hours, or while working from home because often, the employers are not aware of their religious practices, and they unintentionally hurt their feelings.

Post-pandemic measures:

- The first step for employers is recognizing existing injustices and declaring an intention to improve. Employers must back up words with actions, or they will remain hollow promises. They can achieve this by instigating productive and respectful conversations, forming employee resource groups, providing training on averting harassment and discrimination, and establishing secure channels for employees to discuss racial issues.
- In addition to conversations, employers can raise awareness by providing educational resources on the history of various ethnicities and the culture of prejudice. Most people are oblivious to racial injustice and their insensitive remarks to their BIPOC (Black, Indigenous, and People of Color) co-workers.
- The purpose of anti-racism training should never be to mark a box but to educate and inspire positive change. Training alone is insufficient to change people's perspectives. Due to implicit bias, racism exists in attitudes, cultural

messages, stereotypes, and beliefs. Companies can actively reduce bias through training and incorporating processes, policies, and expectations that contribute to developing a culture based on diversity and inclusion.

- The company should make sure that it respects every minority community, which includes Muslims. In order to make sure that the employers respect their religious practices when working in a WFH model, they could arrange online meets and give a time when Muslim employees can pray together at the same time. This helps reduce the number of breaks given to each employee differently as per their convenience, and this will be a community-building activity for the employees. When the organizations are following Hybrid Work Model or full-time work at the office, the employers should ensure that they provide for religious practices, such as a quiet prayer room or flexible scheduling.

CASE STUDIES

Below are case studies of two large organizations that promoted their employees' well-being by initiating various measures. These measures help both the employees and employers in improving their state of well-being in post-pandemic.

Google

As a result of security restrictions imposed by governments, remote work became increasingly commonplace. This is why Google had to develop new methods to assist their employees in achieving a healthy work-life balance and provide mental health support while they work remotely.

Google was the first major corporation to inform employees that they could work remotely after the lockdown was lifted. However, the company has also stated that the mental health of its employees posed the most significant challenge in the transition of most of its workforce to remote work. Consequently, during the COVID-19 pandemic, Google implemented various strategies to ensure its employees' health and safety. If they cannot report to work, it makes no sense to provide amenities such as gyms and swimming pools.

Reset Days

Reset days, also known as Google global days off, were another method Google used to ensure the well-being of its employees during the pandemic. During the pandemic, this was their way of providing employees with opportunities to restore their mental health. The recharge days enable workers to detach from their duties and prevent exhaustion.

Many people felt hurried and disoriented during the pandemic, so the extra paid days off allowed the employees to recover and calm down. Although restore days are well-intentioned, it would be challenging for employees to return to their regular office routines.

Even so, Google provides these days to simplify their employees' lives and boost their productivity.

Flexible Working Hours

Google also provided employees with flexible working hours and experiences. First, Google expanded its global presence by opening new offices and allowing employees to apply for remote work. This allows their employees to continue working from home even after others have returned to the office.

In addition, employees can work from a temporary location for up to four weeks per year. In addition, the company devised focus hours to minimize the number of internal meetings so that employees have more time to concentrate on projects.

Allowance of $1,000

After announcing that their employees would be working from home, Google announced that they would provide a $1,000 allowance to all their employees to make working from home more convenient. Those laboring outside the United States were granted $1000 or the equivalent in their local currency. This was the initial strategy they employed to promote employee health.

Remote employees must typically set up a home office with comfortable office furniture and equipment. Although employees have access to these amenities while working in an office, working from home is a distinct experience.

In light of this, and in an effort to promote their work culture, an allowance was provided to cover the costs of purchasing furniture and equipment, such as computers, to create a suitable working environment.

24/7 Counseling Over Video or Meeting a Counselor

Google provided mental health counseling before the pandemic and continued to do so after employees were required to work from home. To prevent the spread of the pandemic, they instead made video conference counseling available 24/7 to all employees or permitted them to meet with counselors in a safe and secure location.

Employees could request this session during the lockdown period whenever they felt constrained or anxious. Google is already aware that since the pandemic, workplace tension has become more severe than ever. Therefore, employees' empathy and compassion are crucial for achieving long-term growth objectives.

Resilience Training Videos

Google also provided videos for employee resilience training to promote their health and contentment. Lauren Whitt was recruited as a wellness manager and resilience lead to provide employees with this assistance.

The company expanded its existing programs and produced weekly brief training videos on resilience for its employees. The recordings were created by instructors, athletes, and psychologists, and it was alleged that one of their employees was continually viewing them. The company developed employee wellness initiatives out of concern for their mental health and well-being due to stay-at-home notice and isolation.

New Upcoming Plans

Although the COVID-19 pandemic is not entirely over, it is unlikely that conditions will return to how they were before the quarantine period. Instead, major corporations such as Google are preparing for the new norm. Thus, they can ensure employment fulfillment during the pandemic recovery period.

The first company to announce a hybrid workplace following a pandemic: Google was the first organization to retain the hybrid workplace plan after the pandemic restrictions were lifted in various locations.

The hybrid return-to-work plan initially stated that 60% of employees would work a few days per week in the office, 20% would work from home, and 20% would work in new office locations. According to research, more than half of employees desire a hybrid work schedule after the pandemic.

Collect information and make decisions based on what employees need

Google also organized pulse surveys and sent them to their employees. These surveys determine what employees think about their job-related roles, communication, and relationships. It is also to determine what employees need during and after COVID time and prepare for a new type of employee engagement in a hybrid workplace. Furthermore, the employees' health issues are also considered via these pulse surveys. The management team would know the overall health status of all employees and plan for immediate aid if needed.

Can the plans of google be used by other companies?

Since Google is one of the finest locations to work, it is unsurprising that other companies wish to imitate their strategy and offer employee wellness services during and after the pandemic.

Now that pandemic restrictions are being tightened, and the new normal has been established, many companies, including Google, have made hybrid workplaces and workplace safety the norm.

PAYU

PayU is a payment service provider for online merchants based in the Netherlands. The corporation was established in 2002 and has its main office in Hoofddorp. It permits online businesses to collect and process payments via payment methods that are compatible with web and mobile applications. PayU has launched various work-from-home initiatives to improve the well-being of their employees.

Maintaining Employee Engagement Online

PayU, like many other companies, utilizes Facebook's Workplace platform to facilitate employee collaboration and internal communication. Multiple new communities have been established on their Workplace platform to maintain employee engagement during COVID-19. Communities range from groups serving as information and resource centers to PayUneers sharing both positive and negative personal COVID-19 experiences. Whether venting frustration, sharing a new hobby, or encouraging and supporting one another to maintain a healthy lifestyle, the primary goal is to maintain a constant flow of communication that helps everyone feel more connected and less alone.

An illustration is the Global Coffee Corner group. Under #InItTogether, PayUneers can share their own experiences on highly intimate topics, in addition to other fascinating content. Here, we can discuss the difficulties of homeschooling, parenthood during the pandemic, and moments of loneliness and tedium and how to surmount them, giving this online community a sense of camaraderie and support.

Walking the Talk

At PayU, PayUneers take precedence. They recognize the significance of their employees' and their families' physical and mental health, safety, and well-being. Consequently, the introduction of the Employee Assistance Program was a crucial step towards "walking this talk."

The program provides PayUneers and their dependents with counseling, legal and financial consultation, and crisis intervention services. It is free, purely confidential, and can be utilized for emotional, financial, legal, or work-related issues. This professional service is also intended to assist employees in adjusting to the abrupt changes in their working lifestyles brought about by this year's confinement measures.

"Screen Time Off"

As a response to the abrupt changes brought on by COVID-19, short-term measures can be highly effective, but at PayU, employee wellness is an integral component of their long-term strategy. Employees are encouraged to collaborate with their manager to establish daily screen time off' – two hours per day during which all devices are turned off.

Using adapted PMS to improve employee productivity

The implementation of modifications to their performance management system has resulted in a significant rise in PayU employees' productivity. Quarterly objectives and critical results are broken down into 12-month targets. These short-term OKRs provide a distinct path for measuring productivity, which has a positive impact on employee motivation.

CONCLUSION

Workplace well-being has become an increasingly important topic during and after the pandemic. The pandemic has accentuated the significance of supporting employees' mental and physical health, as well as providing flexibility and remote work support. Employers can implement policies and programs that support employee mental health, promote work-life balance, provide access to resources and support, and encourage open communication and feedback to prioritize workplace wellness. Employers can increase employee satisfaction and retention by prioritizing workplace wellness and boosting overall productivity and business success.

REFERENCES

Bellotti, L., Zaniboni, S., Balducci, C., & Grote, G. (2021). Rapid Review on COVID-19, Work-Related Aspects, and Age Differences. *International Journal of Environmental Research and Public Health*, *18*(10), 5166. doi:10.3390/ijerph18105166 PMID:34068101

Hillebrandt, A., & Barclay, L. J. (2022). How COVID-19 can promote workplace cheating behavior via employee anxiety and self-interest–And how prosocial messages may overcome this effect. *Journal of Organizational Behavior*, *43*(5), 858–877. doi:10.1002/job.2612 PMID:35574191

Kantamneni, N. (2020). The impact of the COVID-19 pandemic on marginalized populations in the United States: A research agenda. *Journal of Vocational Behavior*, *119*, 103439. doi:10.1016/j.jvb.2020.103439 PMID:32390658

Lathabhavan, R. (2022). COVID-19 and mental health concerns among business owners: A cross-sectional study from India. *International Journal of Mental Health and Addiction*, 1–11. doi:10.100711469-022-00824-y PMID:35465028

Mann, S., & Chitranshi, J. (2021). Challenges Faced by Employees in Maintaining Work-Life Balance During Work from Home in Covid-19 Pandemic in India. *Nveo-Natural Volatiles & Essential Oils Journal*, 5504-5519.

Chapter 11
A Detailed Post-Pandemic Perspective of Indian Families

Om Sushil Lande
Vellore Institute of Technology, India

Tanvi Yogesh Daulatabadkar
Sophia College, India

ABSTRACT

Indian households have prioritised health and hygiene since the pandemic. Due to increased awareness of social distancing, handwashing, and mask use, families can protect themselves and their loved ones from infectious diseases. Because of this, people are making healthier choices and appreciating preventative healthcare more. Indian families and households have benefited from the pandemic, despite its many negative effects. Digital technology, family ties, gender equality, and health and hygiene will all benefit Indian society in the long run.

INTRODUCTION

The pandemic of COVID-19 has had a significant effect on the families of Indian residents. The following are some of the consequences:

The pandemic has caused a great deal of anxiety and stress among families due to the fear of getting infected with the virus, which is a concern regarding the health of the population. Concerns have been raised by families across the country about the well-being of their loved ones, particularly elderly relatives, and people with pre-existing medical conditions. Impact on the economy the pandemic has also had a significant impact on families' finances as a result of its spread. It has become

DOI: 10.4018/978-1-6684-7221-7.ch011

difficult for a lot of people to meet their fundamental requirements because they have either lost their jobs or seen a significant drop in their income. This has led to increased levels of stress and anxiety regarding financial matters.

Education has been impacted negatively as a result of the pandemic that has been going on in India. Students have been forced to turn to online education because a significant number of schools and colleges have been forced to close for extended periods of time. This has proven to be difficult for a lot of different households, particularly those that do not have access to modern technology or the internet.

Mental health: A great number of people in India have seen a decline in their mental health as a direct result of the pandemic. Isolation from one's peers, fear of the unknown, and uncertainty have all contributed to an uptick in the incidence of depression, anxiety, and other mental health conditions. As the pandemic has progressed, there has been a discernible increase in the number of instances of domestic violence. This can be attributed to the stress and tension caused by the pandemic, as well as the lockdowns and social distancing measures that have forced families to spend more time together as a result of the pandemic.

Figure 1. Percentage of people who say mental health is one of the top health problems facing people in their county today
(Ipsos Global Health Monitor)

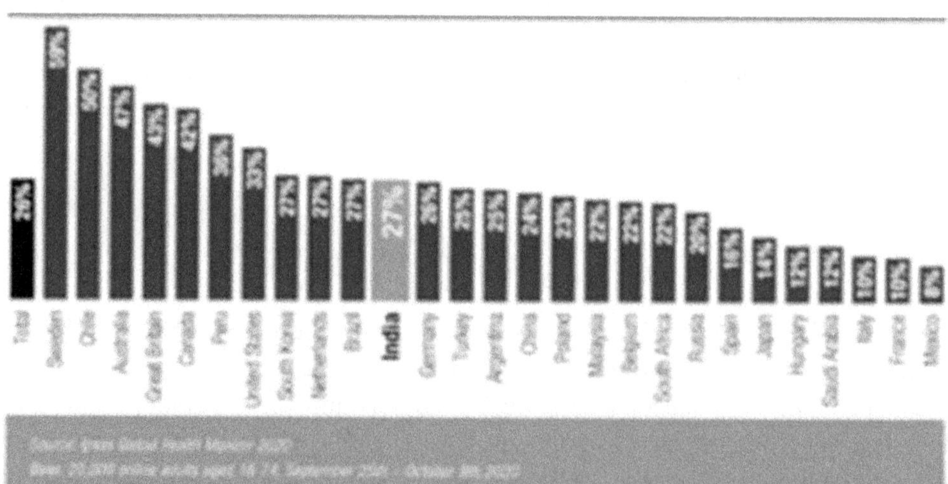

CHANGES IN PARENTING STYLES IN INDIA POST PANDEMIC

The widespread spread of the COVID-19 virus has had a significant impact on the parenting styles and mental health of Indian parents. As a result of the pandemic, families have been compelled to devote more attention and energy to parenting and to spend more time together as a unit. The following is a list of some changes in parenting practices that have been observed in India since the pandemic, along with an explanation of how these changes may affect mental health:

As a consequence of the pandemic, parents are now more aware of the significance of maintaining their mental health and are placing a greater emphasis on providing their children with emotional support and maintaining open lines of communication with them. This trend toward emotionally supportive parenting may be beneficial to children's mental health because it may encourage greater feelings of self-worth, self-assurance, and resiliency in children.

Spending more time online to further one's education: As a direct consequence of the prolonged closure of schools, parents have been forced to take a more active role in their children's educational pursuits, including providing frequent assistance with online learning. These days, parents have to deal with a greater amount of stress and work than ever before, which can be detrimental to their mental health.

As a direct result of the pandemic, parenting styles have evolved, with some parents adopting more poorly enforced or permissive approaches to the management of their children's behavior. It's possible that this is happening because parents are making an effort to create a less tense and more nurturing environment for their children in spite of the additional stress and uncertainty that the pandemic has brought about. However, research has shown that being overly permissive can lead to behavioral problems in children and has a detrimental effect not only on the mental health of children but also on the mental health of their parents.

As a consequence of schools closing and there being fewer opportunities for outdoor recreation, more time is being spent by children in front of screens. Because excessive time spent in front of screens has been associated with negative mental health outcomes in children, such as depression, anxiety, and poor sleep quality, parents and mental health professionals are concerned about this trend. (Strassberger, July 13, 2022)

In conclusion, the pandemic has had a significant impact on the parenting styles and mental health of Indians. While some of these shifts have been positive, such as placing a greater emphasis on emotional well-being, those around, such as increased screen time and altered methods of discipline, have led to concerns regarding the impact they will have on children's mental health in the future. It is essential for parents to be aware of these shifts and how they may impact the mental health of their children in order to cultivate positive outcomes for the entire family. This awareness can help parents foster positive outcomes that will benefit all members of the family. Additionally, they should look for support and resources whenever they are required to do so.

People's ways of living, working, and bringing up their children have been significantly impacted as a result of the pandemic. Because of the pandemic in India, many families have been forced to spend more time together, which has had a significant impact on the ways in which parents' parent and the bonding that occurs within families.

There has been a significant shift recently in parenting styles, with more of an emphasis being placed on providing emotional support and maintaining mental health. Everyone has been under a lot of stress as a result of the pandemic, and parents have had to make adjustments in order to meet the psychological requirements of their children. A growing number of parents are increasingly concerned about the mental well-being of their children and have made it a priority to spend quality time with their kids.

The pandemic has brought to light, once again, the significance of spending time together as a family in order to strengthen bonds. Due to the closure of schools and other activities, families have been forced to come up with ways to entertain themselves inside the home. This has resulted in an increase in game nights, movie nights, and other activities that bring the family closer together.

In addition to the movement toward an approach that is more malleable and adaptable, there has also been a shift in the styles of parenting that are used. As a result of the pandemic's impact on work and school schedules, parents have been forced to develop parenting strategies that are more flexible. As a result of having to juggle work and parenting responsibilities simultaneously, many people have developed a parenting style that is more collaborative.

Concerning the reorganization of priorities, the pandemic brought to light the significance of maintaining one's health and safety. Many parents are now more concerned about the health of their children and have taken measures to ensure their safety, such as adhering to stringent hygiene practices and limiting their children's social interactions. One example of this trend is that many parents are now vaccinating their children. This has also led to a greater appreciation for the straightforward joys that can be found in everyday life, such as spending time with one's family and engaging in activities that take place outside.

The pandemic has had a significant impact on parenting practices in India, resulting in a renewed emphasis on emotional support, family bonding, and the ability to adapt. It has also resulted in a reordering of values, with a greater emphasis placed on health and safety, as well as a recognition of the value of spending quality time with family members.

EFFECTS OF PANDEMIC AND LOCKDOWN ON CHILD PARENT RELATIONSHIP

The COVID-19 pandemic and the associated lockdowns have had significant effects on the relationships between children and their parents, particularly in regard to increased togetherness and increased reliance on digital technologies. These effects have had a significant impact on the relationships between children and their parents. The following are some of the outcomes that could occur:

Stronger reliance on various forms of digital technology children is currently more dependent on technology than they have ever been before as a direct result of educational institutions and other organizations moving their operations online. This can lead to a breakdown in communication between parents and children, an increase in the amount of time spent in front of screens, and possibly the development of a dependency on technological devices.

On the other hand, lockdowns have made it necessary for families to spend more time together, which can help to fortify the bonds that exist between parents and their children. Because of this increased proximity, there is a greater potential for the formation of interpersonal bonds, the communication of ideas, and the exchange of experiences.

When parents are working from home and attempting to juggle childcare and other responsibilities at the same time, the stress caused by the pandemic and the lockdowns can also create tension and strain in the family relationships. This is especially true when the pandemic was caused by the lockdowns. This can lead to increased conflict and stress, both of which can have a negative impact on the relationships between a child and their parents. This can have a negative impact on the relationships between a child and their parents.

It is possible that the traditional roles that are played within the family will shift as a result of the increased amount of time spent together by parents and children. This is because parents and children are spending more time together. For example, parents may find themselves with additional teaching and caregiving responsibilities, whereas children may find themselves with additional responsibilities around the house. Both groups of people may find themselves with additional responsibilities. This may present new opportunities for the cultivation of mutual respect and understanding; however, it may also present difficulties for some families. This may present new opportunities for the cultivation of mutual respect and understanding.

The pandemic and the subsequent lockdown have had a broad range of effects that have made things more difficult for the relationships that children have with their parents. There is a possibility of unfavorable outcomes, such as increased digital dependence and strain on relationships. On the other hand, there is also the possibility of favorable outcomes, such as increased togetherness and the possibility of new roles and responsibilities within the context of the family. Both of these outcomes are possible.

The COVID-19 pandemic and the subsequent lockdown measures have had a significant impact on the relationships that exist between children and their parents. It has also been shown that these measures cause both children and their parents to experience increased levels of stress and anxiety.

Children are more likely to experience anxiety and stress when their normal daily routines are disrupted, when they are socially isolated, and when they are uncertain about the future. The sudden shift to learning through remote means and the accompanying reduction in opportunities for social interaction can both contribute to feelings of annoyance and alienation. These changes may be followed by modifications in behavior, such as increased clinginess, mood swings, and acting out.

Because of the additional demands of homeschooling, working from home, and managing household responsibilities, parents may experience high levels of stress and anxiety in their daily lives. It is possible for parents to experience additional stress as a result of the financial pressures brought on by the pandemic, which may hinder their capacity to be present with their children and sensitive to their requirements.

In spite of these challenges, the pandemic and the lockdown have provided an opportunity for families to strengthen their bonds with one another. Relationships between parents and children can be improved by increasing the amount of time spent together, taking advantage of opportunities for shared activities, and developing a sense of shared purpose in the fight against the pandemic.

In order to mitigate the negative effects of the pandemic and the lockdown on the relationships between children and their parents, parents need to make self-care a priority, communicate openly and honestly with their children, and establish routines and structures to assist in the maintenance of a sense of normalcy. In this trying time, it can be helpful to seek assistance from community resources or mental health professionals in order to manage stress and anxiety.

It has been determined that one of the primary contributors to the negative effects that the pandemic has had on family relationships is the financial strain.

The negative effects of financial strain can surface in a number of different ways, including the loss of a job, a decrease in income, an increase in expenses, or an uncertainty regarding the future. These factors can have an effect on a parent's ability to provide for their children, which can lead to tension and conflict in the relationship between the parent and child.

Children may experience anxiety and stress as a result of the pandemic and the changes it has brought to their day-to-day lives as a result of the pandemic. It's possible that they are worried about their own health, the health of the people they care about, and the unknown future. These stresses can make things more difficult for the relationship that exists between a parent and their child.

In addition, as a result of the pandemic, people are staying inside their homes for longer periods of time, which can result in a deficiency of personal space and privacy for both children and their parents. This can result in increased tension and conflict within the household, placing additional strain on the already strained relationship between the parent and child.

The stress on the family's finances brought on by the pandemic and the subsequent lockdowns has had a significant influence on the overall nature of the parent-child relationship. It's possible that parents are having trouble providing for their children, and that those children are fretting about their own futures. It is essential for families to look for assistance and resources in order to alleviate the strain that is caused by financial difficulties and to foster healthy relationships between parents and children.

CALL ON DOMESTIC VIOLENCE DURING AND AFTER PANDEMIC

Even though it has been an issue for as long as anyone can remember in India, the COVID-19 pandemic has brought it more to the forefront. There has been a general rise in the number of reported incidents of domestic violence across the nation as a direct result of the restrictions and lockdowns imposed as a result of the pandemic.

Many abused women were compelled to spend the pandemic confined inside their homes with their abusers as a consequence of lockdowns and other restrictions on movement that were imposed during the pandemic. This led to an increase in cases of domestic violence, with many women reporting that their abusers became more violent and abusive during the pandemic. This led to an increase in the number of cases of domestic violence. Because of this, there was a rise in the total number of instances of violence in the home. In India in the year 2020, the National Commission for Women reported a fifty percent increase in the number of cases of domestic violence during the first week of the lockdown. This increase occurred during the first week of the lockdown.

When compared to the same time period in the previous year, the number of complaints of domestic violence in India increased by more than 200% during the COVID19 lockdowns. The National Commission on the Status of Women is the source of this information. The reports (Mitali Nikore in Irrational Economics, November 24, 2020,)This is due to the fact that a large number of incidents do not get reported due to the fear of social stigma and repercussions. (Cattaneo, 2021)

During the pandemic, gaining access to support services was one of the most significant challenges that victims of domestic violence needed to surmount in order to escape their abusive relationships. Many victims had a difficult time gaining access to justice as a result of the pandemic's effects, which included the closure of courts and a reduction in the number of police personnel.

On the other hand, the pandemic also provided a window of opportunity for a large number of organizations and individuals to step up and offer support to victims of domestic violence. This support came in the form of shelters, counselling services, and other forms of assistance. A number of programs that were initiated by NGOs and other types of organizations made it possible for victims of domestic violence to have access to counselling as well as other forms of support, including assistance in obtaining legal representation. A large number of organizations came to the aid of victims of domestic violence who were compelled to flee their homes and were subsequently forced to seek refuge elsewhere. These victims received assistance in the form of food, shelter, and other necessities. (Verma, 2021 Mar 10)

The strain of the economy, increased rates of unemployment, and close proximity to violent partners in intimate relationships are some of the factors that have contributed to the rise in domestic violence that has occurred during the pandemic. [The chain of causation] Because of the pandemic, services and support networks for victims of domestic violence have been disrupted, making it more difficult for these victims to get the assistance they need. The government of India has established hotlines and safe houses for people who have been affected by the issue of domestic violence as part of its efforts to address the issue. These measures were taken as part of the government's efforts to address the issue of domestic violence. However, additional actions are required to be taken in order to address the underlying issues that have led to this problem and to provide assistance to those who have survived it. This problem was brought about as a result of a combination of a number of factors. In addition to addressing the issue of gender inequality, this entails increasing the economic opportunities available to women, improving access to healthcare for survivors, and strengthening the legal system.

In conclusion, the pandemic brought on by COVID-19 has had a significant impact on the level of domestic violence that is prevalent in India. The fact that there was an increase in the number of cases brought attention to the fact that there ought to be more support services available for people who are the victims of domestic violence. [Cause and effect] The fact that there was an increase in the number of cases brought attention to the fact that there ought to be more.

BIRTH OF A BABY DURING AND AFTER PANDEMIC IN INDIAN FAMILIES

The COVID-19 pandemic has impacted India's healthcare access and delivery system, including maternal and newborn care. In terms of healthcare access, the following are some of the key factors to consider in Indian families when having a baby during and after the pandemic:

Care During Pregnancy: Pregnant women may have had difficulty accessing prenatal care due to limited mobility and the closure of some healthcare facilities during the pandemic. Furthermore, some women may have avoided going to hospitals or clinics for fear of contracting COVID-19. This could lead to delayed or inadequate prenatal care, affecting both the mother's and the baby's health.

Home births are uncommon in India, where hospital deliveries are still preferred. However, during the pandemic, some hospitals may have limited their services or refused to admit patients who did not have COVID-19 symptoms. This could lead to delivery delays or dangerous home births.

Postpartum Care: Following delivery, both the mother and the baby require postpartum care to ensure their health and well-being. During the pandemic, however, some healthcare facilities may have limited their postpartum services, leaving new mothers and babies without the necessary support and care. (Neurol., 2022)

Access to Vaccines: Vaccines are critical for protecting both mothers and babies from infectious diseases. Vaccine distribution, on the other hand, may have been disrupted or delayed during the pandemic. This could have an effect on the health and ability of newborns to fight infections. (Milstone, 2022)

To summarize, the COVID-19 pandemic has had a significant impact on pregnant women and newborns' access to healthcare in India. During these difficult times, healthcare providers must continue to provide safe and accessible care to ensure the health and well-being of mothers and their babies.

The pandemic has slowed the economy and resulted in job losses, putting many families in financial jeopardy. Childbirth can be costly, including medical costs, and many families may find it difficult to afford it during the pandemic. Furthermore, the pandemic has caused many businesses to close, resulting in income loss and additional financial stress.

During the pandemic, families may have been unable to provide the same level of support that they would have in normal circumstances. Due to social distancing and lockdown restrictions, family members may have been prevented from visiting and supporting new parents, which can be especially difficult for first-time parents. Furthermore, the pandemic has increased the prevalence of mental health issues such as anxiety and depression, which can have a negative impact on family support.

Despite these challenges, many Indian families have joined forces to assist one another during the pandemic. In some cases, extended family members have stepped in to provide financial assistance, while in others, virtual support has been provided through online platforms.

To summarize, the COVID-19 pandemic has had a significant financial and family support impact on Indian families during and after the birth of a child. Despite these significant obstacles, families have discovered ways to support one another and adapt to changing circumstances.

The pandemic has slowed the economy and resulted in job losses, putting many families in financial jeopardy. Childbirth can be costly, including medical costs, and many families may find it difficult to afford it during the pandemic. Furthermore, the pandemic has caused many businesses to close, resulting in income loss and additional financial stress.

During the pandemic, families may have been unable to provide the same level of support that they would have in normal circumstances. Due to social distancing and lockdown restrictions, family members may have been prevented from visiting and supporting new parents, which can be especially difficult for first-time parents. Furthermore, the pandemic has increased the prevalence of mental health issues such as anxiety and depression, which can have a negative impact on family support.

Despite these challenges, many Indian families have joined forces to assist one another during the pandemic. In some cases, extended family members have stepped in to provide financial assistance, while in others, virtual support has been provided through online platforms.

To summarize, the COVID-19 pandemic has had a significant financial and family support impact on Indian families during and after the birth of a child. Despite these significant obstacles, families have discovered ways to support one another and adapt to changing circumstances.

Figure 2. Hospitalized pregnant women with Covid-19 can have severe illness (CDC)

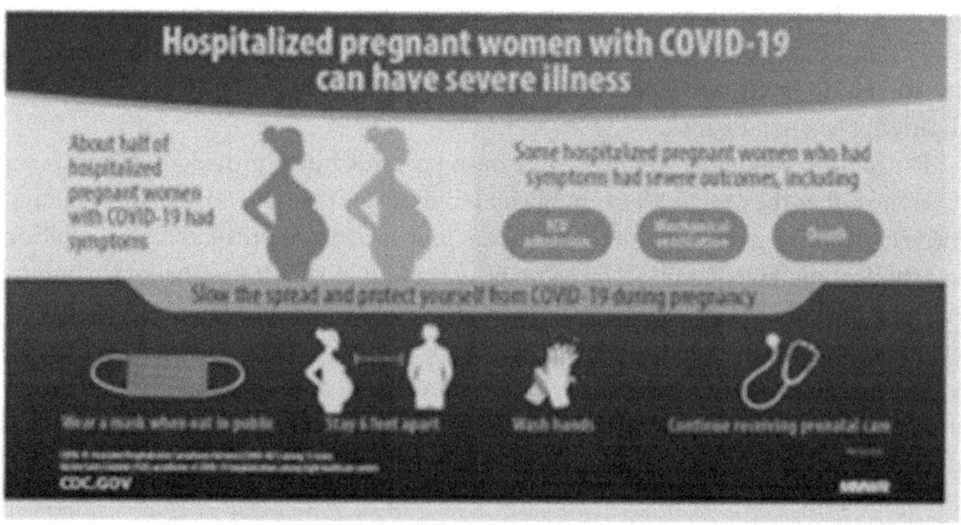

In Indian culture, a baby's birth is a significant event that is usually marked by various customs and rituals. The COVID-19 pandemic, on the other hand, has altered how people celebrate this holiday. Here are some cultural customs associated with childbirth in Indian families, as well as how the pandemic has affected them:

Ceremonial naming: The naming of a child is a significant event in Indian culture. It is usually held on the 11th or 12th day after the baby is born. Due to the pandemic, however, many families have chosen a virtual naming ceremony to avoid large crowds.

A baby shower is a traditional Indian event in which friends and family come together to celebrate the baby's impending arrival. To avoid infection during the pandemic, many families cancelled or postponed the baby shower.

In Indian culture, postnatal care is considered essential for both the mother and the baby. Traditionally, the mother and baby would spend a few weeks with extended family members after the birth. However, because of the pandemic, many families have chosen to isolate themselves and care for the mother and baby at home.

Breastfeeding is regarded as the best way to provide nutrition to a baby in Indian culture. However, due to the stress and anxiety of the pandemic, many mothers had difficulty breastfeeding during the pandemic.

Rituals and customs: In Indian culture, there are numerous traditions and customs associated with the birth of a baby. However, due to the pandemic, many families have had to modify or postpone these traditions in order to avoid large crowds and reduce the risk of infection.

To summarize, the COVID-19 pandemic has had a significant impact on the cultural customs of Indian families surrounding the birth of a child. While many families altered or postponed their customs to ensure their safety during the pandemic, the importance of these customs has not changed.

DEATH OF LOVED ONES DURING PANDEMIC

The COVID-19 pandemic has wreaked havoc in India, causing the deaths of a great number of people's loved ones. The emotional and psychological toll has been significant due to the fact that families and friends are mourning the loss of their loved ones while simultaneously coping with the ongoing effects of the pandemic.

Many people in India who have suffered the loss of loved ones as a result of the pandemic have experienced emotional anguish and distress, including feelings of depression, fear, and uncertainty regarding the future. They may also be dealing with feelings of guilt, regret, and helplessness, especially if they were unable to be with their loved ones during their final moments or properly say goodbye due to restrictions. This is especially likely if they were unable to be with their loved ones during their final moments.

In addition to the emotional toll, there may also be a significant financial toll associated with losing a loved one as a result of the pandemic. After the passing of a loved one, many families are forced to deal with unforeseen medical bills, funeral expenses, and other costs associated with the loss of a family member or friend. This burden can be especially difficult for families who have already been struggling financially as a result of the pandemic's effects on the economy or who have already lost their primary breadwinner as a result of the pandemic.

In general, the loss of loved ones as a result of the pandemic in India has been a traumatic experience for a great number of families and has had significant psychological and financial repercussions. It is imperative that individuals and communities come together to provide those who are grieving with support and resources that will assist them in coping with the aftermath of their loss.

A significant number of Indian families have been left broken by the pandemic as a result of the loss of loved ones. Unfortunately, discrimination and stigma have added to the anguish and suffering of those who have lost loved ones.

One of the problems is the unfavourable view that people have of COVID-19. Those who have been infected with the virus or have passed away as a result of its effects are frequently subjected to stigma and discrimination, which leaves their families feeling embarrassed and alone. This stigma can make it difficult for people to seek help or support when they are going through a difficult time in their lives. (Pappas)

Discrimination is an additional challenge that certain communities in India must overcome. Because of their caste or religion, members of marginalized communities, such as Dalits, have been denied access to cremation or burial grounds, making it difficult for their families to properly mourn the loss of a loved one.

In addition, there have been reports of communities turning their backs on families after a member of the family passed away as a result of COVID-19, which adds to the trauma and sense of isolation that those who have lost loved ones have experienced.

To provide a brief summary, for many Indian families, the loss of loved ones as a result of the pandemic has been a trying and traumatic experience, and discrimination and stigma have only added to their pain and suffering as a result. It is absolutely necessary to find solutions to these problems and offer assistance and resources to those who have been impacted by the pandemic. (Delhi: April month of grim anniversaries; families cope with loss of loved ones to Covid, May 1, 2022)

Particularly challenging for many families has been the administrative work involved in coping with the loss of a family member or close friend who passed away as a result of the pandemic.

The arrangement of funeral services, the acquisition of death certificates, the management of insurance claims, and the resolution of financial and legal matters pertaining to the deceased are some of the administrative challenges that may arise. It has been reported that there have been significant delays and difficulties in completing these tasks as a result of the overwhelming number of deaths that have occurred as a result of the pandemic.

Figure 3. How much higher are excess deaths than official covid deaths? (World Health Organization)

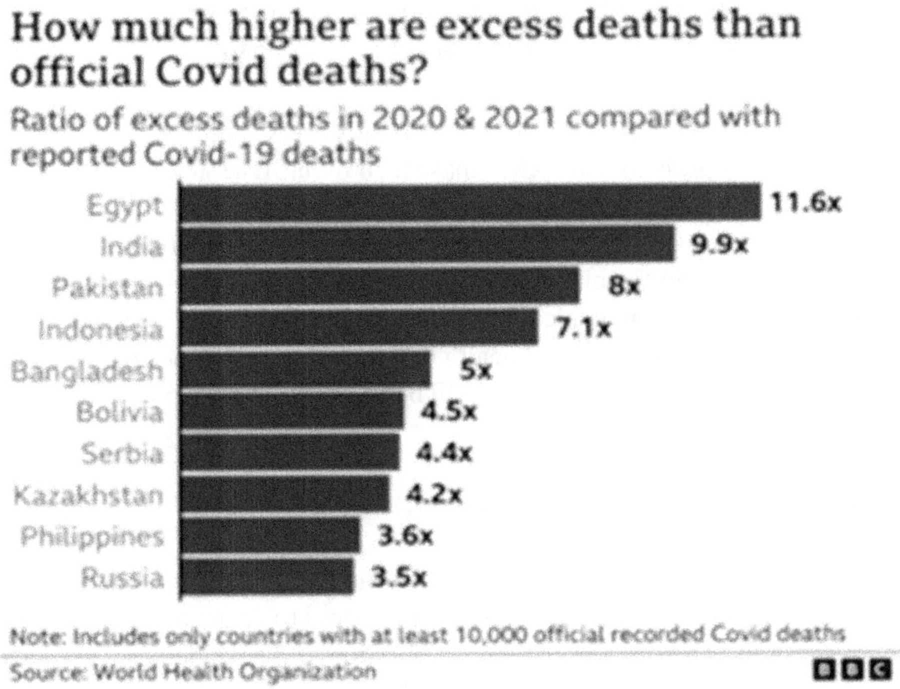

In addition to this, the burden has become even heavier as a result of a lack of clarity and consistency in the guidelines and procedures of the government. Families who are attempting to navigate the process can find themselves in a state of confusion and frustration due to the fact that different states have different regulations regarding how to handle deaths caused by COVID-19.

In addition, the emotional toll of losing a loved one during the pandemic has resulted in enormous stress and hardship for families. This is compounded by the administrative burden that has been placed on them. During this challenging time, many people have expressed the feeling that they have been abandoned by the government and that they are not receiving support from the healthcare system.

In conclusion, the administrative burden of managing the death of a loved one in India during the pandemic has been significant, and families have been forced to face a number of challenges and frustrations as a result. It will be necessary for government agencies and healthcare providers to improve their coordination and communication in order to meet the challenge of providing families with more effective support and direction during this challenging time.

COMPARISON BETWEEN DIFFERENT OCCUPATIONAL MEANS OF INDIAN SOCIETY DURING PANDEMIC

The COVID-19 pandemic has had an effect on virtually every aspect of life, including the ways in which people in Indian society make their living. One such aspect that has been affected is the ability of people to make a living. The pandemic has brought with it a variety of challenges for people working in a variety of occupations, and these challenges have had a significant impact on the mental health of the individuals who have been affected by the pandemic. In this essay, we will compare the effects that the pandemic had on people's mental health based on the various occupations that make up Indian society. This comparison will be based on how people experienced the pandemic.

Those Who Work in the Healthcare Industry

Workers in the healthcare industry have been at the forefront of the fight against COVID-19. As a consequence, they have been required to cope with a significant amount of stress and pressure throughout the duration of the pandemic. They have been working long hours, frequently in very difficult conditions, and have been exposed to the virus on a daily basis. This has put them in a position where they are more likely to contract the illness. Because of this, their likelihood of becoming ill has significantly increased. As a result of the detrimental effects on their mental health, a sizeable number of people who are employed in the healthcare industry have reported experiencing high levels of anxiety, depression, and burnout. Some people who work in healthcare have mentioned that they feel stigmatized due to their line of work, with some people avoiding them or treating them differently because of the perception that they pose a greater risk of carrying the virus. This perception is based on the fact that some people believe that healthcare workers are more likely to be infected with the virus.

Individuals Who Have Obtained Their Degrees in the Fields of Teaching and Education

In India, teaching and education professionals have also been significantly impacted by the pandemic in a significant way. This is because of the country's high population density. Due to the fact that schools and colleges have been closed for the majority of the year, educators, along with other education professionals, have been compelled to adapt to online teaching, which has proven to be a significant challenge for many of them. Because teaching online has required them to learn new technologies and methods of instruction, it has been difficult for them to connect with their students in the same way that they would in a traditional classroom setting. This has made it more difficult for them to connect with their students. In addition to that, it is required of them to become familiar with new forms of instruction as well as technological advancements. Many educators have mentioned that they are experiencing a great deal of stress and anxiety as a direct result of this, and many others have mentioned that they are also experiencing feelings of being overwhelmed and exhausted.

Office Staff and Professionals in a Commercial Establishment

Because of the pandemic, people who work in offices and professionals have also been required to learn new ways to perform their duties in order to continue doing their jobs. As a result of this, a great number of people have been compelled to work from home, which brings with it its own special set of difficulties. Working from home has required them to become familiar with new technologies and has made it difficult for them to strike a healthy balance between their personal and professional lives. Working from home has also required them to become familiar with emerging technologies. People have mentioned that they are putting in significantly more hours of work than they normally would if they were in an office setting. People have also mentioned that they have the impression that they are cut off from their co-workers and live in isolation. Because of this, the amount of stress and anxiety that office workers and professionals experience has significantly increased, which has led many of them to report feelings of mental exhaustion and burnout.

Those Who are Self-Employed in Addition to Those Who Own and Manage Small Businesses

Those who own and operate small businesses and entrepreneurial ventures have been hit particularly hard by the pandemic's negative effects due to the pandemic's disproportionately negative impact on them. Many business owners have been forced to close their establishments because of lockdowns and other restrictions that have been placed on the operations of businesses, and the income of many more business owners has suffered significantly as a direct result of these restrictions. Small business owners and entrepreneurs are experiencing a great deal of stress and anxiety as a result of this, with many of them fretting about their own personal financial futures in addition to the futures of their companies. Some of them have also reported feeling a sense of isolation and loneliness, which may be due to the fact that they frequently work by themselves and do not have the same level of social support as employees who work for larger organizations. This is as a result of the fact that they frequently perform their work independently.

CONCLUSION

To provide a brief summary, the COVID-19 pandemic has had a significant impact on the mental health of individuals working in a wide variety of occupational capacities within the Indian society. Workers in the healthcare industry, professionals in teaching and education, office workers and professionals, as well as owners and entrepreneurs of small businesses are all examples of groups that have been adversely affected by the pandemic. Members of all of these groups have reported high levels of stress, anxiety, and burnout as a result of the pandemic. It is essential for those in positions of authority and employers to acknowledge the mental health effects that the pandemic is having on a variety of occupational settings and to take measures to mitigate those effects, such as making mental health support services more accessible and fostering a better work-life balance. It is essential for businesses to acknowledge the effects the pandemic will have on their employees' mental health due to the various occupational risks. By doing so, we can help to ensure that people working in different occupational means in Indian society will be able to cope with the mental health impacts of the pandemic and emerge from it stronger and more resilient than they were before it. This will help to ensure that people working in different occupational means in Indian society will be able to cope with the mental health impacts of the pandemic.

IMPACT ON GAMERS DURING COVID 19

The COVID-19 pandemic has had a significant effect on the world, as evidenced by the fact that millions of people have been compelled to remain indoors and reduce the amount of time they spend engaging in social activities. As a direct consequence of this, there has been a sizable rise in the number of individuals who participate in online gaming for the purpose of engaging in social activity and obtaining their source of entertainment. Even though playing video games online can be a fun way to relieve some of the tension caused by the pandemic, there is a risk that it could have negative psychological effects if not managed properly. In this essay, I will discuss the psychological effects of playing video games online during the COVID-19 pandemic and provide some solutions to mitigate these effects. I will also provide some context for these effects.

The development of an addiction to playing video games online during the COVID-19 pandemic was one of the most significant psychological effects. Because people spend so much time at home, it can be simple for them to become disorganised and lose track of time while playing video games online for long periods of time. When a person is unable to play their addictive game, they may experience withdrawal symptoms, which include feelings of depression, anxiety, and irritability. Addiction can have a significant impact on a person's mental health. This addiction can also lead to other negative behaviours, such as neglecting responsibilities, losing interest in other activities, and isolating oneself from family and friends. [Case in point:] (Koo, 14 June 2021)

During the COVID-19 pandemic, playing video games online can have the additional psychological effect of isolating players from their peers. Although playing video games online can provide a sense of social interaction, it is not a replacement for actual face-to-face interaction with other people. People who spend an unhealthy amount of time playing video games online may neglect their relationships with family and friends, which can result in feelings of loneliness and isolation for those individuals. This may have a negative impact on mental health, potentially leading to feelings of depression, anxiety, and other unfavourable states of mind.

During the COVID-19 pandemic, one of the psychological effects of playing video games online is an increase in aggressive behaviour. The experience of playing video games online can be both competitive and intense, leading some players to become overly invested in the outcome of their matches. When things do not go their way, this can lead to feelings of anger and frustration, which can manifest in aggressive behaviour both online and in real life. This can lead to feelings of anger and frustration. This increased hostility can have a detrimental effect on mental health, potentially leading to feelings of depression, anxiety, and other unfavourable states of being. (MIshra, 2021)

During the COVID-19 pandemic, what are some solutions that can be implemented to reduce the potentially negative psychological effects of participating in online gaming? The first step in solving the problem is to set clear boundaries. It is essential for people to establish boundaries regarding the amount of time they spend playing video games online and to place a higher priority on engaging in other pursuits, such as going to the gym, spending time with their loved ones and friends, and pursuing their passions. This can help to prevent individuals from becoming addicted to online gaming and ensure that they maintain a healthy balance between gaming and other activities in their lives.

The second approach is to put an emphasis on actual, face-to-face human connection. Although playing video games online can provide a sense of social interaction, it is essential for individuals to place a priority on human connection that takes place in real life. Activities such as spending time with family and friends, engaging in outdoor pursuits, and joining social clubs or organisations can all fall under this category. The prevention of social isolation and the maintenance of healthy relationships can both be facilitated when individuals make genuine human connection a priority in their lives.

The third solution is to develop an awareness of the present moment. Individuals who practise mindfulness may find that it assists them in becoming more aware of their own thoughts and feelings, as well as in more effectively managing their own emotions. People who experience aggression or other negative emotions while playing video games online may find this aspect of the experience particularly beneficial. Individuals can learn to recognise when they are becoming overly invested in winning and can then take steps to manage their emotions in a healthier way by cultivating the skill of mindfulness and applying it to their lives.

In conclusion, participating in online gaming can be an entertaining and satisfying way to pass the time while the COVID-19 pandemic is in full swing. However, it is essential for individuals to be aware of the potential negative psychological effects of excessive participation in online gaming, including addiction, social isolation, and increased aggressiveness. Individuals can mitigate these effects and maintain a healthy balance between online gaming and other activities by setting boundaries, placing a priority on real-life human connection, and practising mindfulness.

EFFECTS ON SUICIDAL PRACTICES DURING COVID 19 PANDEMIC

The COVID-19 pandemic has had an effect on every facet of our lives, from our personal relationships to our professional and academic pursuits. Because of the pandemic and the subsequent lockdowns, there has been a significant rise in the number of people taking their own lives across the world. According to the World Health Organization (WHO), suicide is a global public health issue that results in approximately 800,000 deaths each year. Furthermore, it is the second leading cause of death among young adults between the ages of 15 and 29.

Both the pandemic itself and the subsequent lockdowns have had a significant influence on people's mental health. Anxiety, depression, and other mental illnesses have been on the rise in recent years, and social isolation, financial strain, and unpredictability about the future are all factors that have contributed to this trend. Individuals who were already struggling with mental health issues have seen their conditions worsen as a result of the pandemic, which has led to an increase in the number of individuals having suicidal thoughts and attempting suicide.

During the COVID-19 lockdown, engaging in suicidal behaviours can have a number of negative psychological effects, one of which is a sense of hopelessness. When individuals have access to socially isolating practises, they may experience feelings of disconnection from their loved ones and the world around them. It's possible that they have the impression that they have no control over their lives, which can lead to a sense of hopelessness and an increase in suicidal ideation.

The stigma that is attached to having a mental health problem is an additional negative effect that can be attributed to suicidal behaviours that occurred during the lockdown. Many people are embarrassed or ashamed to admit they have issues with their mental health because they are afraid of being labelled as weak or unstable if they seek help for those issues. This stigma can discourage individuals from seeking the assistance they require, which can then lead to an increase in suicidal behaviour among those affected.

Figure 4. Rise in suicide deaths, by profession and growth in major crimes in 2021 (Hindustan Times)

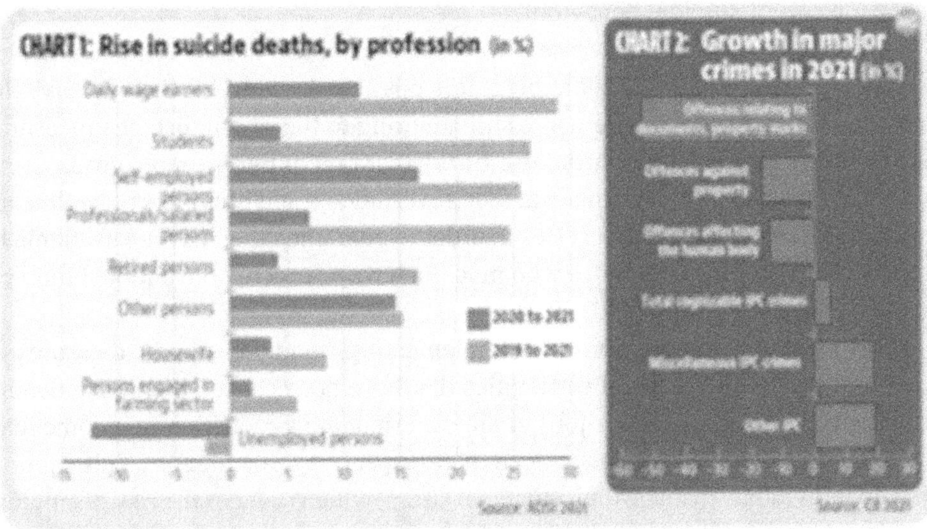

Many people have found themselves in difficult financial situations as a direct consequence of the COVID-19 pandemic, which is a factor that can contribute to suicidal behaviour. Increased stress and anxiety can worsen pre-existing mental health conditions and lead to suicidal behaviour. Loss of employment, reduced income, and financial insecurity are all factors that can lead to increased stress and anxiety.

Additionally, during the pandemic, individuals have had a more difficult time gaining access to mental health services, which has made it more challenging for them to receive the support they require. Face-to-face therapy sessions may not be possible when social distancing measures are in place, and individuals may not have access to virtual therapy either. Those who are struggling with mental health issues and do not have access to mental health services may exhibit an increase in suicidal behaviour as a result of this lack of access.

During the COVID-19 lockdown, there is a variety of options available to address the potentially damaging psychological effects that may be caused by suicidal behaviours.

To begin, it is necessary to educate more people about the significance of maintaining mental health and to eliminate the shame that is often connected to mental health problems. Education campaigns, public awareness programmes, and community outreach initiatives are some examples of activities that can be undertaken to accomplish this goal. These efforts can encourage individuals who are struggling with mental health issues to seek help for those issues, which can reduce the risk of suicidal behaviour.

Second, it is absolutely necessary to broaden people's access to mental health services while the pandemic is ongoing. It is possible for individuals to receive the necessary support they require while still adhering to the social distance measures that they have chosen through the use of teletherapy, online support groups, and virtual therapy sessions. It is important for governments and providers of healthcare to make investments in these services in order to guarantee that they are available to all individuals, particularly those who may not have access to conventional therapy services. (Suzannah Stuijfzand, 2020)

Thirdly, there is the possibility of implementing financial support measures in order to alleviate the financial difficulties that have been caused by the pandemic. Individuals who have lost their jobs or are experiencing a reduction in income may be eligible for financial assistance from their respective governments. This support can help individuals manage their financial stress, which reduces the risk of suicidal behaviour being exhibited by the individual.

The importance of social connections to one's physical and mental well-being is the subject of our fourth point. While individuals should be encouraged to adhere to social distance measures, it is also important to encourage them to maintain social connections. It is possible for individuals to feel less isolated and more connected to others through the use of virtual social events, online support groups, and phone calls with friends and family.

Last but not least, individuals who may be experiencing suicidal thoughts should have access to suicide prevention hotlines as well as crisis centres. People who are going through difficult times can receive immediate support and assistance from these resources, which will lower their risk of taking their own life.

To summarize, the COVID-19 pandemic and the subsequent lockdowns have had a significant influence on people's mental health.

CHANGES IN POLITICAL IDEOLOGIES DURING COVID 19 PANDEMIC IN INDIAN FAMILIES

During the period of the lockdown, the COVID-19 pandemic has had a significant influence on the political ideologies that are held within Indian families. During the course of this article, we are going to discuss the various political ideologies that have surfaced inside of Indian households as a result of the pandemic.

First and foremost, the pandemic has highlighted the significance of public health and the role that the government plays in ensuring the wellbeing of its citizens. In response to the government's slow response to the pandemic, many families have voiced their support for a healthcare system that is both stronger and more efficient, and they have criticised the government for its response. This has resulted in an increase in discontentment with the party in power and a demand for elected officials to be held to a higher standard of accountability.

Second, the pandemic has brought attention to the problem of economic inequality in India. [Citation needed] During the lockdown, many families have had a difficult time making ends meet, and as a result, there has been a growing demand for the government to provide more assistance in the form of social welfare programmes and economic support. As a consequence of this, there has been a rise in support for leftist ideologies, such as those that advocate for increased social welfare programmes and greater government intervention in the economy.

On the other hand, there are households that have voiced their approval of right-wing ideologies, which place an emphasis on personal accountability and the unfettered operation of free markets. They believe that individuals should be responsible for their own financial well-being, and that the government should stay out of the economy entirely. They have levelled criticism at the government for enacting stringent lockdown measures that have had a detrimental effect on both the economy as a whole and small businesses specifically.

In addition to this, the pandemic has brought the problem of communalism in India to the forefront of public discourse. There has been an increase in hate crimes committed against minority communities, and many families have voiced their support for inclusivity and secularism in response to this trend. As a result, there has been a rise in the number of people demanding that the government implement stringent measures to combat have crimes and to foster communal harmony. (Bieber, 27 April 2020)

In addition to this, the pandemic has also sparked a discussion regarding the issues of surveillance and privacy. Many families have voiced their concerns about the possibility of the government abusing its power as a result of the use of technology by the government to track cases of COVID-19 and to enforce lockdown procedures. Because of this, there has been a growing call for increased transparency and accountability in the surveillance methods used by the government.

The COVID-19 pandemic has, in conclusion, had a significant impact on the political ideologies held within Indian families. It has shed light on the significance of issues such as economic inequality, communalism, privacy, and surveillance. the importance of public health. It will be fascinating to observe how these ideologies develop and how they affect the political climate of India as the country continues to struggle with the pandemic.

The pandemic caused by COVID-19 was a global crisis that had never been seen before and had an effect on every facet of life. There have been some positive effects on Indian families and households, despite the fact that the pandemic has had many negative repercussions, such as the loss of life, the disruption of the economy, and the social isolation of people.

The pandemic has had some positive effects on Indian families, one of the most significant of which has been a strengthening of the bonds that bind the family together. Because of the lockdowns and the restrictions placed on travel, families have been compelled to spend more time together, which has led to improved communication, increased mutual understanding, and increased support for one another. It has also been possible for families to rediscover the joys of simple activities such as gardening, cooking, and playing games together, all of which have contributed to a greater sense of togetherness and shared experiences.

Additionally, as a result of the pandemic, traditional gender roles in Indian households have begun to shift. Because there are now so many people working from home and children attending online classes, both men and women are required to share the responsibilities of caring for their families and running their households. This has led to a more equitable distribution of household chores and childcare, which is a positive step towards gender equality in the country. This has been a step in the right direction towards achieving gender equality in the country.

One of the things that has turned out to be a positive consequence of the pandemic is the increased use of digital technology in Indian homes. Families are now able to maintain connections with their loved ones and gain access to necessary goods and services without having to leave the comfort of their own homes thanks to the proliferation of online communication tools and e-commerce platforms. The elderly and other vulnerable members of the community, who might have been isolated in the absence of this initiative, have benefited tremendously from it.

As a result of the pandemic, there has been an increased emphasis placed on health and hygiene in Indian households. Families have been able to take preventative measures to protect themselves and the people they care about from infectious diseases thanks to the increased awareness of the significance of social distancing, washing one's hands frequently, and wearing masks. Because of this, there has been a shift towards making more choices that are beneficial to one's health and a greater appreciation for preventative healthcare.

In conclusion, although the pandemic has had a great deal of unfavourable effects, it has also had some positive effects on the families and households in India. The adoption of digital technology, the strengthening of family ties, the shift towards more equitable gender roles, and the increased emphasis on health and hygiene are all positive developments that will have long-term benefits for Indian society as a whole.

REFERENCES

Bieber, F. (2020). *Global Nationalism in Times of the COVID-19 Pandemic.* Cambridge Press.

Cattaneo, C. (2021). *Violence against women in the Covid-19 pandemic: A review of the literature and a call for shared strategies to tackle health and social emergencies.* Elsevier.

Koo, J. W. (2021). *Problematic Use of Alcohol and Online Gaming as Coping Strategies During the COVID-19 Pandemic: A Mini Review.* Frontiers..

Milstone, A. (2022). *COVID in Babies and Kids: Symptoms and Prevention.* Johns Hopkins Medicine.

Mishra, S. (2021). *Effects of video games on children.* IEA.

Mitali, N. (November 24, 2020,). *With Covid-19, comes the "Shadow Pandemic": How the surge of domestic violence gripped India's women in 2020.* TOI.

Neurol., S. P. (2022). *The COVID-19 Pandemic and Pregnancy: Impact on Mothers and Newborns.* NIH.

Pappas, S. (n.d.). *Helping patients cope with COVID-19* . APA.

Strassberger, M. (2022). *"We Live One Day at a Time": Families' Stories from the Early Months of the COVID-19 Pandemic.*

Stuijfzand, S. C. D.-T. (2020). *Psychological impact of an epidemic/pandemic on the mental health of healthcare professionals: a rapid review.* Commonwealth Fund.

Verma, A. K. (2021). *Understanding Domestic Violence in India During COVID-19: a Routine Activity Approach.* NIH.

Compilation of References

Acuti Martellucci, C., Flacco, M. E., Cappadona, R., Bravi, F., Mantovani, L., & Manzoli, L. (2020). SARS-CoV-2 pandemic: An overview. *Advances in Biological Regulation*, *77*, 100736. doi:10.1016/j.jbior.2020.100736 PMID:32773099

Ahmad, I., Donia, M. B. L., Khan, A., & Waris, M. (2018). Do as I say, and do as I do? The mediating role of psychological contract fulfillment in the relationship between ethical leadership and employee extra-role performance. *Personnel Review*.

al Khajeh, E. H. (2018). Impact of leadership styles on organizational performance. *Journal of Human Resources Management Research*, *2018*, 1–10. doi:10.5171/2018.687849

Al-Ali, N. (2020). Covid-19 and feminism in the Global South: Challenges, initiatives and dilemmas. *European Journal of Women's Studies*, *27*(4), 333–347. doi:10.1177/1350506820943617

Almeida, M., Shrestha, A. D., Stojanac, D., & Miller, L. J. (2020). The impact of the COVID-19 pandemic on women's mental health. *Archives of Women's Mental Health*, *23*(6), 741–748. doi:10.100700737-020-01092-2 PMID:33263142

Alradhawi, M., Shubber, N., Sheppard, J., & Ali, Y. (2020). Effects of the COVID-19 pandemic on mental well-being amongst individuals in society. In International Journal of Surgery, 78, 147–148. Elsevier Ltd. doi:10.1016/j.ijsu.2020.04.070

Al-Shargie, F., & GOH, C. M. (2019). Cognitive Enhancement Techniques and Their Impact on Performance Improvements. *RE:view*.

American Psychological Association (APA). (2020). *Stress in America, 2020: A National Mental Health Crisis*. APA. https://www.apa.org/news/press/releases/stress/2020/report-october

Andersson, G., Carlbring, P., & Furmark, T.SOFIE Research Group. (2012). Therapist experience and knowledge acquisition in internet-delivered CBT for social anxiety disorder: A randomized controlled trial. *PLoS One*, *7*(5), e37411. doi:10.1371/journal.pone.0037411 PMID:22649526

Andersson, G., Carlbring, P., & Hadjistavropoulos, H. D. (2017). Internet-based cognitive behavior therapy. In S. G. Hofmann & G. J. G. Asmundson (Eds.), *The science of cognitive behavioral therapy* (pp. 531–549). Academic Press. doi:10.1016/B978-0-12-803457-6.00021-0

Antoinette Bargagliotti, L. (2012). Work engagement in nursing: A concept analysis. *Journal of Advanced Nursing*, *68*(6), 1414–1428. doi:10.1111/j.1365-2648.2011.05859.x PMID:22044047

Ardelt, M., & Grunwald, S. (2018). The importance of self-reflection and awareness for human development in hard times. *Research in Human Development*, *15*(3–4), 187–199. doi:10.1080/15427609.2018.1489098

Arghode, V., Lathan, A., Alagaraja, M., Rajaram, K., & McLean, G. N. (2021). Empathic organizational culture and leadership: Conceptualizing the framework. *European Journal of Training and Development*.

Armour, R. (2020). *Transformational versus servant leadership: Their role on employee eudaimonic well-being*.

Arya, J., & Mali, P. C. (2021). Influence of COVID-19 Pandemic on Assisted Reproductive Techniques Services in India: A Review. *Journal of Life Science*, *7*(6S), 9S–16S.

ASRM. (2020). *ASRM Patient Management and Clinical Recommendations During the Coronavirus (COVID-19) Pandemic*. ASRM. https://www.asrm.org/news-and-publications/news-and-research/announcements/update-1-released-to-the-asrm-patient-management-and-clinical-recommendations-during-the-coronavirus-covid-19-pandemic/

Athota, V. S. (2021). Lessons from failures. In *Mind over Matter and Artificial Intelligence* (pp. 49–56). Springer. doi:10.1007/978-981-16-0482-9_5

Avey, J. B., Avolio, B. J., & Luthans, F. (2011). Experimentally analyzing the impact of leader positivity on follower positivity and performance. *The Leadership Quarterly*, *22*(2), 282–294. doi:10.1016/j.leaqua.2011.02.004

Avey, J. B., Reichard, R. J., Luthans, F., & Mhatre, K. H. (2011). Meta-analysis of the impact of positive psychological capital on employee attitudes, behaviors, and performance. *Human Resource Development Quarterly*, *22*(2), 127–152. doi:10.1002/hrdq.20070

Avolio, B. J., & Gardner, W. L. (2005). Authentic leadership development: Getting to the root of positive forms of leadership. *The Leadership Quarterly*, *16*(3), 315–338. doi:10.1016/j.leaqua.2005.03.001

Ayala, E. E., Omorodion, A. M., Nmecha, D., Winseman, J. S., & Mason, H. R. C. (2017). What do medical students do for self-care? A student-centered approach to well-being. *Teaching and Learning in Medicine*, *29*(3), 237–246. doi:10.1080/10401334.2016.1271334 PMID:28632007

Azim Premji University. (2021). State of Working India 2021. Azim Premji University.

Baec, C.-Y., & Shin, J.-G. (2017). The Differential Effects of Transformational Leadership and Organizational Justice on Work Engagement: The Mediating Role of Psychological Contract Breach. *The Journal of The Korea Contents Association*, *17*(1), 299–336. doi:10.5392/JKCA.2017.17.01.299

Bakioğlu, F., Korkmaz, O., & Ercan, H. (2020). Fear of COVID-19 and Positivity: Mediating Role of Intolerance of Uncertainty, Depression, Anxiety, and Stress. *International Journal of Mental Health and Addiction, 1*. doi:10.100711469-020-00331-y PMID:32837421

Bakker, D., Kazantzis, N., Rickwood, D., & Rickard, N. (2016). Mental Health Smartphone Apps: Review and Evidence-Based Recommendations for Future Developments. *JMIR Mental Health, 3*(1), e7. doi:10.2196/mental.4984 PMID:26932350

Bakouri, M., & Staerklé, C. (2015). Coping with structural disadvantage: Overcoming negative effects of perceived barriers through bonding identities. *British Journal of Social Psychology, 54*(4), 648–670. doi:10.1111/bjso.12102 PMID:25683895

Baluku, M. M., Kikooma, J. F., & Kibanja, G. M. (2016). Psychological capital and the startup capital–entrepreneurial success relationship. *Journal of Small Business and Entrepreneurship, 28*(1), 27–54. doi:10.1080/08276331.2015.1132512

Barrot, J. S., Llenares, I. I., & del Rosario, L. S. (2021). Students' online learning challenges during the pandemic and how they cope with them: The case of the Philippines. *Education and Information Technologies, 26*(6), 7321–7338. doi:10.100710639-021-10589-x PMID:34075300

Basadur, M. (2004). Leading others to think innovatively together: Creative leadership. *The Leadership Quarterly, 15*(1), 103–121. doi:10.1016/j.leaqua.2003.12.007

Basak, S. (2021). Factors affecting work-life balance of women in Bangladesh: A study during COVID-19 pandemic. *Canadian Journal of Business and Information Studies, 3*(3), 38–48.

Baumel, A., Muench, F., Edan, S., & Kane, J. M. (2019). Objective User Engagement With Mental Health Apps: Systematic Search and Panel-Based Usage Analysis. *Journal of Medical Internet Research, 21*(9), e14567. doi:10.2196/14567 PMID:31573916

Bau, N., Khanna, G., Low, C., Shah, M., Sharmin, S., & Voena, A. (2022). Women's Well-being During a Pandemic and its Containment. *Journal of Development Economics, 156*, 102839. doi:10.1016/j.jdeveco.2022.102839 PMID:35221446

Beck, J. S., & Beck, A. (2011). *Cognitive behavior therapy*. Guilford Publication.

Becker, S., Miron-Shatz, T., Schumacher, N., Krocza, J., Diamantidis, C., & Albrecht, U. V. (2014). mHealth 2.0: Experiences, Possibilities, and Perspectives. *JMIR mHealth and uHealth, 2*(2), e24. doi:10.2196/mhealth.3328 PMID:25099752

Bellotti, L., Zaniboni, S., Balducci, C., & Grote, G. (2021). Rapid Review on COVID-19, Work-Related Aspects, and Age Differences. *International Journal of Environmental Research and Public Health, 18*(10), 5166. doi:10.3390/ijerph18105166 PMID:34068101

Ben-Kimhy, R., Youngster, M., Medina-Artom, T. R., Avraham, S., Gat, I., Marom Haham, L., Hourvitz, A., & Kedem, A. (2020). Fertility patients under COVID-19: Attitudes, perceptions, and psychological reactions. *Human Reproduction (Oxford, England), 2020*(12), 2774–2783. doi:10.1093/humrep/deaa248 PMID:32877507

Ben-Zeev, D. (2017). CrossCheck: Integrating self-report, behavioral sensing, and smartphone use to identify digital indicators of psychotic relapse. *Psychiatric rehabilitation journal, 40*(3) 266.

Bernerth, J. B., & Hirschfeld, R. R. (2016). The subjective well-being of group leaders as explained by the quality of leader–member exchange. *The Leadership Quarterly, 27*(4), 697–710. doi:10.1016/j.leaqua.2016.04.003

Berry, H. L. (2021). Enabling a youth-and mental health-sensitive greener post-pandemic recovery. *World Psychiatry; Official Journal of the World Psychiatric Association (WPA), 20*(2), 152–153. doi:10.1002/wps.20843 PMID:34002504

Berry, N., Lobban, F., Emsley, R., & Bucci, S. (2016). Acceptability of Interventions Delivered Online and Through Mobile Phones for People Who Experience Severe Mental Health Problems: A Systematic Review. *Journal of Medical Internet Research, 18*(5), e121. doi:10.2196/jmir.5250 PMID:27245693

Bhatnagar, J. (2007). Talent management strategy of employee engagement in Indian ITES employees: Key to retention. *Employee Relations, 29*(6), 640–663. doi:10.1108/01425450710826122

Bhosale, J. (2020). *Prices of agricultural commodities drop 20% post COVID-19 outbreak.* Economic Times. https://economictimes.indiatimes.com/news/economy/agriculture/prices-of-agricultural-commodities-drop-20-post-covid-19-outbreak/articleshow/74705537.cms

Bieber, F. (2020). *Global Nationalism in Times of the COVID-19 Pandemic.* Cambridge Press.

Bjørnnes, A. K. (2022). *Fighting the waves; COVID-19 family life interference in a neurodevelopmental disorder-caregiver.*

Blanchard, K., & Hodges, P. (2008). *Lead like Jesus: Lessons from the greatest leadership role model of all time.* Thomas Nelson.

Boivin, J., Harrison, C., Mathur, R., Burns, G., Pericleous-Smith, A., & Gameiro, S. (2020). Patient experiences of fertility clinic closure during the COVID-19 pandemic: Appraisals, coping and emotions. *Human Reproduction (Oxford, England), 35*(11), 2556–2566. doi:10.1093/humrep/deaa218 PMID:32761248

Bonanno, G. A., Galea, S., Bucciarelli, A., & Vlahov, D. (2007). What Predicts Psychological Resilience After Disaster? The Role of Demographics, Resources, and Life Stress. *Journal of Consulting and Clinical Psychology, 75*(5), 671–682. doi:10.1037/0022-006X.75.5.671 PMID:17907849

Bondade, S., Iyengar, R. S., Shivakumar, B. K., & Karthik, K. N. (2018). Intimate Partner Violence and Psychiatric Comorbidity in Infertile Women - A Cross-Sectional Hospital Based Study. *Indian Journal of Psychological Medicine, 40*(6), 540–546. doi:10.4103/IJPSYM.IJPSYM_158_18 PMID:30533950

Boniol, M., McIsaac, M., Xu, L., Wuliji, T., Diallo, K., & Campbell, J. (2019). *Gender equity in the health workforce: analysis of 104 countries.* World Health Organization.

Britt, T. W., Shen, W., Sinclair, R. R., Grossman, M. R., & Klieger, D. M. (2016). How much do we really know about employee resilience? *Industrial and Organizational Psychology: Perspectives on Science and Practice*, *9*(2), 378–404. doi:10.1017/iop.2015.107

Broad, J. D., & Luthans, F. (2017). Leading and developing health and safety through collective psychological capital. *Leading to Occupational Health and Safety: How Leadership Behaviours Impact Organizational Safety and Well-Being, 255.*

Brown, K. W., & Ryan, R. M. (2003). The Benefits of Being Present: Mindfulness and Its Role in Psychological Well-Being. In Journal of Personality and Social Psychology, 84(4). doi:10.1037/0022-3514.84.4.822

Brown, K. W., & Ryan, R. M. (2004). Fostering healthy self-regulation from within and without: A self-determination theory perspective. *Positive Psychology in Practice*, 105–124.

Brown, K. W., & Ryan, R. M. (2015). A self-determination theory perspective on fostering healthy self-regulation from within and without. *Positive Psychology in Practice: Promoting Human Flourishing in Work, Health, Education, and Everyday Life*, *2*, 139–157. doi:10.1002/9781118996874.ch9

Brown, K. W., Ryan, R. M., & Creswell, J. D. (2007). Mindfulness: Theoretical foundations and evidence for its salutary effects. *Psychological Inquiry*, *18*(4), 211–237. doi:10.1080/10478400701598298

Burleson, W. (2005). Developing creativity, motivation, and self-actualization with learning systems. *International Journal of Human-Computer Studies*, *63*(4), 436–451. doi:10.1016/j.ijhcs.2005.04.007

Burnett, D., Masi, A., Diaz, A. M., Rizzo, R., Lin, P. I., & Eapen, V. (2021). Distress levels of parents of children with neurodevelopmental disorders during the COVID-19 pandemic: A comparison between Italy and Australia. *International Journal of Environmental Research and Public Health*, *18*(21), 11066. doi:10.3390/ijerph182111066 PMID:34769585

Caldwell, C., & Hasan, Z. (2016). Covenantal leadership and the psychological contract: Moral insights for the modern leader. *Journal of Management Development*, *35*(10), 1302–1312. doi:10.1108/JMD-02-2016-0027

Cao, J. (2022). Exploration on the Cultivation of Undergraduates' Entrepreneurship Ability from the Perspective of Mental Health Education. *Journal of Healthcare Engineering*, *2022*, 1–9. doi:10.1155/2022/9668220 PMID:35340258

Cao, L. B., Hao, Q., Liu, Y., Sun, Q., Wu, B., Chen, L., & Yan, L. (2021). Anxiety Level During the Second Localized COVID-19 Pandemic Among Quarantined Infertile Women: A Cross-Sectional Survey in China. *Frontiers in Psychiatry*, *12*, 647483. doi:10.3389/fpsyt.2021.647483 PMID:34366908

Carey, M. A. (2016). Comment: Concerns in the Analysis of Focus Group Data. *Sage, 5*(4), 487–495. doi:10.1177/104973239500500409

Carleton, E. L., Barling, J., & Trivisonno, M. (2018). Leaders' trait mindfulness and transformational leadership: The mediating roles of leaders' positive affect and leadership self-efficacy. *Canadian Journal of Behavioural Science/Revue Canadienne Des Sciences Du Comportement, 50*(3), 185.

Caron, J., Asselin, H., Beaudoin, J.-M., & Muresanu, D. (2019). Promoting perceived insider status of indigenous employees: A review within the psychological contract framework. *Cross Cultural & Strategic Management, 26*(4), 609–638. doi:10.1108/CCSM-02-2019-0031

Carp-Veliscu, A., Mehedintu, C., Frincu, F., Bratila, E., Rasu, S., Iordache, I., Bordea, A., et al. (2022). The Effects of SARS-CoV-2 Infection on Female Fertility: A Review of the Literature. *International Journal of Environmental Research and Public Health, 19*(2), 984. MDPI AG. doi:10.3390/ijerph19020984

Cathy, A. (2003). *The consortium for entrepreneurship education.*

Cattaneo, C. (2021). *Violence against women in the Covid-19 pandemic: A review of the literature and a call for shared strategies to tackle health and social emergencies.* Elsevier.

Chakraborty, K., & Chatterjee, M. (2020). Psychological impact of COVID-19 pandemic on general population in West Bengal: A cross-sectional study. *Indian Journal of Psychiatry, 62*(3), 266–272. doi:10.4103/psychiatry.IndianJPsychiatry_276_20 PMID:32773869

Charoensukmongkol, P., & Suthatorn, P. (2018). Salespeople's trait mindfulness and emotional exhaustion: The mediating roles of optimism, resilience, and self-efficacy. *International Journal of Services. Economics and Management, 9*(2), 125–142.

Chatterji, S., McDougal, L., Johns, N., Ghule, M., Rao, N., & Raj, A. (2021). COVID-19-Related Financial Hardship, Job Loss, and Mental Health Symptoms: Findings from a Cross-Sectional Study in a Rural Agrarian Community in India. *International Journal of Environmental Research and Public Health, 18*(16), 8647. doi:10.3390/ijerph18168647 PMID:34444394

Chemers, M. M., Watson, C. B., & May, S. T. (2000). Dispositional affect and leadership effectiveness: A comparison of self-esteem, optimism, and efficacy. *Personality and Social Psychology Bulletin, 26*(3), 267–277. doi:10.1177/0146167200265001

Chen, Z. X., Tsui, A. S., & Zhong, L. (2008). Reactions to psychological contract breach: A dual perspective. *Journal of Organizational Behavior: The International Journal of Industrial. Occupational and Organizational Psychology and Behavior, 29*(5), 527–548. doi:10.1002/job.481

Christie, H., Hiscox, L. V., Halligan, S. L., & Creswell, C. (2022). Examining harmful impacts of the COVID-19 pandemic and school closures on parents and carers in the United Kingdom: A rapid review. *JCPP Advances, 2*(3). doi:10.1002/jcv2.12095 PMID:36247724

Chully, A. A., Jose, J., & Luthufi, M. (2022). Authentic leadership in a pandemic world: an exploratory study in the Indian context. *Journal of Management Development.*

Cito, G., Pizzarelli, C., Zurkirch, V., Basile, V., Ruggiero, M., & Coccia, M. E. (2022). Parenthood in Infertile Couples Attending Assisted Reproductive Technologies (ARTs) Centers: What Has Changed During the COVID-19 Pandemic? *Journal of Reproduction & Infertility*, *23*(2), 120–127. doi:10.18502/jri.v23i2.8997 PMID:36043127

Copeland, W. E., McGinnis, E., Bai, Y., Adams, Z., Nardone, H., Devadanam, V., Rettew, J., & Hudziak, J. J. (2021). Impact of COVID-19 pandemic on college student mental health and wellness. *Journal of the American Academy of Child and Adolescent Psychiatry*, *60*(1), 134–141. doi:10.1016/j.jaac.2020.08.466 PMID:33091568

Cornaglia, F., Crivellaro, E., & McNally, S. (2015). Mental health and education decisions. *Labour Economics*, *33*, 1–12. doi:10.1016/j.labeco.2015.01.005

Cousins, S. (2020). COVID-19 has "devastating" effect on women and girls. *Lancet*, *396*(10247), 301–302. doi:10.1016/S0140-6736(20)31679-2 PMID:32738942

Coyle, D., Doherty, G., & Sharry, J. (2012). An evaluation of a solution focused computer game in adolescent interventions. *Clinical Child Psychology and Psychiatry*, *17*(2), 225–242. doi:10.1177/1359104511417264 PMID:19515752

Cullinane, N., & Dundon, T. (2006). The psychological contract: A critical review. *International Journal of Management Reviews*, *8*(2), 113–129. doi:10.1111/j.1468-2370.2006.00123.x

Currie, G., Finlay, B., Seth, A., Roth, C., Elsabbagh, M., Hudon, A., Hunt, M., Jodoin, S., Lach, L., Lencucha, R., Nicholas, D. B., Shakako, K., & Zwicker, J. (2022). Mental health challenges during COVID-19: Perspectives from parents with children with neurodevelopmental disabilities. *International Journal of Qualitative Studies on Health and Well-being*, *17*(1), 2136090. doi:10.1080/17482631.2022.2136090 PMID:36309898

Dalal, P. K., Roy, D., Choudhary, P., Kar, S. K., & Tripathi, A. (2020). Emerging mental health issues during the COVID-19 pandemic: An Indian perspective. *Indian Journal of Psychiatry*, *62*(9, Suppl 3), S354. doi:10.4103/psychiatry.IndianJPsychiatry_372_20 PMID:33227050

Dalgard, O. S., Dowrick, C., Lehtinen, V., Vazquez-Barquero, J. L., Casey, P., Wilkinson, G., Ayuso-Mateos, J. L., Page, H., & Dunn, G. (2006). Negative life events, social support and gender difference in depression. *Social Psychiatry and Psychiatric Epidemiology*, *41*(6), 444–451. doi:10.1007/s00127-006-0051-5

Darr, W., & Johns, G. (2008). Work strain, health, and absenteeism: A meta-analysis. *Journal of Occupational Health Psychology*, *13*(4), 293–318. doi:10.1037/a0012639 PMID:18837626

Das, N. (2020). Psychiatrist in post-COVID-19 era – Are we prepared? *Asian Journal of Psychiatry*, *51*, 102082. doi:10.1016/j.ajp.2020.102082 PMID:32283513

Dawson, L., Einboden, R., McCloughen, A., & Buus, N. (2021). Beyond polyphony: Open Dialogue in a Women's Shelter in Australia as a possibility for supporting violence-informed practice. *Journal of Marital and Family Therapy*, *47*(1), 136–149. doi:10.1111/jmft.12457 PMID:32990992 de Bruin, E. I., Zijlstra, B. J. H., & Bögels, S. M. (2014). The meaning of mindfulness in children and adolescents: Further validation of the Child and Adolescent Mindfulness Measure (CAMM) in two independent samples from the Netherlands. *Mindfulness*, *5*(4), 422–430.

de Haldevang, M. (2020). *Coronavirus has crippled global protest movements*. Quartz.

De', R., Pandey, N., & Pal, A. (2020). Impact of digital surge during Covid-19 pandemic: A viewpoint on research and practice. *International Journal of Information Management*, *55*, 102171. doi:10.1016/j.ijinfomgt.2020.102171 PMID:32836633

Demir, A., & Budur, T. (2019). Roles of leadership styles in corporate social responsibility to non-governmental organizations (NGOs). *International Journal of Social Sciences & Educational Studies*, *5*(4), 174–183.

Denis, A. V., Shah, J. S., Penzia, A. S., Domar, A. D., & Toth, T. L. (2020). Infertility remains a top stressor despite the COVID-19 pandemic. *Reproductive Biomedicine Online*, *41*(3), 425–427. doi:10.1016/j.rbmo.2020.05.015 PMID:32600945

Densten, I. L. (2005). The relationship between visioning behaviours of leaders and follower burnout. *British Journal of Management*, *16*(2), 105–118. doi:10.1111/j.1467-8551.2005.00428.x

Depp, C. A., Perivoliotis, D., Holden, J., Dorr, J., & Granholm, E. L. (2019). Single-Session Mobile-Augmented Intervention in Serious Mental Illness: A Three-Arm Randomized Controlled Trial. *Schizophrenia Bulletin*, *45*(4), 752–762. doi:10.1093chbulby135 PMID:30281086

Dimas, I. D., Rebelo, T., Lourenço, P. R., & Pessoa, C. I. P. (2018). Bouncing back from setbacks: On the mediating role of team resilience in the relationship between transformational leadership and team effectiveness. *The Journal of Psychology*, *152*(6), 358–372. doi:10.1080/00223980.2018.1465022 PMID:30089085

Dominiak, M., Kaczmarek-Majer, K., Antosik-Wójcińska, A. Z., Opara, K. R., Olwert, A., Radziszewska, W., Hryniewicz, O., Święcicki, Ł., Wojnar, M., & Mierzejewski, P. (2022). Behavioral and Self-reported Data Collected From Smartphones for the Assessment of Depressive and Manic Symptoms in Patients With Bipolar Disorder: Prospective Observational Study. *Journal of Medical Internet Research*, *24*(1), e28647. doi:10.2196/28647 PMID:34874015

Donker, T., Petrie, K., Proudfoot, J., Clarke, J., Birch, M. R., & Christensen, H. (2013). Smartphones for smarter delivery of mental health programs: A systematic review. *Journal of Medical Internet Research*, *15*(11), e247. doi:10.2196/jmir.2791 PMID:24240579

Dsouza, D. D., Quadros, S., Hyderabadwala, Z. J., & Mamun, M. A. (2020). Aggregated COVID-19 suicide incidences in India: Fear of COVID-19 infection is the prominent causative factor. *Psychiatry Research*, *290*, 113145. doi:10.1016/j.psychres.2020.113145 PMID:32544650

du Plessis, Y., & Barkhuizen, N. (2012). Psychological capital, a requisite for organisational performance in South Africa. *Suid-Afrikaanse Tydskrif vir Ekonomiese en Bestuurswetenskappe*, *15*(1), 16–30. doi:10.4102ajems.v15i1.122

Duan, L., & Zhu, G. (2020). Psychological interventions for people affected by the COVID-19 epidemic. *The Lancet. Psychiatry*, *7*(4), 300–302. doi:10.1016/S2215-0366(20)30073-0 PMID:32085840

Elkholy, H., Tawfik, F., Ibrahim, I., Salah El-din, W., Sabry, M., Mohammed, S., Hamza, M., Alaa, M., Fawzy, A. Z., Ashmawy, R., Sayed, M., & Omar, A. N. (2021). Mental health of frontline healthcare workers exposed to COVID-19 in Egypt: A call for action. *The International Journal of Social Psychiatry*, *67*(5), 522–531. doi:10.1177/0020764020960192 PMID:32972298

Engzell, P., Frey, A., & Verhagen, M. D. (2021). Learning loss due to school closures during the COVID-19 pandemic. *Proceedings of the National Academy of Sciences of the United States of America*, *118*(17), e2022376118. Advance online publication. doi:10.1073/pnas.2022376118 PMID:33827987

Epitropaki, O. (2013). A multi-level investigation of psychological contract breach and organizational identification through the lens of perceived organizational membership: Testing a moderated–mediated model. *Journal of Organizational Behavior*, *34*(1), 65–86. doi:10.1002/job.1793

Erkkilä, K. (2000). Entrepreneurial education: mapping the debates in the United States, the United Kingdom, and Finland. Taylor & Francis.

Erkutlu, H., & Chafra, J. (2013). Effects of trust and psychological contract violation on authentic leadership and organizational deviance. *Management Research Review*, *36*(9), 828–848. doi:10.1108/MRR-06-2012-0136

Etzelmueller, A., Vis, C., Karyotaki, E., Baumeister, H., Titov, N., Berking, M., Cuijpers, P., Riper, H., & Ebert, D. D. (2020). Effects of Internet-Based Cognitive Behavioral Therapy in Routine Care for Adults in Treatment for Depression and Anxiety: Systematic Review and Meta-Analysis. *Journal of Medical Internet Research*, *22*(8), e18100. doi:10.2196/18100 PMID:32865497

Evans, T. M., Bira, L., Gastelum, J. B., Weiss, L. T., & Vanderford, N. L. (2018). Evidence for a mental health crisis in graduate education. *Nature Biotechnology*, *36*(3), 282–284. doi:10.1038/nbt.4089 PMID:29509732

Fehr, E., & Falk, A. (2002). Psychological foundations of incentives. *European Economic Review*, *46*(4–5), 687–724. doi:10.1016/S0014-2921(01)00208-2

Firth, J., Cotter, J., Torous, J., Bucci, S., Firth, J. A., & Yung, A. R. (2016). Mobile Phone Ownership and Endorsement of "mHealth" AmongPeople With Psychosis: A Meta-analysis of Cross-sectional Studies. *Schizophrenia Bulletin*, *42*(2), 448–455. doi:10.1093chbulbv132 PMID:26400871

Firth, J., Torous, J., Nicholas, J., Carney, R., Pratap, A., Rosenbaum, S., & Sarris, J. (2017). The efficacy of smartphone-based mental health interventions for depressive symptoms: A meta-analysis of randomized controlled trials. *World Psychiatry; Official Journal of the World Psychiatric Association (WPA)*, *16*(3), 287–298. doi:10.1002/wps.20472 PMID:28941113

Firth, J., Torous, J., Nicholas, J., Carney, R., Rosenbaum, S., & Sarris, J. (2017). Can smartphone mental health interventions reduce symptoms of anxiety? A meta-analysis of randomized controlled trials. *Journal of Affective Disorders*, *218*, 15–22. doi:10.1016/j.jad.2017.04.046 PMID:28456072

Fontanesi, L., Marchetti, D., Mazza, C., Di Giandomenico, S., Roma, P., & Verrocchio, M. C. (2020). The effect of the COVID-19 lockdown on parents: A call to adopt urgent measures. *Psychological Trauma: Theory, Research, Practice, and Policy*, *12*(S1), S79–S81. doi:10.1037/tra0000672 PMID:32525382

Frasquilho, D., Matos, M. G., Salonna, F., Guerreiro, D., Storti, C. C., Gaspar, T., & Caldas-De-Almeida, J. M. (2016). Mental health outcomes in times of economic recession: A systematic literature review. *BMC Public Health*, *16*(1), 115. Advance online publication. doi:10.118612889-016-2720-y PMID:26847554

Frederiksen, Y., Farver-Vestergaard, I., Skovgård, N. G., Ingerslev, H. J., & Zachariae, R. (2015). Efficacy of psychosocial interventions for psychological and pregnancy outcomes in infertile women and men: A systematic review and meta-analysis. *BMJ Open*, *5*(1), e006592. doi:10.1136/bmjopen-2014-006592 PMID:25631310

Frisch, M. B. (2005). *Quality of life therapy: Applying a life satisfaction approach to positive psychology and cognitive therapy*. John Wiley & Sons.

Ganjiwale, D., Ganjiwale, J., Sharma, B., & Mishra, B. (2016). Quality of life and coping strategies of caregivers of children with physical and mental disabilities. *Journal of Family Medicine and Primary Care*, *5*(2), 343. doi:10.4103/2249-4863.192360 PMID:27843839

Gao, J., Zheng, P., Jia, Y., Chen, H., Mao, Y., Chen, S., Wang, Y., Fu, H., & Dai, J. (2020). Mental health problems and social media exposure during COVID-19 outbreak. *PLoS One*, *15*(4), e0231924. doi:10.1371/journal.pone.0231924 PMID:32298385

Gillespie-Smith, K., McConachie, D., Ballantyne, C., Auyeung, B., & Goodall, K. (2021). The impact of COVID-19 restrictions on psychological distress in family caregivers of children with neurodevelopmental disability in the UK. *Journal of Autism and Developmental Disorders*. doi:10.100710803-021-05132-3 PMID:34286392

Giota, K., & Kleftaras, G. (2014). Mental Health Apps: Innovations, Risks and Ethical Considerations. *E-Health Telecommunication Systems and Networks*, *3*(03), 19–23. doi:10.4236/etsn.2014.33003

Gleicher, N. (2020). The COVID-19 pandemic through the eyes of an NYC fertility center: A unique learning experience with often unexpected results. *Reproductive Biology and Endocrinology*, *18*(1), 1–16. doi:10.118612958-020-00663-3 PMID:33148264

Glomb, T. M., Duffy, M. K., Bono, J. E., & Yang, T. (2011). Mindfulness at work. In *Research in personnel and human resources management*. Emerald Group Publishing Limited. doi:10.1108/S0742-7301(2011)0000030005

Gonzalez, M. (2012). *Mindful leadership: The 9 ways to self-awareness, transforming yourself, and inspiring others*. John Wiley & Sons.

Gonzalez, T., De la Rubia, M. A., Hincz, K. P., Comas-Lopez, M., Subirats, L., Fort, S., & Sacha, G. M. (2020). Influence of COVID-19 confinement on students' performance in higher education. *PLoS One*, *15*(10), e0239490. doi:10.1371/journal.pone.0239490 PMID:33035228

Goodwin, V. L., Wofford, J. C., & Whittington, J. L. (2001). A theoretical and empirical extension to the transformational leadership construct. *Journal of Organizational Behavior: The International Journal of Industrial. Occupational and Organizational Psychology and Behavior*, *22*(7), 759–774. doi:10.1002/job.111

Gordon, J. L., & Balsom, A. A. (2020). The psychological impact of fertility treatment suspensions during the COVID-19 pandemic. *PLoS One*, *15*(9), e0239253. doi:10.1371/journal.pone.0239253 PMID:32946479

Graham, D. W. (2021). Heraclitus. In E. N. Zalta (Ed.), Stanford Encyclopedia of Philosophy (Summer2021 ed.). Metaphysics Research Lab, Stanford University.

Grant, J. E., Drummond, L., Nicholson, T. R., Fagan, H., Baldwin, D. S., Fineberg, N. A., & Chamberlain, S. R. (2022). Obsessive-compulsive symptoms and the Covid-19 pandemic: A rapid scoping review. *Neuroscience and Biobehavioral Reviews*, *132*, 1086–1098. doi:10.1016/j.neubiorev.2021.10.039 PMID:34740755

Greene, P. G., & Brush, C. (2014a). *Teaching entrepreneurship: A practice-based approach*. Edward Elgar Publishing.

Griggs, R. A. (2014). Coverage of the Stanford Prison Experiment in Introductory Psychology Textbooks. *Teaching of Psychology*, *41*(3), 195–203. doi:10.1177/0098628314537968

Grist, R., Porter, J., & Stallard, P. (2017). Mental Health Mobile Apps for Preadolescents and Adolescents: A Systematic Review. *Journal of Medical Internet Research*, *19*(5), e176. doi:10.2196/jmir.7332 PMID:28546138

Grossmeier, J., Fabius, R., Flynn, J. P., Noeldner, S. P., Fabius, D., Goetzel, R. Z., & Anderson, D. R. (2016). Linking workplace health promotion best practices and organizational financial performance. *Journal of Occupational and Environmental Medicine*, *58*(1), 16–23. doi:10.1097/JOM.0000000000000631 PMID:26716844

Grover, S., Dua, D., Sahoo, S., Mehra, A., Nehra, R., & Chakrabarti, S. (2020). Why all COVID-19 hospitals should have mental health professionals: The importance of mental health in a worldwide crisis! *Asian Journal of Psychiatry*, *51*, 102147. doi:10.1016/j.ajp.2020.102147 PMID:32473537

Grumi, S., Provenzi, L., Gardani, A., Aramini, V., Dargenio, E., Naboni, C., Vacchini, V., & Borgatti, R. (2020). Rehabilitation services lockdown during the COVID-19 emergency: The mental health response of caregivers of children with neurodevelopmental disabilities. *Disability and Rehabilitation*, *43*(1), 27–32. doi:10.1080/09638288.2020.1842520 PMID:33167738

Gualano, M. R., Bert, F., Martorana, M., Voglino, G., Andriolo, V., Thomas, R., & Siliquini, R. (2020). How digital health technologies facilitate the implementation of the principles of person-centered healthcare. *Health Policy and Technology*, *9*(4), 361–367.

Gumley, A., Bradstreet, S., Ainsworth, J., Allan, S., Alvarez-Jimenez, M., Beattie, L., Bell, I., Birchwood, M., Briggs, A., Bucci, S., Castagnini, E., Clark, A., Cotton, S. M., Engel, L., French, P., Lederman, R., Lewis, S., Machin, M., MacLennan, G., ... Gleeson, J. (2020). Early Signs Monitoring to Prevent Relapse in Psychosis and Promote Well-Being, Engagement, and Recovery: Protocol for a Feasibility Cluster Randomized Controlled Trial Harnessing Mobile Phone Technology Blended With Peer Support. *JMIR Research Protocols*, *9*(1), e15058. doi:10.2196/15058 PMID:31917372

Gupta, M., Jaiswal, P., Bansiwal, R., Sethi, A., Vanamail, P., Kachhawa, G., Kumari, R., & Mahey, R. (2021). Anxieties and apprehensions among women waiting for fertility treatments during the COVID-19 pandemic. *International Journal of Gynaecology and Obstetrics: the Official Organ of the International Federation of Gynaecology and Obstetrics*, *152*(3), 441–443. doi:10.1002/ijgo.13468 PMID:33155288

Gupta, V., & Singh, S. (2014). Psychological capital as a mediator of the relationship between leadership and creative performance behaviors: Empirical evidence from the Indian R&D sector. *International Journal of Human Resource Management*, *25*(10), 1373–1394. doi:10.1080/09585192.2013.870311

Hager, E., Odetokun, I. A., 2, I. D., Bolarinwa Id, O., Zainab, A., Okechukwu, O., & Al-Mustaphaid, A. I. (2020). *Knowledge, attitude, and perceptions towards the 2019 Coronavirus Pandemic: A bi-national survey in Africa*. PLOS Research. doi:10.1371/journal.pone.0236918

Hägg, G., & Gabrielsson, J. (2019). A systematic literature review of the evolution of pedagogy in entrepreneurial education research. *International Journal of Entrepreneurial Behaviour & Research*, *26*(5), 829–861. doi:10.1108/IJEBR-04-2018-0272

Halder, A. (2021). Salient Yet Silent: A Need for Strategies to Cope with Violence against Infertile Women during COVID-19 Pandemic. *EC Gynaecology*, *10*, 29–31.

Harari, G. M., Lane, N. D., Wang, R., Crosier, B. S., Campbell, A. T., & Gosling, S. D.(2016, November). Using Smartphones to Collect Behavioral Data in Psychological Science: Opportunities, Practical Considerations, and Challenges. *Perspectives on Psychological Science*, *11*(6), 838–854. doi:10.1177/1745691616650285 PMID:27899727

Hasan, S. D., Osborn, D. R., & Chauhan, A. (2022). Myths About COVID Vaccines. *KnowsWhy.com*. https://www.knowswhy.com/myths-about-covid-vaccines/

Hasan, S. M., Khan, E. A., & Nabi, M. N. U. (2017). Entrepreneurial education at university level and entrepreneurship development. *Education + Training*, *59*(7/8), 888–906. doi:10.1108/ET-01-2016-0020

Haslam, S. A., O'Brien, A., Jetten, J., Vormedal, K., & Penna, S. (2005). Taking the strain: Social identity, social support, and the experience of stress. *British Journal of Social Psychology, 44*(3), 355–370. doi:10.1348/014466605X37468 PMID:16238844

Hassed, C., & Chambers, R. (2014). *Mindful Learning: Reduce stress and improve brain performance for effective learning* (Vol. 3). Exisle Publishing.

Hatak, I. (2021). *Mental health in entrepreneurship. In the World Encyclopaedia of Entrepreneurship*. Edward Elgar Publishing.

Henderson, D. J., Wayne, S. J., Shore, L. M., Bommer, W. H., & Tetrick, L. E. (2008). Leader—member exchange, differentiation, and psychological contract fulfillment: A multilevel examination. *The Journal of Applied Psychology, 93*(6), 1208–1219. doi:10.1037/a0012678 PMID:19025243

Henson, P., Wisniewski, H., Hollis, C., Keshavan, M., & Torous, J. (2019). Digital mental health apps and the therapeutic alliance: Initial review. *BJPsych Open, 5*(1), e15. doi:10.1192/bjo.2018.86 PMID:30762511

Herholdt, M. D. (2008). An integrated approach to human existence with spirituality as a facet of wellness: spirituality and well-being. *Practical Theology in South Africa= Praktiese Teologie in Suid-Afrika, 23*(1), 183–200.

Hew, K. F., Jia, C., Gonda, D. E., & Bai, S. (2020). Transitioning to the "new normal" of learning in unpredictable times: Pedagogical practices and learning performance in fully online flipped classrooms. *International Journal of Educational Technology in Higher Education, 17*(1), 1–22. doi:10.118641239-020-00234-x PMID:34778516

Hillebrandt, A., & Barclay, L. J. (2022). How COVID-19 can promote workplace cheating behavior via employee anxiety and self-interest–And how prosocial messages may overcome this effect. *Journal of Organizational Behavior, 43*(5), 858–877. doi:10.1002/job.2612 PMID:35574191

Hizam-Hanafiah, M., Yousaf, S. U., & Usman, B. (2017). The influence of psychological capital on the growth intentions of entrepreneurs: A study on Malaysian SME entrepreneurs. *Business and Economic Horizons (BEH), 13*(1232-2019–722), 556–569.

Hoffman, C. D., Sweeney, D. P., Hodge, D., Lopez-Wagner, M. C., & Looney, L. (2009). Parenting Stress and Closeness: Mothers of Typically Developing Children and Mothers of Children With Autism. *Sage, 24*(3), 178–187. doi:10.1177/1088357609338715

Hofmann, S. G., & Smits, J. A. (2008). Cognitive-behavioral therapy for adult anxiety disorders: A meta-analysis of randomized placebo-controlled trials. *The Journal of Clinical Psychiatry, 69*(4), 621–632. doi:10.4088/JCP.v69n0415 PMID:18363421

Hooda, S. (2020). *Stress and coping strategies in Primary caregivers of children with intellectual disability* [Doctoral dissertation]. Shodhganga: a reservoir of Indian theses.

Hopkins, N., & Reicher, S. (2016). The psychology of health and well-being in mass gatherings: A review and a research agenda. In Journal of Epidemiology and Global Health, 6(2), 49–57). Elsevier Ltd. doi:10.1016/j.jegh.2015.06.001

Horesh, D., Kapel Lev-Ari, R., & Hasson-Ohayon, I. (2020). Risk factors for psychological distress during the COVID-19 pandemic in Israel: Loneliness, age, gender, and health status play an important role. *British Journal of Health Psychology, 25*(4), 925–933. doi:10.1111/bjhp.12455 PMID:32656926

Hosseinpanahi, M., Mirghafourvand, M., Farshbaf-Khalili, A., Esmaeilpour, K., Rezaei, M., & Malakouti, J. (2020). The effect of counseling based on acceptance and commitment therapy on mental health and quality of life among infertile couples: A randomized controlled trial. *Journal of Education and Health Promotion, 9*(1), 251. doi:10.4103/jehp.jehp_512_20 PMID:33224995

Howell, J. M., & Shamir, B. (2005). The role of followers in the charismatic leadership process: Relationships and their consequences. *Academy of Management Review, 30*(1), 96–112. doi:10.5465/amr.2005.15281435

Huang, C., Wang, Y., Li, X., Ren, L., Zhao, J., Hu, Y., Zhang, L., Fan, G., Xu, J., Gu, X., Cheng, Z., Yu, T., Xia, J., Wei, Y., Wu, W., Xie, X., Yin, W., Li, H., Liu, M., & Cao, B. (2020). Clinical features of patients infected with 2019 novel coronavirus in Wuhan, China. *Lancet, 395*(10223), 497–506. doi:10.1016/S0140-6736(20)30183-5 PMID:31986264

Huang, Y., & Zhao, N. (2020). Generalized anxiety disorder, depressive symptoms and sleep quality during COVID-19 outbreak in China: A web-based cross-sectional survey. *Psychiatry Research, 288*, 112954. doi:10.1016/j.psychres.2020.112954 PMID:32325383

Humphrey, R. H. (2002). The many faces of emotional leadership. *The Leadership Quarterly, 13*(5), 493–504. Advance online publication. doi:10.1016/S1048-9843(02)00140-6

Hyland, T. (2015). On the contemporary applications of mindfulness: Some implications for education. *Journal of Philosophy of Education, 49*(2), 170–186. doi:10.1111/1467-9752.12135

Hyland, T. (2016). The limits of mindfulness: Emerging issues for education. *British Journal of Educational Studies, 64*(1), 97–117. doi:10.1080/00071005.2015.1051946

Ihme, K. R. M., & Sundstrom, P. (2021). The mindful shield: The effects of mindfulness training on resilience and leadership in military leaders. *Perspectives in Psychiatric Care, 57*(2), 675–688. doi:10.1111/ppc.12594 PMID:32740947

Insel, T. R. (2017). Digital Phenotyping: Technology for a New Science of Behavior. *Journal of the American Medical Association, 318*(13), 1215–1216. doi:10.1001/jama.2017.11295 PMID:28973224

Jacobson, D. (2004). Indian Society and Ways of Living. *Asia Society*. https://asiasociety.org/education/indian-society-and-ways-living

Jaiswal, P., Mahey, R., Singh, S., Vanamail, P., Gupta, M., Cheluvaraju, R., Sharma, J. B., & Bhatla, N. (2022). *The psychological impact of suspension/postponement of fertility treatments on infertile women waiting during the COVID pandemic*. Psychological Impact of Suspension/ Postponement of Fertility Treatments on Infertile Women Waiting During COVID Pandemic. doi:10.5468/ogs.21254

Jalili Nikoo, S., Ghasemi Jobaneh, R., & Taghvaeinia, A. (2018). Effectiveness of Mindfulness Training on Emotional Maturity and Occupational Stress of Nurses. *Reviews in Health Care, 4*(1), 20–25.

Jena, L. K., Pradhan, S., & Panigrahy, N. P. (2018). Pursuit of organisational trust: Role of employee engagement, psychological well-being, and transformational leadership. *Asia Pacific Management Review, 23*(3), 227–234. doi:10.1016/j.apmrv.2017.11.001

Jones, C. N., You, S., & Furlong, M. J. (2013). A preliminary examination of covitality as integrated well-being in college students. *Social Indicators Research, 111*(2), 511–526. doi:10.100711205-012-0017-9

Jorm, A. F., Griffiths, K. M., Christensen, H., Parslow, R. A., & Rogers, B. (2004). Actions taken to cope with depression at different levels of severity: A community survey. *Psychological Medicine, 34*(2), 293–299. doi:10.1017/S003329170300895X PMID:14982135

Joseph, T. (2016). Developing the Leader-Follower Relationship: Perceptions of Leaders and Followers. *Journal of Leadership, Accountability and Ethics, 13*(1).

Kamath, M. S., Joseph, T., Karuppusami, R., Chinta, P., Pal, A., Nallamilli, S. R., Sarkar, S., Poobalan, A. & Kunjummen, A. T. (2021). Knowledge, anxiety levels and attitudes of infertile couples towards COVID-19 and its impact on self-funded fertility treatment: a cross-sectional questionnaire survey. *Human reproduction open, 2021*(4).

Kämpfen, F., Kohler, I. V., Ciancio, A., Bruine de Bruin, W., Maurer, J., & Kohler, H. P. (2020). Predictors of mental health during the Covid-19 pandemic in the US: Role of economic concerns, health worries, and social distancing. *PLoS One, 15*(11), e0241895. doi:10.1371/journal.pone.0241895 PMID:33175894

Kantamneni, N. (2020). The impact of the COVID-19 pandemic on marginalized populations in the United States: A research agenda. *Journal of Vocational Behavior, 119*, 103439. doi:10.1016/j.jvb.2020.103439 PMID:32390658

Kappagoda, U., Othman, P., Zainul, H., & Alwis, G. (2014). Psychological capital and job performance: The mediating role of work attitudes. *Dr. Hohd. Zainul and Alwis, Gamini, Psychological Capital, and Job Performance: The Mediating Role of Work Attitudes (June 27, 2014). Journal of Human Resource and Sustainability Studies.*

Kessing, L. V., Hansen, H. V., Christensen, E. M., Dam, H., Gluud, C., & Wetterslev, J. (2014). Do young adults with bipolar disorder benefit from early intervention? *Journal of Affective Disorders, 152–154*, 403–408. doi:10.1016/j.jad.2013.10.001 PMID:24268595

Khalil, R., Mansour, A. E., Fadda, W. A., Almisnid, K., Aldamegh, M., Al-Nafeesah, A., Alkhalifah, A., & Al-Wutayd, O. (2020). The sudden transition to synchronized online learning during the COVID-19 pandemic in Saudi Arabia: A qualitative study exploring medical students' perspectives. *BMC Medical Education, 20*(1), 1–10. doi:10.118612909-020-02208-z PMID:32859188

Khan, F. M. (2018). *A Study of Perceived Stress Quality of Life and Coping Strategies of Parents of Children with Special Needs* [Master's thesis]. Shodhganga: a reservoir of Indian theses.

Khan, N., Ahmad, N., Beg, A. H., Ismail, E. I., Abd Alla, A. N., & Nubli, M. (2010). Epilepsy control by prayer type Yoga exercise. *2010 Second International Conference on Computer Research and Development*, 391–395. 10.1109/ICCRD.2010.61

Khan, S. S., Hopkins, N., Tewari, S., Srinivasan, N., Reicher, S. D., & Ozakinci, G. (2014). Efficacy and well-being in rural north India: The role of social identification with a large-scale community identity. *European Journal of Social Psychology, 44*(7), 787–798. doi:10.1002/ejsp.2060 PMID:26160989

Kim, B.-J. (2019). Unstable jobs cannot cultivate good organizational citizens: The sequential mediating role of organizational trust and identification. *International Journal of Environmental Research and Public Health, 16*(7), 1102. doi:10.3390/ijerph16071102 PMID:30934804

Kim, M., Kim, A. C. H., Newman, J. I., Ferris, G. R., & Perrewé, P. L. (2019). The antecedents and consequences of positive organizational behavior: The role of psychological capital for promoting employee well-being in sport organizations. *Sport Management Review, 22*(1), 108–125. doi:10.1016/j.smr.2018.04.003

King-Dowling, S., Proudfoot, N. A., & Obeid, J. (2019). Comorbidity Among Chronic Physical Health Conditions and Neurodevelopmental Disorders in Childhood. *Current Developmental Disorders Reports, 6*(4), 248–258. doi:10.100740474-019-00173-x

King, E., & Haar, J. M. (2017). Mindfulness and job performance: A study of Australian leaders. *Asia Pacific Journal of Human Resources, 55*(3), 298–319. doi:10.1111/1744-7941.12143

Kluger, J. (2022). Pandemic Anxiety Is Fueling a Rise in OCD Symptoms. *Time Magizine*. https://time.com/6140256/ocd-covid-19-anxiety/

Knapp, S., Gottlieb, M. C., & Handelsman, M. M. (2017). Enhancing professionalism through self-reflection. *Professional Psychology, Research and Practice, 48*(3), 167–174. doi:10.1037/pro0000135

Kong, M. (2020). What COVID-19 means for non-neurotypical children and their families. *Pediatric Research, 89*(3), 396–397. doi:10.1038/s41390-020-0913-7

Kong, X., Kong, F., Zheng, K., Tang, M., Chen, Y., Zhou, J., Li, Y., Diao, L., Wu, S., Jiao, P., Su, T., & Dong, Y. (2020). Effect of psychological–behavioral intervention on the depression and anxiety of COVID-19 patients. *Frontiers in Psychiatry, 11*, 586355. doi:10.3389/fpsyt.2020.586355 PMID:33329130

Koning, L. F., & van Kleef, G. A. (2015). How leaders' emotional displays shape followers' organizational citizenship behavior. *The Leadership Quarterly*, *26*(4), 489–501. doi:10.1016/j.leaqua.2015.03.001

Konte, A. G. (2021). Mindfulness and its impacts on managers: A pilot study. *Human Systems Management*, *40*(4), 605–617. doi:10.3233/HSM-201016

Koo, J. W. (2021). *Problematic Use of Alcohol and Online Gaming as Coping Strategies During the COVID-19 Pandemic: A Mini Review.* Frontiers..

Koprowski, K., Meyer, D., Stanfill, T., & Tivis, L. J. (2021). Cultivating joy: Improving nurse resilience through use of a practice playbook. *Applied Nursing Research*, *62*, 151484. doi:10.1016/j.apnr.2021.151484 PMID:34814992

Kotzé, M. (2018). The influence of psychological capital, self-leadership, and mindfulness on work engagement. *South African Journal of Psychology. Suid-Afrikaanse Tydskrif vir Sielkunde*, *48*(2), 279–292. doi:10.1177/0081246317705812

Kotzé, M. (2021). The relationship between public service employees' personal resources and psychological well-being. *International Review of Administrative Sciences*, 0020852320985926.

Kramer, A., & Kramer, K. Z. (2020). The potential impact of the Covid-19 pandemic on occupational status, work from home, and occupational mobility. In *Journal of Vocational Behavior* (Vol. 119, p. 103442). Academic Press Inc. doi:10.1016/j.jvb.2020.103442

Krippendorff, K. (2005). *The semantic turn: A new foundation for design.* CRC Press.

Kulkarni, C. A., Telang, P., & Wane, M. (2021). Efficacy of Mindfulness Meditation on Emotional Maturity of Mothers of Cerebral Palsy Children. *Journal of Pharmaceutical Research International*, 615–622.

Kumar, A., & Nayar, K. R. (2020). COVID 19 and its mental health consequences. doi:10.1080/09638237.2020.1757052

Kumar, D. (2021). School mental health program in India: Need to shift from a piecemeal approach to a long-term comprehensive approach with strong intersectoral coordination. *Indian Journal of Psychiatry*, *63*(1), 91. doi:10.4103/psychiatry.IndianJPsychiatry_204_20 PMID:34083828

Kurt, N., & Demirbolat, A. O. (2018). Investigation of the Relationship Between Psychological Capital Perception, Psychological Well-Being and Job Satisfaction of Teachers. *Journal of Education and Learning*, *8*(1), 87. doi:10.5539/jel.v8n1p87

La Rosa, V. L., Barra, F., Chiofalo, B., Platania, A., Di Guardo, F., & Conway, F. (2019). An overview on the relationship between endometriosis and infertility: The impact on sexuality and psychological well-being. *Journal of Psychosomatic Obstetrics and Gynaecology*, 1–5. PMID:31466493

Lai, J., Ma, S., Wang, Y., Cai, Z., Hu, J., Wei, N., Wu, J., Du, H., Chen, T., Li, R., Tan, H., Kang, L., Yao, L., Huang, M., Wang, H., Wang, G., Liu, Z., & Hu, S. (2020). Factors associated with mental health outcomes among health care workers exposed to coronavirus disease 2019. *JAMA Network Open, 3*(3), e203976–e203976. doi:10.1001/jamanetworkopen.2020.3976 PMID:32202646

Larsen, L., Helland, M. S., & Holt, T. (2022). The impact of school closure and social isolation on children in vulnerable families during COVID-19: A focus on children's reactions. *European Child & Adolescent Psychiatry, 31*(8), 1–11. doi:10.100700787-021-01758-x PMID:33770275

Lathabhavan, R. (2022). COVID-19 and mental health concerns among business owners: A cross-sectional study from India. *International Journal of Mental Health and Addiction*, 1–11. doi:10.100711469-022-00824-y PMID:35465028

Lattie, E. G., Adkins, E. C., Winquist, N., Stiles-Shields, C., Wafford, Q. E., & Graham, A. K. (2019). Digital Mental Health Interventions for Depression, Anxiety, and Enhancement of Psychological Well-Being Among College Students: Systematic Review. *Journal of Medical Internet Research, 21*(7), e12869. doi:10.2196/12869 PMID:31333198

Leal Filho, W., Wall, T., Rayman-Bacchus, L., Mifsud, M., Pritchard, D. J., Lovren, V. O., Farinha, C., Petrovic, D. S., & Balogun, A. L. (2021). Impacts of COVID-19 and social isolation on academic staff and students at universities: A cross-sectional study. *BMC Public Health, 21*(1), 1213. doi:10.118612889-021-11040-z PMID:34167494

Leana, C. R., & Feldman, D. C. (1991). Gender differences in responses to unemployment. *Journal of Vocational Behavior, 38*(1), 65–77. doi:10.1016/0001-8791(91)90018-H

Lechner, L., Bolman, C., & van Dalen, A. (2007). Definite involuntary childlessness: Associations between coping, social support, and psychological distress. *Human Reproduction (Oxford, England), 22*(1), 288–294. doi:10.1093/humrep/del327 PMID:16920722

Lee, D., Choi, Y., Youn, S., & Chun, J. U. (2017). Ethical Leadership and Employee Moral Voice: The Mediating Role of Moral Efficacy and the Moderating Role of Leader–Follower Value Congruence. *Journal of Business Ethics, 141*(1), 47–57. doi:10.100710551-015-2689-y

Lee, V., Albaum, C., Tablon Modica, P., Ahmad, F., Gorter, J. W., Khanlou, N., McMorris, C., Lai, J., Harrison, C., Hedley, T., Johnston, P., Putterman, C., Spoelstra, M., & Weiss, J. A. (2021). The impact of <scp>COVID</scp> -19 on the mental health and wellbeing of caregivers of autistic children and youth: A scoping review. *Autism Research, 14*(12), 2477–2494. doi:10.1002/aur.2616 PMID:34591373

Lekamwasam, R., & Lekamwasam, S. (2020). Effects of covid-19 pandemic on health and wellbeing of older people: A comprehensive review. *Annals of Geriatric Medicine and Research, 24*(3), 166–172. doi:10.4235/agmr.20.0027 PMID:32752587

Li, M., Chen, J., & Deng, Y. (2020). *Scaling features in the spreading of COVID-19*. Ming Li.

Loayza, N. & Pennings, S. M. (2020). Macroeconomic Policy in the Time of COVID-19: A Primer for Developing Countries. *Our World in Data*. https://ourworldindata.org/coronavirus-source-data

Lokeshvar, R., Deepa, N., Madhivadhani, K., Divya, P., & Asuvathaman, M. (2021). Evaluating the Impact of COVID-19 on Mental Health problems in Indian context. *J Pharm Adv Res*, *4*(6), 1296–1301.

Low, C. H., Bordia, P., & Bordia, S. (2016). What do employees want and why? An exploration of employees' preferred psychological contract elements across career stages. *Human Relations*, *69*(7), 1457–1481. doi:10.1177/0018726715616468

Luthans, F. (2002). Positive organizational behavior: Developing and managing psychological strengths. *The Academy of Management Perspectives*, *16*(1), 57–72. doi:10.5465/ame.2002.6640181

Luthans, F., Avey, J. B., Avolio, B. J., Norman, S. M., & Combs, G. M. (2006). Psychological capital development: toward a micro-intervention. *Journal of Organizational Behavior: The International Journal of Industrial. Occupational and Organizational Psychology and Behavior*, *27*(3), 387–393. doi:10.1002/job.373

Luthans, F., Avey, J. B., Avolio, B. J., & Peterson, S. J. (2010). The development and resulting performance impact of positive psychological capital. *Human Resource Development Quarterly*, *21*(1), 41–67. doi:10.1002/hrdq.20034

Luthans, F., Avey, J. B., Clapp-Smith, R., & Li, W. (2008). More evidence on the value of Chinese workers' psychological capital: A potentially unlimited competitive resource? *International Journal of Human Resource Management*, *19*(5), 818–827. doi:10.1080/09585190801991194

Luthans, F., Avey, J. B., & Patera, J. L. (2008). Experimental analysis of a web-based training intervention to develop positive psychological capital. *Academy of Management Learning & Education*, *7*(2), 209–221. doi:10.5465/amle.2008.32712618

Luthans, F., & Avolio, B. J. (2003). Authentic leadership development. *Positive Organizational Scholarship*, *241*, 258.

Luthans, F., Avolio, B. J., Avey, J. B., & Norman, S. M. (2007). Positive psychological capital: Measurement and relationship with performance and satisfaction. *Personnel Psychology*, *60*(3), 541–572. doi:10.1111/j.1744-6570.2007.00083.x

Luthans, F., & Broad, J. D. (2022). Positive psychological capital to help combat the mental health fallout from the pandemic and VUCA environment. *Organizational Dynamics*, *51*(2), 100817. doi:10.1016/j.orgdyn.2020.100817 PMID:35719171

Luthans, F., & Peterson, S. J. (2002). Employee engagement and manager self-efficacy. *Journal of Management Development*, *21*(5), 376–387. doi:10.1108/02621710210426864

Luthans, F., Vogelgesang, G. R., & Lester, P. B. (2006). Developing the psychological capital of resiliency. *Human Resource Development Review*, *5*(1), 25–44. doi:10.1177/1534484305285335

Luthans, F., Youssef, C. M., & Avolio, B. J. (2007). Psychological capital: Investing and developing positive organizational behavior. *Positive Organizational Behavior*, *1*(2), 9–24. doi:10.4135/9781446212752.n2

Luxton, D. D., McCann, R. A., Bush, N. E., Mishkind, M. C., & Reger, G. M. (2011). mHealth for Mental Health: Integrating Smartphone Technology in Behavioral Healthcare. *Professional Psychology, Research and Practice*, *42*(6), 505–512. doi:10.1037/a0024485

Lyvers, M., Makin, C., Toms, E., Thorberg, F. A., & Samios, C. (2014). Trait mindfulness in relation to emotional self-regulation and executive function. *Mindfulness*, *5*(6), 619–625. doi:10.100712671-013-0213-y

Magnano, P., Craparo, G., & Paolillo, A. (2016). Resilience and Emotional Intelligence: Which role in achievement motivation. *International Journal of Psychological Research*, *9*(1), 9–20. doi:10.21500/20112084.2096

Mahey, R., Sharma, A., Kumari, A., Kachhawa, G., Gupta, M., Meena, J., & Bhatla, N. (2020). The impact of a segregated team roster on obstetrics and gynecology services in response to the COVID-19 pandemic in a tertiary care center in India. *International Journal of Gynaecology and Obstetrics: the Official Organ of the International Federation of Gynaecology and Obstetrics*, *151*(3), 341–346. doi:10.1002/ijgo.13408 PMID:33011974

Mahfouz, J. (2018). Mindfulness training for school administrators: Effects on well-being and leadership. *Journal of Educational Administration*, *56*(6), 602–619. doi:10.1108/JEA-12-2017-0171

Majumdar, P., Biswas, A., & Sahu, S. (2020). COVID-19 pandemic and lockdown: Cause of sleep disruption, depression, somatic pain, and increased screen exposure of office workers and students of India. *Chronobiology International*, *37*(8), 1191–1200. doi:10.1080/07420528.2020.1786107 PMID:32660352

Makwana, N. (2019). Disaster and its impact on mental health: A narrative review. *Journal of Family Medicine and Primary Care*, *8*(10), 3090. doi:10.4103/jfmpc.jfmpc_893_19 PMID:31742125

Malhotra, N., Shah, D., & Pai, R. (2013). Assisted reproductive technology in India: A 3-year retrospective data analysis. *Journal of Human Reproductive Sciences*, *6*(4), 235–240. doi:10.4103/0974-1208.126286 PMID:24672161

Malhotra, S., & Shah, R. (2015). Women and mental health in India: An overview. *Indian Journal of Psychiatry*, *57*(6, Suppl 2), S205. doi:10.4103/0019-5545.161479 PMID:26330636

Malik, N., & Dhar, R. L. (2017). Authentic leadership and its impact on extra role behaviour of nurses: The mediating role of psychological capital and the moderating role of autonomy. *Personnel Review*, *46*(2), 277–296. doi:10.1108/PR-05-2015-0140

Malinowski, P., & Lim, H. J. (2015). Mindfulness at work: Positive affect, hope, and optimism mediate the relationship between dispositional mindfulness, work engagement, and well-being. *Mindfulness*, *6*(6), 1250–1262. doi:10.100712671-015-0388-5

Malla, A., & Shaw, T. (1987). Attitudes towards mental illness: The influence of education and experience. *The International Journal of Social Psychiatry*, *33*(1), 33–41. doi:10.1177/002076408703300105 PMID:3583603

Man as a social animal. (2012). The Hindu. https://www.thehindu.com/features/education/research/man-as-a-social-animal/article2988145.ece

MarakasG. M. (2013). *Abnormal Psych*.

Margerison-Zilko, C., Goldman-Mellor, S., Falconi, A., & Downing, J. (2016). Health Impacts of the Great Recession: A Critical Review. *Current Epidemiology Reports*, *3*(1), 81–91. doi:10.100740471-016-0068-6 PMID:27239427

Marshall, M. N. (1996). Sampling for qualitative research. *Family Practice © Oxford University Press, 13*(6). http://fampra.oxfordjournals.org/

Martinsone, B., & Tzivian, L. (2021). Differences in stress and coping during the COVID-19 pandemic in families with and without children with developmental disorders or chronic conditions. *Frontiers in Public Health*, *9*, 704577. doi:10.3389/fpubh.2021.704577 PMID:34490186

Masi, A., Mendoza Diaz, A., Tully, L., Azim, S. I., Woolfenden, S., Efron, D., & Eapen, V. (2021). Impact of the COVID-19 pandemic on the well-being of children with neurodevelopmental disabilities and their parents. *Journal of Paediatrics and Child Health*, *57*(5), 631–636. doi:10.1111/jpc.15285 PMID:33426739

Mathe, K., Scott-Halsell, S., Kim, S., & Krawczyk, M. (2017). Psychological capital in the quick service restaurant industry: A study of unit-level performance. *Journal of Hospitality & Tourism Research (Washington, D.C.)*, *41*(7), 823–845. doi:10.1177/1096348014550923

Maunder, R., Hunter, J., Vincent, L., Bennett, J., Peladeau, N., Leszcz, M., Sadavoy, J., Verhaeghe, L. M., Steinberg, R., & Mazzulli, T. (2003). The immediate psychological and occupational impact of the 2003 SARS outbreak in a teaching hospital. *Canadian Medical Association Journal*, *168*(10), 1245–1251. PMID:12743065

McDermott, A. M., Conway, E., Rousseau, D. M., & Flood, P. C. (2013). Promoting effective psychological contracts through leadership: The missing link between HR strategy and performance. *Human Resource Management*, *52*(2), 289–310. doi:10.1002/hrm.21529

Meda, N., Pardini, S., Slongo, I., Bodini, L., Zordan, M. A., Rigobello, P., Visioli, F., & Novara, C. (2021). Students' mental health problems before, during, and after the COVID-19 lockdown in Italy. *Journal of Psychiatric Research*, *134*, 69–77. doi:10.1016/j.jpsychires.2020.12.045 PMID:33360865

Mellor, N., & Webster, J. (2013). Enablers and challenges in implementing a comprehensive workplace health and well-being approach. *International Journal of Workplace Health Management*, *6*(2), 129–142. doi:10.1108/IJWHM-08-2011-0018

Milstone, A. (2022). *COVID in Babies and Kids: Symptoms and Prevention.* Johns Hopkins Medicine.

Mishra, S. (2021). *Effects of video games on children.* IEA.

Mitali, N. (November 24, 2020,). *With Covid-19, comes the "Shadow Pandemic": How the surge of domestic violence gripped India's women in 2020.* TOI.

Mitrović, M., Kostić, J. O., & Ristić, M. (2022). Intolerance of uncertainty and distress in women with delayed IVF treatment due to the COVID-19 pandemic: The mediating role of situation appraisal and coping strategies. *Journal of Health Psychology, 27*(11), 2515–2528. doi:10.1177/13591053211049950 PMID:34670414

Modrek, S., Stuckler, D., McKee, M., Cullen, M. R., & Basu, S. (2013). A Review of Health Consequences of Recessions Internationally and a Synthesis of the US Response during the Great Recession. *Public Health Reviews, 35*(1), 1–33. doi:10.1007/BF03391695

Mohr, D. C., Lyon, A. R., Lattie, E. G., Reddy, M., & Schueller, S. M. (2017). Accelerating Digital Mental Health Research From Early Design and Creation to Successful Implementation and Sustainment. *Journal of Medical Internet Research, 19*(5), e153. doi:10.2196/jmir.7725 PMID:28490417

Mojtabai, R., Olfson, M., & Mechanic, D. (2002). Perceived need and help-seeking in adults with mood, anxiety, or substance use disorders. *Archives of General Psychiatry, 59*(1), 77–84. doi:10.1001/archpsyc.59.1.77 PMID:11779286

Mowrer, O. H. (1947). On the dual nature of learning—A re-interpretation of "conditioning" and "problem-solving.". *Harvard Educational Review, 17*, 102–148.

Muhaidat, N., Alshrouf, M. A., Karam, A. M., & Elfalah, M. Jnr. (2021). Infertility Management Disruption During the COVID-19 Outbreak in a Middle-Income Country: Patients' Choices, Attitudes, and Concerns. *Patient Preference and Adherence, 15*, 2279–2288. doi:10.2147/PPA.S327055 PMID:34675492

Mukhtar, S. (2020). Psychological health during the coronavirus disease 2019 pandemic outbreak. *The International Journal of Social Psychiatry, 66*(5), 512–516. doi:10.1177/0020764020925835 PMID:32434402

Mulliner, J. (2018). *Employee engagement, motivation, resilience, and leadership: An exploration of relationships within a higher education institution.*

Murdia K, (2021) Covid-19 and IVF: Long wait for women trying to be mothers through Assisted Reproductive Technology. NEWS 18.COM.Last update, 2021; 16:14 IST

Murphy, S. (2021). The Role of Self-Efficacy and Multiple Intelligences. In Multiple Intelligences and Leadership. doi:10.4324/9781410606495-18

Murphy, S. E., & Ensher, E. A. (2008). A qualitative analysis of charismatic leadership in creative teams: The case of television directors. *The Leadership Quarterly, 19*(3), 335–352. doi:10.1016/j.leaqua.2008.03.006

Murthy, R. S. (2014). Mental health initiatives in India (1947-2010). *Social Work in Mental Health: Contexts and Theories for Practice, 5*, 28.

Murthy, R. S. (2017). National Mental Health Survey of India 2015-2016. *Indian Journal of Psychiatry*, *59*(1), 21–26. doi:10.4103/psychiatry.IndianJPsychiatry_102_17 PMID:28529357

Naidoo, V., Abarantyne, I., & Rugimbana, R. (2019). The impact of psychological contracts on employee engagement at a university of technology. *SA Journal of Human Resource Management*, *17*. doi:10.4102ajhrm.v17i0.1039

Naser, A. Y., Dahmash, E. Z., Al-Rousan, R., Alwafi, H., Alrawashdeh, H. M., Ghoul, I., Abidine, A., Bokhary, M. A., AL-Hadithi, H. T., Ali, D., Abuthawabeh, R., Abdelwahab, G. M., Alhartani, Y. J., Al Muhaisen, H., Dagash, A., & Alyami, H. S. (2020). Mental health status of the general population, healthcare professionals, and university students during 2019 coronavirus disease outbreak in Jordan: A cross-sectional study. *Brain and Behavior*, *10*(8). doi:10.1002/brb3.1730 PMID:32578943

Nayak, S., & Shenoi, S. (2013). Synopsis of training programme for dermatologists in non-pharmacological (Psychological) interventions in dermatology. *Indian Journal of Dermatology, Venereology and Leprology*, *79*(2), 275.

Neurol., S. P. (2022). *The COVID-19 Pandemic and Pregnancy: Impact on Mothers and Newborns*. NIH.

Newman, A., Ucbasaran, D., Zhu, F. E. I., & Hirst, G. (2014). Psychological capital: A review and synthesis. *Journal of Organizational Behavior*, *35*(S1), S120–S138. doi:10.1002/job.1916

Nicola, M., Alsafi, Z., Sohrabi, C., Kerwan, A., Al-Jabir, A., Iosifidis, C., Agha, M., & Agha, R. (2020). The socio-economic implications of the coronavirus pandemic (COVID-19): A review. In International Journal of Surgery, 78, 185–193. Elsevier Ltd. doi:10.1016/j.ijsu.2020.04.018

Nisha, S. I., & Bakul, F. (2022). Parents/primary caregivers' perspectives on the well-being, and home-based learning of children with neurodevelopmental disorders during COVID-19 in Bangladesh. *International Journal of Developmental Disabilities*, 1–10. doi:10.1080/20473869.2022.2121140

Norris, S. L., & Currieri, M. (1999). Performance enhancement training through neurofeedback. In *Introduction to quantitative EEG and neurofeedback* (pp. 223–240). Elsevier. doi:10.1016/B978-012243790-8/50011-0

Nüchter, V., Abson, D. J., von Wehrden, H., & Engler, J. O. (2021). The concept of resilience in recent sustainability research. *Sustainability (Switzerland)*, *13*(5), 1–21. doi:10.3390u13052735

Nylén-Eriksen, M., Lara-Cabrera, M. L., Grov, E. K., Skarsvaag, H., Lie, I., Dahl-Michelsen, T., Sæterstrand, T. M., Mandahl, A., Hafstad, H., Lersveen, M. B., & United Nations Children's Fund (2020). *6 ways parents can support their kids through the COVID-19 outbreak*. UNICEF. https://www.unicef.org/coronavirus/6-ways-parents-can-support-their-kids-through-coronavirus-covid-19

Oakman, J., Kinsman, N., Stuckey, R., Graham, M., & Weale, V. (2020). A rapid review of mental and physical health effects of working at home: How do we optimise health? *BMC Public Health*, *20*(1), 1–13. doi:10.118612889-020-09875-z PMID:33256652

Oladapo, V. (2014). The impact of talent management on retention. *Journal of Business Studies Quarterly*, *5*(3), 19.

Pappas, S. (n.d.). *Helping patients cope with COVID-19* . APA.

Park, J. G., Kim, J. S., Yoon, S. W., & Joo, B.-K. (2017). The effects of empowering leadership on psychological well-being and job engagement: The mediating role of psychological capital. *Leadership and Organization Development Journal*.

Parto, M., & Besharat, M. A. (2011). Mindfulness, psychological well-being, and psychological distress in adolescents: Assessing the mediating variables and mechanisms of autonomy and self-regulation. *Procedia: Social and Behavioral Sciences*, *30*, 578–582. doi:10.1016/j.sbspro.2011.10.112

Paternite, C. E. (2005). School-based mental health programs and services: Overview and introduction to the special issue. *Journal of Abnormal Child Psychology*, *33*(6), 657–663. doi:10.100710802-005-7645-3 PMID:16328742

Patnaik, S., Mishra, U. S., & Mishra, B. B. (2021). Can psychological capital reduce stress and job insecurity? An experimental examination with indian evidence. *Asia Pacific Journal of Management*, 1–26.

Paulauskaite, L., Farris, O., Spencer, H. M., & Hassiotis, A.EPICC-ID group. (2021). My son can't socially distance or wear a mask: How families of preschool children with severe developmental delays and challenging behavior experienced the COVID-19 pandemic. *Journal of Mental Health Research in Intellectual Disabilities*, *14*(2), 225–236. doi:10.1080/19315864.2021.1874578

Paul, K. I., & Moser, K. (2009). Unemployment impairs mental health: Meta-analyses. *Journal of Vocational Behavior*, *74*(3), 264–282. doi:10.1016/j.jvb.2009.01.001

Pecor, K. W., Barbayannis, G., Yang, M., Johnson, J., Materasso, S., Borda, M., Garcia, D., Garla, V., & Ming, X. (2021). Quality of Life Changes during the COVID-19 Pandemic for Caregivers of Children with ADHD and/or ASD. *International Journal of Environmental Research and Public Health 2021, 18*(7), 3667. doi:10.3390/ijerph18073667

Peng, J. C., Jien, J.-J., & Lin, J. (2016). Antecedents and consequences of psychological contract breach. *Journal of Managerial Psychology*, *31*(8), 1312–1326. doi:10.1108/JMP-10-2015-0383

Peoquin, K., & Lafontaine, M. F. (2010). What are the correlates of infertility-related clinical anxiety? A literature review and the presentation of a conceptual model. *Marriage & family review, 46*(8), 580-620.

Pericleous-Smith, A., Dark, S., McCluskey, G., Mizen, L., & Crawshaw, M. (2021). Survey of fertility counseling provision in UK licensed treatment centers during the first phase of the COVID-19 pandemic. *Human Fertility*, 1–11. doi:10.1080/14647273.2021.1898053 PMID:33749479

Peterson, S. J., & Luthans, F. (2003). The positive impact and development of hopeful leaders. *Leadership and Organization Development Journal*, *24*(1), 26–31. doi:10.1108/01437730310457302

Petzold, M. B., Bendau, A., Plag, J., Pyrkosch, L., Mascarell Maricic, L., Betzler, F., Rogoll, J., Große, J., & Ströhle, A. (2020). Risk, resilience, psychological distress, and anxiety at the beginning of the COVID-19 pandemic in Germany. *Brain and Behavior*, *10*(9), e01745. doi:10.1002/brb3.1745 PMID:32633464

Piper, K. (2020). The devastating consequences of coronavirus lockdowns in poor countries. *VOX*. https://www.vox.com/future-perfect/2020/4/18/21212688/coronavirus-lockdowns-developing-world

Pitanatri, P. D. S., Pitana, I. G., & Valeri, M. (2022). Natural and Man-Made Crisis Management in a Small Island Tourism Destination: The Case of Bali. *Tourism Risk*, 61–79. doi:10.1108/978-1-80117-708-520221005

Plomp, J., Tims, M., Akkermans, J., Khapova, S. N., Jansen, P. G. W., & Bakker, A. B. (2016). Career competencies and job crafting: How proactive employees influence their well-being. *Career Development International*, *21*(6), 587–602. doi:10.1108/CDI-08-2016-0145

Proudfoot, J., Parker, G., Hadzi Pavlovic, D., Manicavasagar, V., Adler, E., & Whitton, A. (2010). Community attitudes to the appropriation of mobile phones for monitoring and managing depression, anxiety, and stress. *Journal of Medical Internet Research*, *12*(5), e64. doi:10.2196/jmir.1475 PMID:21169174

Punit, I. S. (2020). India school teachers grapple unruly online classes amid lockdown. *Quartz India*. https://qz.com/india/1851939/india-school-teachers-grapple-unruly-online-classes-amid-lockdown/

Rabenu, E., & Tziner, A. (2021). Back to routine after the coronavirus pandemic lockdown: A proposal from a psychological perspective. *Industrial and Organizational Psychology: Perspectives on Science and Practice*, *14*(1–2), 178–183. doi:10.1017/iop.2021.23

Rahman, U. U., Rehman, Ch. A., Imran, M. K., & Aslam, U. (2017). Does team orientation matter? Linking work engagement and relational psychological contract with performance. *Journal of Management Development*, *36*(9), 1102–1113. doi:10.1108/JMD-10-2016-0204

Ramirez, P. T., Chiva, L., Eriksson, A. G. Z., Frumovitz, M., Fagotti, A., Martin, A. G., Jhingran, A., & Pareja, R. (2020). COVID-19 global pandemic: Options for management of gynecologic cancers. [). BMJ Specialist Journals.]. *International Journal of Gynecological Cancer*, *30*(5), 561–563. doi:10.1136/ijgc-2020-001419 PMID:32221023

Rasekh Jahromi, A., Daroneh, E., Jamali, S., Ranjbar, A., & Rahmanian, V. (2022). Impact of COVID-19 pandemic on depression and hopelessness in infertile women. *Journal of Psychosomatic Obstetrics & Gynecology*, 1-7.

Rayton, B. A., Brammer, S. J., & Millington, A. I. (2015). Corporate social performance and the psychological contract. *Group & Organization Management*, *40*(3), 353–377. doi:10.1177/1059601114561476

Rego, A., Sousa, F., Marques, C., & Cunha, M. P. (2012). Optimism predicting employees' creativity: The mediating role of positive affect and the positivity ratio. *European Journal of Work and Organizational Psychology*, *21*(2), 244–270. doi:10.1080/1359432X.2010.550679

Rego, P., Lopes, M. P., & Nascimento, J. L. (2016). Authentic leadership and organizational commitment: The mediating role of positive psychological capital. [JIEM]. *Journal of Industrial Engineering and Management*, *9*(1), 129–151. doi:10.3926/jiem.1540

Reiner, M. (2019). Emerging technologies for sport performance enhancement: Embodied cognition and manipulation of brain rhythms. Handbook of Embodied Cognition and Sport Psychology, 333–355.

Rezapour, M., Dehzangi, A., & Saadati, F. (2022). Students' negative emotions and their rational and irrational behaviors during COVID-19 outbreak. *PLoS One*, *17*(3), e0264985. doi:10.1371/journal.pone.0264985 PMID:35255106

Riasudeen, S., & Singh, P. (2021). Leadership effectiveness and psychological well-being: The role of workplace spirituality. *Journal of Human Values*, *27*(2), 109–125. doi:10.1177/0971685820947334

Rifai, H. A. (2005). A test of the relationships among perceptions of justice, job satisfaction, affective commitment, and organizational citizenship behavior. *Gadjah Mada International Journal of Business*, *7*(2), 131–154. doi:10.22146/gamaijb.5574

Rigby, C. S., Schultz, P. P., & Ryan, R. M. (2014). Mindfulness, interest-taking, and self-regulation. The Wiley Blackwell Handbook of Mindfulness, 1, 216–235.

Roche, M., Haar, J. M., & Luthans, F. (2014). The role of mindfulness and psychological capital on the well-being of leaders. *Journal of Occupational Health Psychology*, *19*(4), 476–489. doi:10.1037/a0037183 PMID:24933594

Rogers, Y., Hazlewood, W. R., Marshall, P., Dalton, N., & Hertrich, S. (2010). Ambient influence: Can twinkly lights lure and abstract representations trigger behavioral change? *UbiComp'10 - Proceedings of the 2010 ACM Conference on Ubiquitous Computing*, (pp. 261–270). ACM.10.1145/1864349.1864372

Romate, J., & Rajkumar, E. (2022). Exploring the experiences, psychological well-being and needs of frontline healthcare workers of government hos-pitals in India: A qualitative study. *Humanit Soc Sci Commun.*, *9*(1), 89. doi:10.105741599-022-01093-9

Ronchi, A., Pagliuca, F., Zito Marino, F., Montella, M., Franco, R., & Cozzolino, I. (2020). Interventional cytopathology in the COVID-19 era. *Cytopathology*, *31*(6), 509–513. doi:10.1111/cyt.12886 PMID:32654199

Rooney, K. L., & Domar, A. D. (2018). The relationship between stress and infertility. *Dialogues in Clinical Neuroscience*, *20*(1), 41–47. doi:10.31887/DCNS.2018.20.1/klrooney PMID:29946210

Rothwell, W. (2010). *Effective succession planning: Ensuring leadership continuity and building talent from within*. Amacom.

Roy, A., Singh, A. K., Mishra, S., Chinnadurai, A., Mitra, A., & Bakshi, O. (2021). Mental health implications of COVID-19 pandemic and its response in India. *The International Journal of Social Psychiatry*, *67*(5), 587–600. doi:10.1177/0020764020950769 PMID:32873106

Roy, D., Tripathy, S., Kar, S. K., Sharma, N., Verma, S. K., & Kaushal, V. (2020). Prevalence of stress, anxiety, depression among the general population during the COVID-19 pandemic: A systematic review and meta-analysis. *Asian Journal of Psychiatry*, *51*, 102083. doi:10.1016/j.ajp.2020.102083 PMID:32283510

Rust, A. A., & Koketso, L. P. (2012). *Perceived challenges to talent management in the South African public service: An exploratory study of the City of Cape Town municipality*.

Saadatkhah, M., Narimani, M., Mousazadeh, T., & Varniyab, S. T. (2021). *Comparison of the efficacy of mindfulness-based cognitive therapy and acceptance and commitment therapy on emotional maturity in people with substance abuse disorders*.

Sarkar, A., Saha, P. K., & Arora, A. (2021). COVID-19 Pandemic and infertility: Gynecological Dilemma from an Indian perspective. *Reproductive Sciences (Thousand Oaks, Calif.)*, *28*(4), 1020–1022. doi:10.100743032-021-00474-w PMID:33544338

Schabracq, M. J. (2003). What an organisation can do about its employees' well-being and health: An overview. The Handbook of Work and Health Psychology, 585.

Scheier, M. F., & Carver, C. S. (1992). Effects of optimism on psychological and physical well-being: Theoretical overview and empirical update. *Cognitive Therapy and Research*, *16*(2), 201–228. doi:10.1007/BF01173489

Schellong, J., Lorenz, P., & Weidner, K. (2019). Proposing a standardized, step-by-step model for creating post-traumatic stress disorder (PTSD) related mobile mental health apps in a framework based on technical and medical norms. *European Journal of Psychotraumatology*, *10*(1), 1611090. doi:10.1080/20008198.2019.1611090 PMID:31143412

Schultz, P. P., & Ryan, R. M. (2015). The "why,""what," and "how" of healthy self-regulation: Mindfulness and well-being from a self-determination theory perspective. In *Handbook of mindfulness and self-regulation* (pp. 81–94). Springer. doi:10.1007/978-1-4939-2263-5_7

Schwartz, D. A., & Graham, A. L. (2020). Potential maternal and infant outcomes from coronavirus 2019-NCOV (SARS-CoV-2) infecting pregnant women: Lessons from SARS, MERS, and other human coronavirus infections. In Viruses, 12(2). MDPI AG. doi:10.3390/v12020194

Seifer, D. B., Petok, W. D., Agrawal, A., Glenn, T. L., Bayer, A. H., Witt, B. R., Burgin, B. D., & Lieman, H. J. (2021). Psychological experience and coping strategies of patients in the Northeast US delaying care for infertility during the COVID-19 pandemic. *Reproductive Biology and Endocrinology*, *19*(1), 1–16. PMID:33397418

Seligman, M. E. P., & Csikszentmihalyi, M. (2014). Positive psychology: An introduction. In *Flow and the foundations of positive psychology* (pp. 279–298). Springer. doi:10.1007/978-94-017-9088-8_18

Semo, B., & Frissa, S. M. (2020). The mental health impact of the COVID-19 pandemic: Implications for sub-Saharan Africa. *Psychology Research and Behavior Management*, *13*, 713–720. doi:10.2147/PRBM.S264286 PMID:32982500

Shanbehzadeh, S., Tavahomi, M., Zanjari, N., Ebrahimi-Takamjani, I., & Amiri-Arimi, S. (2021). Physical and mental health complications post-COVID-19: Scoping review. *Journal of Psychosomatic Research*, *147*, 110525. doi:10.1016/j.jpsychores.2021.110525 PMID:34051516

Sharma, A. (2021). Retention and Engagement of Human Capital: Causal Contribution of Perceived Organi/alional Prestige and Job Characteristics. *The Journal of Applied Business and Economics*, *23*(2), 68–82.

Sharma, A., Tiwari, S., Deb, M. K., & Marty, J. L. (2020). Severe acute respiratory syndrome coronavirus-2 (SARS-CoV-2): A global pandemic and treatment strategies. *International Journal of Antimicrobial Agents*, *56*(2), 106054. doi:10.1016/j.ijantimicag.2020.106054 PMID:32534188

Sharma, N., & Vaish, H. (2020). Impact of COVID–19 on mental health and physical load on women professionals: An online cross-sectional survey. *Health Care for Women International*, *41*(11–12), 1255–1272. doi:10.1080/07399332.2020.1825441 PMID:33021925

Sharma, S., & Sharma, S. K. (2016). Team resilience: Scale development and validation. *Vision (Basel)*, *20*(1), 37–53. doi:10.1177/0972262916628952

Shorey, S., Lau, L. S. T., Tan, J. X., Ng, E. D., & Aishworiya, R. (2021). Families With Children With Neurodevelopmental Disorders During COVID-19: A Scoping Review. *Journal of Pediatric Psychology*, *46*(5), 514–525. doi:10.1093/jpepsy/jsab029 PMID:33758930

Simon, G. E., & Ludman, E. J. (2009). It's time for disruptive innovation in psychotherapy. *Lancet*, *374*(9690), 594–595. doi:10.1016/S0140-6736(09)61415-X PMID:19699995

Singh, S., Roy, D., Sinha, K., Parveen, S., Sharma, G., & Joshi, G. (2020). Impact of COVID-19 and lockdown on mental health of children and adolescents: A narrative review with recommendations. *Psychiatry Research*, *293*, 113429. doi:10.1016/j.psychres.2020.113429 PMID:32882598

Smit, B., & Wandel, J. (2006). Adaptation, adaptive capacity and vulnerability. *Global Environmental Change*, *16*(3), 282–292. doi:10.1016/j.gloenvcha.2006.03.008

Snyder, R., Shapiro, S., & Treleaven, D. (2012). Attachment theory and mindfulness. *Journal of Child and Family Studies*, *21*(5), 709–717. doi:10.100710826-011-9522-8

Soltani, M., Shairi, M. R., Roshan, R., & Rahimi, C. R. (2014). The impact of emotionally focused therapy on emotional distress in infertile couples. *International Journal of Fertility & Sterility*, *7*(4), 337. PMID:24520504

Speed, E. (2006). Patients, consumers, and survivors: A case study of mental health service user discourses. *Social Science & Medicine*, *62*(1), 28–38. doi:10.1016/j.socscimed.2005.05.025 PMID:15993529

Spialek, M. L., Czlapinski, H. M., & Houston, J. B. (2016). Disaster communication ecology and community resilience perceptions following the 2013 central Illinois tornadoes. *International Journal of Disaster Risk Reduction*, *17*, 154–160. doi:10.1016/j.ijdrr.2016.04.006

Stanisławski, K. (2019). The coping circumplex model: An integrative model of the structure of coping with stress. *Frontiers in Psychology*, *10*, 694. doi:10.3389/fpsyg.2019.00694 PMID:31040802

Steinberg, A., & Elmer, J. (2022). Public perceptions on post-cardiac arrest care and outcomes. In Resuscitation (Vol. 170). doi:10.1016/j.resuscitation.2021.11.011

Steinke, J., Bolunmez, B., Fletcher, L., Wang, V., Tomassetti, A. J., Repchick, K. M., Zaccaro, S. J., Dalal, R. S., & Tetrick, L. E. (2015). Improving cybersecurity incident response team effectiveness using teams-based research. *IEEE Security and Privacy*, *13*(4), 20–29. doi:10.1109/MSP.2015.71

Stinson, B., & Arthur, D. (2013). A novel EEG for alpha brain state training, neurobiofeedback and behavior change. *Complementary Therapies in Clinical Practice*, *19*(3), 114–118. doi:10.1016/j.ctcp.2013.03.003 PMID:23890456

Strassberger, M. (2022). *"We Live One Day at a Time": Families' Stories from the Early Months of the COVID-19 Pandemic.*

Stuijfzand, S. C. D.-T. (2020). *Psychological impact of an epidemic/pandemic on the mental health of healthcare professionals: a rapid review.* Commonwealth Fund.

Suzuki, K., & Hiratani, M. (2021). The association of mental health problems with preventive behavior and caregivers' anxiety about COVID-19 in children with neurodevelopmental disorders. *Frontiers in Psychiatry*, *12*, 713834. doi:10.3389/fpsyt.2021.713834 PMID:34335341

Tang, W., Hu, T., Hu, B., Jin, C., Wang, G., Xie, C., Chen, S., & Xu, J. (2020). Prevalence and correlates of PTSD and depressive symptoms one month after the outbreak of the COVID-19 epidemic in a sample of home-quarantined Chinese university students. *Journal of Affective Disorders*, *274*, 1–7. doi:10.1016/j.jad.2020.05.009 PMID:32405111

Tanjung, S. R., Syahrizal, & Abror. (2021). *The Influence of Organizational Climate Support on Psychological Well-Being and Employee Loyalty with Psychological Capital as Mediating Variables.* Proceedings of the Sixth Padang International Conference On Economics Education, Economics, Business and Management, Accounting and Entrepreneurship (PICEEBA 2020). Atlantis Press. 10.2991/aebmr.k.210616.078

Tanoue, Y., Nomura, S., Yoneoka, D., Kawashima, T., Eguchi, A., Shi, S., Harada, N., & Miyata, H. (2020). Mental health of family, friends, and co-workers of COVID-19 patients in Japan. *Psychiatry Research*, *291*, 113067. doi:10.1016/j.psychres.2020.113067 PMID:32535504

Taylor, S., Landry, C. A., Paluszek, M. M., Fergus, T. A., McKay, D., & Asmundson, G. J. G. (2020). Development and initial validation of the COVID Stress Scales. *Journal of Anxiety Disorders*, *72*, 102232. Advance online publication. doi:10.1016/j.janxdis.2020.102232 PMID:32408047

The Lancet. (2020). The gendered dimensions of COVID-19. *Lancet*, *395*(10231), 1168. doi:10.1016/S0140-6736(20)30823-0 PMID:32278370

Thibaut, F., & van Wijngaarden-Cremers, P. J. M. (2020). Women's mental health in the time of Covid-19 pandemic. *Frontiers in Global Women's Health*, *1*, 588372. doi:10.3389/fgwh.2020.588372 PMID:34816164

Times, T. E. (2020). Work from home burnout: Stress, insomnia, anxiety becoming the new normal. *The Economic Times*. https://economictimes.indiatimes.com/magazines/panache/work-from-home-burnout-stress-insomnia-anxiety-becoming-the-new-n ormal/articleshow/75425733.cms

Tippett, A. (2022). Life on pause: An analysis of UK fertility patients' coping mechanisms after the cancellation of fertility treatment due to COVID-19. *Journal of Health Psychology*, *27*(7), 1583–1600. doi:10.1177/1359105321999711 PMID:33685265

Tokgoz, V. Y., Kaya, Y., & Tekin, A. B. (2022). The level of anxiety in infertile women whose ART cycles are postponed due to the COVID-19 outbreak. *Journal of Psychosomatic Obstetrics and Gynaecology*, *43*(2), 114–121. doi:10.1080/0167482X.2020.1806819 PMID:32812477

Torales, J., O'Higgins, M., Castaldelli-Maia, J. M., & Ventriglio, A. (2020). The outbreak of COVID-19 coronavirus and its impact on global mental health. *The International Journal of Social Psychiatry*, *66*(4), 317–320. doi:10.1177/0020764020915212 PMID:32233719

Torous, J., Bucci, S., Bell, I. H., Kessing, L. V., Faurholt-Jepsen, M., Whelan, P., Carvalho, A. F., Keshavan, M., Linardon, J., & Firth, J. (2021). The growing field of digital psychiatry: Current evidence and the future of apps, social media, chatbots, and virtual reality. *World Psychiatry; Official Journal of the World Psychiatric Association (WPA)*, *20*(3), 318–335. doi:10.1002/wps.20883 PMID:34505369

Torous, J., & Roberts, L. W. (2017). Needed Innovation in Digital Health and Smartphone Applications for Mental Health: Transparency and Trust. *JAMA Psychiatry*, *74*(5), 437–438. doi:10.1001/jamapsychiatry.2017.0262 PMID:28384700

Travis, D. J., Nugent, J. S., & Lengnick-Hall, R. (2019). Cultivating healthy, inclusive workplaces: Why it matters and how organizations make progress. In *Creating psychologically healthy workplaces*. Edward Elgar Publishing. doi:10.4337/9781788113427.00029

Truss, C., Delbridge, R., Alfes, K., Shantz, A., & Soane, E. (2013). *Employee engagement in theory and practice*. Routledge London. doi:10.4324/9780203076965

Turabian, J. L. (2019). Doctor-Patient Relationship in the Case of Infertility: A Vision from General Medicine. [CrossRef]. *Adv. Reprod. Sci. Reprod. Health Infertil, 1*, 104.

Turocy, J. M., Robles, A., Hercz, D., D'Alton, M., Forman, E. J., & Williams, Z. (2020). THE EMOTIONAL IMPACT OF THE ASRM GUIDELINES ON FERTILITY PATIENTS DURING THE COVID-19 PANDEMIC. *Fertility and Sterility, 114*(3), e63. doi:10.1016/j.fertnstert.2020.08.194

Ueda, R., Okada, T., Kita, Y., Ozawa, Y., Inoue, H., Shioda, M., Kono, Y., Kono, C., Nakamura, Y., Amemiya, K., Ito, A., Sugiura, N., Matsuoka, Y., Kaiga, C., Kubota, M., & Ozawa, H. (2021). The quality of life of children with neurodevelopmental disorders and their parents during the Coronavirus disease 19 emergency in Japan. *Scientific Reports, 11*(1), 1–8. doi:10.1038/s41598-021-82743-x

Vaidyam, A. N., Wisniewski, H., Halamka, J. D., Kashavan, M. S., & Torous, J. B. (2019). Chatbots and Conversational Agents in Mental Health: A Review of the Psychiatric Landscape. *Canadian Journal of Psychiatry, 64*(7), 456–464. doi:10.1177/0706743719828977 PMID:30897957

Van Rheenen, T. E., Meyer, D., Neill, E., Phillipou, A., Tan, E. J., Toh, W. L., & Rossell, S. L. (2020). Mental health status of individuals with a mood-disorder during the COVID-19 pandemic in Australia: Initial results from the COLLATE project. *Journal of Affective Disorders, 275*, 69–77. doi:10.1016/j.jad.2020.06.037 PMID:32658826

Varvogli, L., & Darviri, C. (2011). Stress management techniques: Evidence-based procedures that reduce stress and promote health. *Health Science Journal, 5*, 74–89.

Venturella, I., Crivelli, D., Fronda, G., & Balconi, M. (2018). Neurocognitive enhancement: mindfulness practices applied to management. *10th International Scientific Conference on Neuroethics and 5th Conference of the Italian Society for Neuroethics*. N-A.

Venugopal, V. C., Mohan, A., & Chennabasappa, L. K. (2022). Status of mental health and its associated factors among the general populace of India during COVID-19 pandemic. *Asia-Pacific Psychiatry, 14*(2), e12412. doi:10.1111/appy.12412 PMID:32830876

Verma, A. K. (2021). *Understanding Domestic Violence in India During COVID-19: a Routine Activity Approach*. NIH.

Viana, R. B., Dankel, S. J., Loenneke, J. P., Gentil, P., Vieira, C. A., Andrade, M. dos S., Vancini, R. L., & de Lira, C. A. B. (2020). The effects of exergames on anxiety levels: A systematic review and meta-analysis. In Scandinavian Journal of Medicine and Science in Sports, 30(7), pp. 1100–1116. Blackwell Munksgaard. doi:10.1111ms.13654

Vitale, S. G., La Rosa, V. L., Rapisarda, A. M. C., & Laganà, A. S. (2017). Endometriosis and Infertility: The Impact on Quality of Life and Mental Health. *Journal of Endometriosis and Pelvic Pain Disorders, 9*(2), 112–115. doi:10.5301/je.5000274

Vitale, S. G., La Rosa, V. L., Rapisarda, A. M., & Lagana, A. S. (2017). Psychology of infertility and assisted reproductive treatment: The Italian situation. *Journal of Psychosomatic Obstetrics and Gynaecology*, *38*(1), 1–3. doi:10.1080/0167482X.2016.1244184 PMID:27750491

Vohra, M., & Pandey, N. (2018). Effects of mindfulness on psychological well-being among school going children. *IAHRW International Journal of Social Sciences Review*, *6*(5), 952–954.

Wainberg, M. L., Scorza, P., Shultz, J. M., Helpman, L., Mootz, J. J., Johnson, K. A., Neria, Y., Bradford, J. E., Oquendo, M. A., & Arbuckle, M. R. (2017). Challenges and Opportunities in Global Mental Health: A Research-to-Practice Perspective. *Current Psychiatry Reports*, *19*(5), 28. doi:10.100711920-017-0780-z PMID:28425023

Walker, A., & Hutton, D. M. (2006). The application of the psychological contract to workplace safety. *Journal of Safety Research*, *37*(5), 433–441. doi:10.1016/j.jsr.2006.06.001 PMID:17125794

Walker, E. R., Moore, E., Tapscott, S., Alperin, M., Cummings, J. R., & Druss, B. G. (2021). Developing Regional Mental Health Priorities: Mixed-Methods Needs Assessment of Eight States in the Southeastern United States. *Psychiatric Services (Washington, D.C.)*, *72*(3), 358–361. doi:10.1176/appi.ps.202000141 PMID:33234050

Walumbwa, F. O., Luthans, F., Avey, J. B., & Oke, A. (2011). Retracted: Authentically leading groups: The mediating role of collective psychological capital and trust. *Journal of Organizational Behavior*, *32*(1), 4–24. doi:10.1002/job.653

Wang, K., Varma, D. S., & Prosperi, M. (2018). A systematic review of the effectiveness of mobile apps for monitoring and management of mental health symptoms or disorders. *Journal of Psychiatric Research*, *107*, 73–78. doi:10.1016/j.jpsychires.2018.10.006 PMID:30347316

Wang, L., Li, D., Pan, S., Zhai, J., Xia, W., Sun, C., & Zou, M. (2021). The relationship between 2019-nCoV and psychological distress among parents of children with autism spectrum disorder. *Globalization and Health*, *17*(1), 1–14. doi:10.118612992-021-00674-8 PMID:33632259

Watts, S. E., & Andrews, G. (2014). Internet access is NOT restricted globally to high income countries: So why are evidenced based prevention and treatment programs for mental disorders so rare? *Asian Journal of Psychiatry*, *10*, 71–74. doi:10.1016/j.ajp.2014.06.007 PMID:25042956

Wegge, J., Van Dick, R., Fisher, G., Wecking, C., & Moltzen, K. (2006). Work motivation, organisational identification, and well-being in call centre work. *Work and Stress*, *20*(1), 60–83. doi:10.1080/02678370600655553

Wells, C. M., & Klocko, B. A. (2018). Principal well-being and resilience: Mindfulness as a means to that end. *NASSP Bulletin*, *102*(2), 161–173. doi:10.1177/0192636518777813

Wenham, C., Smith, J., & Morgan, R. (2020). COVID-19: The gendered impacts of the outbreak. *Lancet*, *395*(10227), 846–848. doi:10.1016/S0140-6736(20)30526-2 PMID:32151325

Wernsing, T. (2014). Psychological capital: A test of measurement invariance across 12 national cultures. *Journal of Leadership & Organizational Studies*, *21*(2), 179–190. doi:10.1177/1548051813515924

WHO. (2004). *Promoting mental health: Concepts, emerging evidence, practice: Summary report*. World Health Organization.

WHO. (2020). *Coronavirus disease (COVID-19), Situation Report*. WHO. https://apps.who.int/iris/handle/10665/332151

Wise, E. H., Hersh, M. A., & Gibson, C. M. (2012). Ethics, self-care, and well-being for psychologists: Reenvisioning the stress-distress continuum. *Professional Psychology, Research and Practice*, *43*(5), 487–494. doi:10.1037/a0029446

Wiweko, B., Ho, T. M., Tanaka, A., Raggio, V., Lee, J. R., Patil, M., Chan, C. C. W., Wutayavanich, T., Diao, F., Nair, S., & Mendiola, R. F. (2021). COVID-19 Pandemic Impacts Decision-Making and Psychosocial Behavior in Women Seeking Fertility Treatment in APAC—An ASPIRE Patient Experience Report. *Fertility & Reproduction*, *3*(03), 58–77. doi:10.1142/S2661318221500080

World Health Organization. (2004). *International Statistical Classification of Diseases and related health problems: Alphabetical index* (Vol. 3). World Health Organization.

World Health Organization. (2018). *Infertility*. International Classification of Diseases, 11th Revision (ICD-11)

World Health Organization. (2019). *International statistical classification of diseases and related health problems* (11th ed.). WHO. https://icd.who.int/

World Health Organization. (2020). *Coronavirus disease (COVID-19) advice for the public: Advocacy*. WHO. https://www.who.int/emergencies/diseases/novel-coronavirus-2019/advice-for-public/healthy-parenting

Wyn, J., Cahill, H., Holdsworth, R., Rowling, L., & Carson, S. (2000). MindMatters, a whole-school approach promoting mental health and well-being. *The Australian and New Zealand Journal of Psychiatry*, *34*(4), 594–601. doi:10.1080/j.1440-1614.2000.00748.x PMID:10954390

Xiang, Y., Li, W., Zhang, Q., Jin, Y., Rao, W., Zeng, L., Lok, G. K. I., Chow, I. H. I., Cheung, T., & Hall, B. J. (2020). Correspondence Timely research papers about COVID-19 in. *Lancet*, *6736*(20), 30375. doi:10.1016/S0140-6736(20)30375-5 PMID:32078803

Yamamoto, T., Tanaka, S., Yoshizaki, A., Yoshimura, Y., Fauzi, A. A., Syarinaz, A., Adlan, A., Jayanath, S., Hamzah, N., Fujino, H., & Tachibana, M. (2022). *Relationship between children with neurodevelopmental disorders and their caregivers and friends during early phase of COVID-19 school closure in Japan: Association with difficulty in implementing infection prevention.*

Yang, J., Lopez Cervera, R., Tye, S. J., Ekker, S. C., & Pierret, C. (2018). Adolescent mental health education InSciEd Out: A case study of an alternative middle school population. *Journal of Translational Medicine*, *16*(1), 1–10. doi:10.118612967-018-1459-x PMID:29615090

Yasmin, H. (2020). Covid 19: Stress Management among Students and its Impact on Their Effective Learning. *International Technology and Education Journal, 4*(2).

Yuan, B., Li, W., Liu, H., Cai, X., Song, S., Zhao, J., Hu, X., Li, Z., Chen, Y., Zhang, K., Liu, Z., Peng, J., Wang, C., Wang, J., & An, Y. (2020). Correlation between immune response and self-reported depression during convalescence from COVID-19. *Brain, Behavior, and Immunity*, *88*, 39–43. doi:10.1016/j.bbi.2020.05.062 PMID:32464158

Yu, S. (2018). Uncovering the hidden impacts of inequality on mental health: A global study. *Translational Psychiatry*, *8*(1), 1–10. doi:10.103841398-018-0148-0 PMID:29777100

Zhai, Y., & Du, X. (2020). Loss and grief amidst COVID-19: A path to adaptation and resilience. *Brain, Behavior, and Immunity*, *87*, 80–81. doi:10.1016/j.bbi.2020.04.053 PMID:32335197

Zhang, J., Shuai, L., Yu, H., Wang, Z., Qiu, M., Lu, L., Cao, X., Xia, W., Wang, Y., & Chen, R. (2020). Acute stress, behavioural symptoms and mood states among school-age children with attention-deficit/hyperactive disorder during the COVID-19 outbreak. *Asian Journal of Psychiatry*, *51*, 102077. doi:10.1016/j.ajp.2020.102077 PMID:32315967

Zhao, M., Wang, M., Zhang, J., Ye, J., Xu, Y., Wang, Z., Ye, D., Liu, J., & Wan, J. (2020). Advances in the relationship between coronavirus infection and cardiovascular diseases. In *Biomedicine and Pharmacotherapy* (Vol. 127). Elsevier Masson SAS., doi:10.1016/j.biopha.2020.110230

Zhao, X., Lin, X., Chen, M., & Mahmood, S. (2022). Research on the influence mechanism of entrepreneurial environment on college students' entrepreneurial performance based on psychology. *Psychiatria Danubina*, *34*(suppl 2), 319–319.

Zhu, N., Zhang, D., & Wang, W. (2019). A novel coronavirus from patients with pneumonia in China. *The New England Journal of Medicine*, *2020*(382), 727–733. PMID:31978945

Zhu, Y., Zhang, L., Zhou, X., Li, C., & Yang, D. (2021). Thc impact of social distancing during COVID-19: A conditional process model of negative emotions, alienation, affective disorders, and post-traumatic stress disorder. *Journal of Affective Disorders*, *281*, 131–137. doi:10.1016/j.jad.2020.12.004 PMID:33316718

Zimbardo, P. G., Haney, C., Banks, W. C., & Jaffe, D. (1973). Interpersonal dynamics in a simulated prison. *International Journal of Criminology and Penology*, *1*, 69–97.

Zineldin, M., & Hytter, A. (2012). Leaders' negative emotions and leadership styles influencing subordinates' well-being. *International Journal of Human Resource Management*, *23*(4), 748–758. doi:10.1080/09585192.2011.606114

Related References

To continue our tradition of advancing academic research, we have compiled a list of recommended IGI Global readings. These references will provide additional information and guidance to further enrich your knowledge and assist you with your own research and future publications.

Ababio, G. K. (2018). Nutraceuticals: The Dose Makes the Difference – It's All in the Dose. In A. Verma, K. Srivastava, S. Singh, & H. Singh (Eds.), *Nutraceuticals and Innovative Food Products for Healthy Living and Preventive Care* (pp. 24–47). Hershey, PA: IGI Global. doi:10.4018/978-1-5225-2970-5.ch002

Adams, M. G. (2018). Systematically Investigating Instructor Impact on Student Satisfaction in Graduate Programs. In D. Polly, M. Putman, T. Petty, & A. Good (Eds.), *Innovative Practices in Teacher Preparation and Graduate-Level Teacher Education Programs* (pp. 200–214). Hershey, PA: IGI Global. doi:10.4018/978-1-5225-3068-8.ch012

Akgül, Y., & Tunca, M. Z. (2018). Proliferating View of Knowledge Management and Balanced Scorecard Outcome Linkage. In N. Baporikar (Ed.), *Global Practices in Knowledge Management for Societal and Organizational Development* (pp. 168–193). Hershey, PA: IGI Global. doi:10.4018/978-1-5225-3009-1.ch008

Alcaraz-Valencia, P. A., Gaytán-Lugo, L. S., & Gallardo, S. C. (2018). An Exploratory Study on the Interaction Beyond Virtual Environments to Improve Listening Ability When Learning English as a Second Language. In F. Cipolla-Ficarra (Ed.), *Optimizing Human-Computer Interaction With Emerging Technologies* (pp. 306–331). Hershey, PA: IGI Global. doi:10.4018/978-1-5225-2616-2.ch013

Altıntaş, F. Ç., & Kavurmacı, C. (2018). Value Statements in Web Pages of Turkish State Universities: A Basic Classification. In U. Thomas (Ed.), *Advocacy in Academia and the Role of Teacher Preparation Programs* (pp. 302–316). Hershey, PA: IGI Global. doi:10.4018/978-1-5225-2906-4.ch017

Amoroso, D. L. (2018). The Importance of Advocacy on Reputation and Loyalty: Comparison of Japanese, Chinese, and the Filipino Consumers. In P. Ordóñez de Pablos (Ed.), *Management Strategies and Technology Fluidity in the Asian Business Sector* (pp. 114–125). Hershey, PA: IGI Global. doi:10.4018/978-1-5225-4056-4.ch007

Atiku, S. O., & Fields, Z. (2018). Organisational Learning Dimensions and Talent Retention Strategies for the Service Industries. In N. Baporikar (Ed.), *Global Practices in Knowledge Management for Societal and Organizational Development* (pp. 358–381). Hershey, PA: IGI Global. doi:10.4018/978-1-5225-3009-1.ch017

Ayoola-Amale, A. (2018). Women in Leadership: Why We Need More Women Leaders. In B. Cook (Ed.), *Handbook of Research on Examining Global Peacemaking in the Digital Age* (pp. 211–222). Hershey, PA: IGI Global. doi:10.4018/978-1-5225-3032-9.ch015

Baran, A. G. (2018). Through the Syrians Refuge in Turkey Towards the Creation of the War Migration Theory. In Ş. Erçetin (Ed.), *Social Considerations of Migration Movements and Immigration Policies* (pp. 178–196). Hershey, PA: IGI Global. doi:10.4018/978-1-5225-3322-1.ch011

Beckett-Camarata, J. (2018). Public Choice and Financing Local Government Fiscal Reform in Albania. In H. Levine & K. Moreno (Eds.), *Positioning Markets and Governments in Public Management* (pp. 197–208). Hershey, PA: IGI Global. doi:10.4018/978-1-5225-4177-6.ch015

Bedford, D. A. (2018). Sustainable Knowledge Management Strategies: Aligning Business Capabilities and Knowledge Management Goals. In N. Baporikar (Ed.), *Global Practices in Knowledge Management for Societal and Organizational Development* (pp. 46–73). Hershey, PA: IGI Global. doi:10.4018/978-1-5225-3009-1.ch003

Benaouda, A., & García-Peñalvo, F. J. (2018). Towards an Intelligent System for the Territorial Planning: Agricultural Case. In F. García-Peñalvo (Ed.), *Global Implications of Emerging Technology Trends* (pp. 158–178). Hershey, PA: IGI Global. doi:10.4018/978-1-5225-4944-4.ch010

Beneventi, P. (2018). When Technology Becomes Popular: A Multimedia, Shared Production for the Information Age. In *Technology and the New Generation of Active Citizens: Emerging Research and Opportunities* (pp. 23–44). Hershey, PA: IGI Global. doi:10.4018/978-1-5225-3770-0.ch002

Bernal, L. D., & Cusi, M. L. (2018). Corporate Entrepreneurship in Colombia: Contrast Cases of Two Colombian Manufacturing SMEs. In R. Perez-Uribe, C. Salcedo-Perez, & D. Ocampo-Guzman (Eds.), *Handbook of Research on Intrapreneurship and Organizational Sustainability in SMEs* (pp. 368–390). Hershey, PA: IGI Global. doi:10.4018/978-1-5225-3543-0.ch017

Berning, S. C., & Ambrosius, J. (2018). How the Human Resource Practices of Chinese MNEs in Africa Create Economic Growth and Livelihood Options. In S. Hipsher (Ed.), *Examining the Private Sector's Role in Wealth Creation and Poverty Reduction* (pp. 85–109). Hershey, PA: IGI Global. doi:10.4018/978-1-5225-3117-3.ch005

Bharti, A., & Mittal, A. (2018). Perishable Goods Supply Cold Chain Management in India. In A. Kumar & S. Saurav (Eds.), *Supply Chain Management Strategies and Risk Assessment in Retail Environments* (pp. 232–246). Hershey, PA: IGI Global. doi:10.4018/978-1-5225-3056-5.ch013

Bhattacharya, S., Kumar, R. V., & Dutta, A. (2018). Exploring Kapferer's Brand Identity Prism Applicability in Indian Political Marketing Aspect With Special Focus to Youth Voters. In Rajagopal, & R. Behl (Eds.), Start-Up Enterprises and Contemporary Innovation Strategies in the Global Marketplace (pp. 136-152). Hershey, PA: IGI Global. doi:10.4018/978-1-5225-4831-7.ch010

Bhattarai, R. K. (2018). Enterprise Immune System. In *Enterprise Resiliency in the Continuum of Change: Emerging Research and Opportunities* (pp. 88–111). Hershey, PA: IGI Global. doi:10.4018/978-1-5225-2627-8.ch003

Bhattarai, R. K. (2018). Enterprise Philosophy. In *Enterprise Resiliency in the Continuum of Change: Emerging Research and Opportunities* (pp. 1–43). Hershey, PA: IGI Global. doi:10.4018/978-1-5225-2627-8.ch001

Bhattarai, R. K. (2018). Enterprise Resiliency. In *Enterprise Resiliency in the Continuum of Change: Emerging Research and Opportunities* (pp. 112–137). Hershey, PA: IGI Global. doi:10.4018/978-1-5225-2627-8.ch004

Bisen, S. S., & Deshpande, Y. (2018). The Impact of the Internet in Twenty-First Century Addictions: An Overview. In B. Bozoglan (Ed.), *Psychological, Social, and Cultural Aspects of Internet Addiction* (pp. 1–19). Hershey, PA: IGI Global. doi:10.4018/978-1-5225-3477-8.ch001

Biswal, S. K. (2018). Branding Culture: A Study of Telugu Film Industry. In S. Dasgupta, S. Biswal, & M. Ramesh (Eds.), *Holistic Approaches to Brand Culture and Communication Across Industries* (pp. 1–23). Hershey, PA: IGI Global. doi:10.4018/978-1-5225-3150-0.ch001

Blake, S., & Burkett, C. M. (2018). Individual Creativity: Predictors and Characteristics. In *Creativity in Workforce Development and Innovation: Emerging Research and Opportunities* (pp. 88–104). Hershey, PA: IGI Global. doi:10.4018/978-1-5225-4952-9.ch005

Blomeley, S., & Hamilton, A. H. (2018). Writing Partners: Bridging the Personal and Social in the Service-Learning Classroom. In O. Delano-Oriaran, M. Penick-Parks, & S. Fondrie (Eds.), *Culturally Engaging Service-Learning With Diverse Communities* (pp. 202–222). Hershey, PA: IGI Global. doi:10.4018/978-1-5225-2900-2.ch012

Bohra, M., & Visen, A. (2018). Nutraceutical Properties in Flowers. In A. Verma, K. Srivastava, S. Singh, & H. Singh (Eds.), *Nutraceuticals and Innovative Food Products for Healthy Living and Preventive Care* (pp. 217–235). Hershey, PA: IGI Global. doi:10.4018/978-1-5225-2970-5.ch010

Boyd, L. N. (2018). Fortifying Parent Partnerships Through the Black Church Space. In K. Norris & S. Collier (Eds.), *Social Justice and Parent Partnerships in Multicultural Education Contexts* (pp. 118–137). Hershey, PA: IGI Global. doi:10.4018/978-1-5225-3943-8.ch007

Bozoglan, B. (2018). The Role of Family Factors in Internet Addiction Among Children and Adolescents: An Overview. In B. Bozoglan (Ed.), *Psychological, Social, and Cultural Aspects of Internet Addiction* (pp. 146–168). Hershey, PA: IGI Global. doi:10.4018/978-1-5225-3477-8.ch008

Briz-Ponce, L., Juanes-Méndez, J. A., & García-Peñalvo, F. J. (2018). Current Situation and Appraisal Tendencies of M-Learning. In F. García-Peñalvo (Ed.), *Global Implications of Emerging Technology Trends* (pp. 115–129). Hershey, PA: IGI Global. doi:10.4018/978-1-5225-4944-4.ch007

Brkljačić, T., Majetić, F., & Wertag, A. (2018). I'm Always Online: Well-Being and Main Sources of Life Dis/Satisfaction of Heavy Internet Users. In B. Bozoglan (Ed.), *Psychological, Social, and Cultural Aspects of Internet Addiction* (pp. 72–89). Hershey, PA: IGI Global. doi:10.4018/978-1-5225-3477-8.ch004

Brown, M. A. Sr. (2018). Defining Your Team. In *Motivationally Intelligent Leadership: Emerging Research and Opportunities* (pp. 1–22). Hershey, PA: IGI Global. doi:10.4018/978-1-5225-3746-5.ch001

Brown, M. A. Sr. (2018). Empowering Leaders With Tools. In *Motivationally Intelligent Leadership: Emerging Research and Opportunities* (pp. 72–96). Hershey, PA: IGI Global. doi:10.4018/978-1-5225-3746-5.ch006

Brown, M. A. Sr. (2018). Sensemaking Theory. In *Motivationally Intelligent Leadership: Emerging Research and Opportunities* (pp. 46–55). Hershey, PA: IGI Global. doi:10.4018/978-1-5225-3746-5.ch004

Brown, S., & Bousalis, R. (2018). Best Practices in K-12 Arts Integration: Curricular Connections. In *Curriculum Integration in Contemporary Teaching Practice: Emerging Research and Opportunities* (pp. 95–124). Hershey, PA: IGI Global. doi:10.4018/978-1-5225-4065-6.ch004

Brown, S., & Bousalis, R. (2018). Interdisciplinary Curriculum in K-12 Schools: Current Practices in the Field. In *Curriculum Integration in Contemporary Teaching Practice: Emerging Research and Opportunities* (pp. 125–143). Hershey, PA: IGI Global. doi:10.4018/978-1-5225-4065-6.ch005

Bullock, C. A. (2018). Collaboration: Academes, Government, and Community to Drive Economic Uplift and Empowerment. In S. Burton (Ed.), *Engaged Scholarship and Civic Responsibility in Higher Education* (pp. 1–24). Hershey, PA: IGI Global. doi:10.4018/978-1-5225-3649-9.ch001

Burdenko, E. V., & Mudrova, S. V. (2018). Indicators System as a Measure of Development Level of Knowledge Economy: Application of World Bank Methodology. In N. Baporikar (Ed.), *Global Practices in Knowledge Management for Societal and Organizational Development* (pp. 74–105). Hershey, PA: IGI Global. doi:10.4018/978-1-5225-3009-1.ch004

Burston, B., & Collier-Stewart, S. (2018). STEM for All: The Importance of Parent/School/Community Partnerships Across the K-12 Pipeline and Beyond. In K. Norris & S. Collier (Eds.), *Social Justice and Parent Partnerships in Multicultural Education Contexts* (pp. 274–288). Hershey, PA: IGI Global. doi:10.4018/978-1-5225-3943-8.ch015

Carboni, M., & Perelli, C. (2018). "Beyond" Religious Tourism: The Case of Fez. In H. El-Gohary, D. Edwards, & R. Eid (Eds.), *Global Perspectives on Religious Tourism and Pilgrimage* (pp. 71–83). Hershey, PA: IGI Global. doi:10.4018/978-1-5225-2796-1.ch005

Cascella, M., Muzio, M. R., Bimonte, S., & Cuomo, A. (2018). Nutraceuticals for Prevention of Chemotherapy-Induced Peripheral Neuropathy. In A. Verma, K. Srivastava, S. Singh, & H. Singh (Eds.), *Nutraceuticals and Innovative Food Products for Healthy Living and Preventive Care* (pp. 236–259). Hershey, PA: IGI Global. doi:10.4018/978-1-5225-2970-5.ch011

Cena, F., Rapp, A., Likavec, S., & Marcengo, A. (2018). Envisioning the Future of Personalization Through Personal Informatics: A User Study. *International Journal of Mobile Human Computer Interaction, 10*(1), 52–66. doi:10.4018/IJMHCI.2018010104

Chandiramani, J., & Airy, A. (2018). Urbanization and Socio-Economic Growth in South Asia Region. In U. Benna & I. Benna (Eds.), *Urbanization and Its Impact on Socio-Economic Growth in Developing Regions* (pp. 130–154). Hershey, PA: IGI Global. doi:10.4018/978-1-5225-2659-9.ch007

Chang, Y., Choi, S. B., Lee, J., & Jin, W. C. (2018). Population Size vs. Number of Crimes: Is the Relationship Superlinear? *International Journal of Information Systems and Social Change, 9*(1), 26–39. doi:10.4018/IJISSC.2018010102

Chaudhary, N. S., & Yadav, R. (2018). Cross-Cultural Conflicts: Concept, Causes, and Elucidations. In N. Sharma, V. Singh, & S. Pathak (Eds.), *Management Techniques for a Diverse and Cross-Cultural Workforce* (pp. 79–96). Hershey, PA: IGI Global. doi:10.4018/978-1-5225-4933-8.ch005

Chirisa, I., Mukarwi, L., & Matamanda, A. R. (2018). Social Costs and Benefits of the Transformation of the Traditional Families in an African Urban Society. In U. Benna & I. Benna (Eds.), *Urbanization and Its Impact on Socio-Economic Growth in Developing Regions* (pp. 179–197). Hershey, PA: IGI Global. doi:10.4018/978-1-5225-2659-9.ch009

Chitima, S. S., & Ndlovu, I. (2018). Incorporating Indigenous Knowledge in the Preservation of Collections at the Batonga Community Museum in Zimbabwe. In P. Ngulube (Ed.), *Handbook of Research on Heritage Management and Preservation* (pp. 396–407). Hershey, PA: IGI Global. doi:10.4018/978-1-5225-3137-1.ch019

Choudhury, D. K., & Rao, P. (2018). Determinants of FDI Inflows in Developing Countries: A Dynamic Panel Approach. In V. Malepati & C. Gowri (Eds.), *Foreign Direct Investments (FDIs) and Opportunities for Developing Economies in the World Market* (pp. 25–45). Hershey, PA: IGI Global. doi:10.4018/978-1-5225-3026-8.ch002

Cipolla-Ficarra, F. V., Carré, J., Quiroga, A., & Ficarra, V. M. (2018). Anti-Models for Architectural Graphic Expression and UX Education. In F. Cipolla-Ficarra, M. Ficarra, M. Cipolla-Ficarra, A. Quiroga, J. Alma, & J. Carré (Eds.), *Technology-Enhanced Human Interaction in Modern Society* (pp. 218–233). Hershey, PA: IGI Global. doi:10.4018/978-1-5225-3437-2.ch011

Cipolla-Ficarra, F. V., Ficarra, V. M., & Cipolla-Ficarra, M. (2018). Inverted Semanteme Into Financial Information Online. In F. Cipolla-Ficarra, M. Ficarra, M. Cipolla-Ficarra, A. Quiroga, J. Alma, & J. Carré (Eds.), *Technology-Enhanced Human Interaction in Modern Society* (pp. 263–283). Hershey, PA: IGI Global. doi:10.4018/978-1-5225-3437-2.ch013

Cipolla-Ficarra, F. V., Quiroga, A., & Ficarra, V. M. (2018). Kernel of the Labyrinths Hypertextuals. In F. Cipolla-Ficarra, M. Ficarra, M. Cipolla-Ficarra, A. Quiroga, J. Alma, & J. Carré (Eds.), *Technology-Enhanced Human Interaction in Modern Society* (pp. 122–142). Hershey, PA: IGI Global. doi:10.4018/978-1-5225-3437-2.ch006

Coffey, S. M. (2018). Unveilings Through Transformative Pedagogy: Striving for Realization of Du Bois' Educational Paradigm. In U. Thomas (Ed.), *Advocacy in Academia and the Role of Teacher Preparation Programs* (pp. 206–224). Hershey, PA: IGI Global. doi:10.4018/978-1-5225-2906-4.ch012

da Rocha, J. P. (2018). Process Outcomes. In *Political Mediation in Modern Conflict Resolution: Emerging Research and Opportunities* (pp. 155–164). Hershey, PA: IGI Global. doi:10.4018/978-1-5225-5118-8.ch004

Dahiya, K., & Dhankhar, R. (2018). Role of Nutraceuticals in Cancer. In A. Verma, K. Srivastava, S. Singh, & H. Singh (Eds.), *Nutraceuticals and Innovative Food Products for Healthy Living and Preventive Care* (pp. 176–194). Hershey, PA: IGI Global. doi:10.4018/978-1-5225-2970-5.ch008

Dasgupta, S., & Kothari, R. (2018). The Impact of Digital Word-of-Mouth Communication on Consumer Decision-Making Processes: With Special Reference to Fashion Apparel Industry. In S. Dasgupta, S. Biswal, & M. Ramesh (Eds.), *Holistic Approaches to Brand Culture and Communication Across Industries* (pp. 176–198). Hershey, PA: IGI Global. doi:10.4018/978-1-5225-3150-0.ch010

Dávila, F. A. (2018). Relationship Lending and Entrepreneurial Behavior: A Game-Theoretic-Based Modeling. In Rajagopal, & R. Behl (Eds.), Start-Up Enterprises and Contemporary Innovation Strategies in the Global Marketplace (pp. 65-86). Hershey, PA: IGI Global. doi:10.4018/978-1-5225-4831-7.ch006 de Sousa, J. C. (2018). Memory. In *Neuromarketing and Big Data Analytics for Strategic Consumer Engagement: Emerging Research and Opportunities* (pp. 92–100). Hershey, PA: IGI Global. doi:10.4018/978-1-5225-4834-8.ch006

de Sousa, J. C. (2018). Sensory and Motor System. In *Neuromarketing and Big Data Analytics for Strategic Consumer Engagement: Emerging Research and Opportunities* (pp. 68–91). Hershey, PA: IGI Global. doi:10.4018/978-1-5225-4834-8.ch005

Deka, D. B., & Jadeja, M. (2018). Childhood Sexual Abuse: Prevention and Intervention. In R. Gopalan (Ed.), *Social, Psychological, and Forensic Perspectives on Sexual Abuse* (pp. 127–146). Hershey, PA: IGI Global. doi:10.4018/978-1-5225-3958-2.ch010

Dobell, E., Herold, S., & Buckley, J. (2018). Spreadsheet Error Types and Their Prevalence in a Healthcare Context. *Journal of Organizational and End User Computing*, *30*(2), 20–42. doi:10.4018/JOEUC.2018040102

Donert, K., & Papoutsis, P. (2018). School on the Cloud: Connecting Education to the Cloud for Digital Citizenship. In K. Koutsopoulos, K. Doukas, & Y. Kotsanis (Eds.), *Handbook of Research on Educational Design and Cloud Computing in Modern Classroom Settings* (pp. 157–182). Hershey, PA: IGI Global. doi:10.4018/978-1-5225-3053-4.ch008

Downton, M. P. (2018). Preparation for Future Teaching: Authentic Activities in a Teacher Education Classroom. In D. Polly, M. Putman, T. Petty, & A. Good (Eds.), *Innovative Practices in Teacher Preparation and Graduate-Level Teacher Education Programs* (pp. 293–305). Hershey, PA: IGI Global. doi:10.4018/978-1-5225-3068-8.ch016

Drivas, G., Sotiriou, C., Bonanou, H., Saliari, S., Balafouti, M., & Tsevi, H. (2018). The Sky Is the Limit! In K. Koutsopoulos, K. Doukas, & Y. Kotsanis (Eds.), *Handbook of Research on Educational Design and Cloud Computing in Modern Classroom Settings* (pp. 101–121). Hershey, PA: IGI Global. doi:10.4018/978-1-5225-3053-4.ch006

Erçetin, Ş. Ş., & Bisaso, S. M. (2018). Migration and Refugee Crisis: Structural and Managerial Implications for Education. In Ş. Erçetin (Ed.), *Educational Development and Infrastructure for Immigrants and Refugees* (pp. 47–71). Hershey, PA: IGI Global. doi:10.4018/978-1-5225-3325-2.ch003

Erçetin, Ş. Ş., & Kubilay, S. (2018). Educational Expectations of Refugee Mothers for Their Children. In Ş. Erçetin (Ed.), *Educational Development and Infrastructure for Immigrants and Refugees* (pp. 171–195). Hershey, PA: IGI Global. doi:10.4018/978-1-5225-3325-2.ch009

Erçetin, Ş. Ş., Potas, N., Açıkalın, Ş. N., Özdemir, N., & Doğan, A. M. (2018). Municipalities and Refugee Crisis: Ansar Policies and Numbers. In Ş. Erçetin (Ed.), *Social Considerations of Migration Movements and Immigration Policies* (pp. 46–57). Hershey, PA: IGI Global. doi:10.4018/978-1-5225-3322-1.ch003

Erkekoğlu, L. C., & Madi, İ. (2018). The Hashemite Kingdom of Jordan. In S. Ozdemir, S. Erdogan, & A. Gedikli (Eds.), *Handbook of Research on Sociopolitical Factors Impacting Economic Growth in Islamic Nations* (pp. 95–121). Hershey, PA: IGI Global. doi:10.4018/978-1-5225-2939-2.ch006

Essien, E. D. (2018). Strengthening Performance of Civil Society Through Dialogue and Critical Thinking in Nigeria: Its Ethical Implications. In S. Chhabra (Ed.), *Handbook of Research on Civic Engagement and Social Change in Contemporary Society* (pp. 82–102). Hershey, PA: IGI Global. doi:10.4018/978-1-5225-4197-4.ch005

Feza, N. N. (2018). The Socioeconomic Status Label Associated With Mathematics. In I. Tshabangu (Ed.), *Global Ideologies Surrounding Children's Rights and Social Justice* (pp. 186–203). Hershey, PA: IGI Global. doi:10.4018/978-1-5225-2578-3.ch012

Fleener, J., Lu, L., Dun, J., & Mingquan, Y. (2018). Sustaining a Teacher Professional Learning Community in China Through Technology. In H. Spires (Ed.), *Digital Transformation and Innovation in Chinese Education* (pp. 80–99). Hershey, PA: IGI Global. doi:10.4018/978-1-5225-2924-8.ch005

Forge, J. (2018). Defence. In *The Morality of Weapons Design and Development: Emerging Research and Opportunities* (pp. 52–77). Hershey, PA: IGI Global. doi:10.4018/978-1-5225-3984-1.ch004

Forge, J. (2018). Justification. In *The Morality of Weapons Design and Development: Emerging Research and Opportunities* (pp. 78–93). Hershey, PA: IGI Global. doi:10.4018/978-1-5225-3984-1.ch005

Forge, J. (2018). Projectile Weapons. In *The Morality of Weapons Design and Development: Emerging Research and Opportunities* (pp. 94–117). Hershey, PA: IGI Global. doi:10.4018/978-1-5225-3984-1.ch006

Forge, J. (2018). Proportionality, Just War Theory, and Weapons Design. In *The Morality of Weapons Design and Development: Emerging Research and Opportunities* (pp. 139–154). Hershey, PA: IGI Global. doi:10.4018/978-1-5225-3984-1.ch008

Forge, J. (2018). Purposes and Means. In *The Morality of Weapons Design and Development: Emerging Research and Opportunities* (pp. 34–51). Hershey, PA: IGI Global. doi:10.4018/978-1-5225-3984-1.ch003

Fudge, M. (2018). The Inequity of User Fees and the Overreliance by Communities to Generate Revenue. In H. Levine & K. Moreno (Eds.), *Positioning Markets and Governments in Public Management* (pp. 147–158). Hershey, PA: IGI Global. doi:10.4018/978-1-5225-4177-6.ch011

Furumoto, R. R. (2018). Mexican-American Parents Using Critical Literacy to Address Climate Change. In K. Norris & S. Collier (Eds.), *Social Justice and Parent Partnerships in Multicultural Education Contexts* (pp. 187–208). Hershey, PA: IGI Global. doi:10.4018/978-1-5225-3943-8.ch010

Gabay, D. (2018). Who's Represented in Canadian Teaching and Learning Centres? In B. Blummer, J. Kenton, & M. Wiatrowski (Eds.), *Promoting Ethnic Diversity and Multiculturalism in Higher Education* (pp. 172–198). Hershey, PA: IGI Global. doi:10.4018/978-1-5225-4097-7.ch010

Garner, G. (2018). Foundations for Yoga Practice in Rehabilitation. In S. Telles & N. Singh (Eds.), *Research-Based Perspectives on the Psychophysiology of Yoga* (pp. 263–307). Hershey, PA: IGI Global. doi:10.4018/978-1-5225-2788-6.ch015

Geethanjali, P. (2018). Bio-Inspired Techniques in Human-Computer Interface for Control of Assistive Devices: Bio-Inspired Techniques in Assistive Devices. In D. Lopez & M. Durai (Eds.), *HCI Challenges and Privacy Preservation in Big Data Security* (pp. 23–46). Hershey, PA: IGI Global. doi:10.4018/978-1-5225-2863-0.ch002

Gharote, M. (2018). Common Features Between Findings in Traditional Texts and Contemporary Science: Yoga Texts and Contemporary Science. In S. Telles & N. Singh (Eds.), *Research-Based Perspectives on the Psychophysiology of Yoga* (pp. 309–315). Hershey, PA: IGI Global. doi:10.4018/978-1-5225-2788-6.ch016

Giosi, A., Zaccaro, E., & Testarmata, S. (2018). Social Responsibility, Shared Value, and Business Modelling: An Integrated Approach. In M. Risso & S. Testarmata (Eds.), *Value Sharing for Sustainable and Inclusive Development* (pp. 100–121). Hershey, PA: IGI Global. doi:10.4018/978-1-5225-3147-0.ch005

Grădinaru, C., Toma, S. I., & Marinescu, P. I. (2018). Entrepreneurial Thinking in the Educational System. In M. Risso & S. Testarmata (Eds.), *Value Sharing for Sustainable and Inclusive Development* (pp. 29–48). Hershey, PA: IGI Global. doi:10.4018/978-1-5225-3147-0.ch002

Güler, A. (2018). PKK-Related Asylum Applications from Turkey: Counter-Terrorism Measures vs. Refugee Status. In Ş. Erçetin (Ed.), *Social Considerations of Migration Movements and Immigration Policies* (pp. 117–142). Hershey, PA: IGI Global. doi:10.4018/978-1-5225-3322-1.ch008

Gupta, S. K. (2018). Sexual Abuse of Children and Adults With Intellectual Disabilities: Preventive, Supportive, and Intervention Strategies for Clinical Practice. In R. Gopalan (Ed.), *Social, Psychological, and Forensic Perspectives on Sexual Abuse* (pp. 197–206). Hershey, PA: IGI Global. doi:10.4018/978-1-5225-3958-2.ch014

Gürcan, Ö. F., & Gümüşsoy, Ç. A. (2018). Factors Influencing Effective Knowledge Transfer in Organizations. In N. Baporikar (Ed.), *Global Practices in Knowledge Management for Societal and Organizational Development* (pp. 271–292). Hershey, PA: IGI Global. doi:10.4018/978-1-5225-3009-1.ch013

Hagen, I., Kofoed, S., & Nayar, U. (2018). Yoga for Psychological Wellbeing in Modern Life and Contexts. In S. Telles & N. Singh (Eds.), *Research-Based Perspectives on the Psychophysiology of Yoga* (pp. 316–334). Hershey, PA: IGI Global. doi:10.4018/978-1-5225-2788-6.ch017

Handayani, B. (2018). The Paradox of Authenticity and Its Implications for Contemporary and "Bizarre" Tourism Campaigns. In S. Sarma (Ed.), *Global Observations of the Influence of Culture on Consumer Buying Behavior* (pp. 48–65). Hershey, PA: IGI Global. doi:10.4018/978-1-5225-2727-5.ch003

Huamaní, G. A., Fernández-López, S., Gómez, I. N., Rey-Ares, L., Rodríguez-Gulías, M. J., & Rodeiro-Pazos, D. (2018). The Role Models as Determinants of New Technology-Based Firms: An Exploratory Study. In A. Carrizo Moreira, J. Guilherme Leitão Dantas, & F. Manuel Valente (Eds.), *Nascent Entrepreneurship and Successful New Venture Creation* (pp. 272–288). Hershey, PA: IGI Global. doi:10.4018/978-1-5225-2936-1.ch013

Hucks, D., Sturtz, T., & Tirabassi, K. (2018). Building, Shaping, and Modeling Tools for Literacy Development and Civic Engagement. In *Fostering Positive Civic Engagement Among Millennials: Emerging Research and Opportunities* (pp. 22–35). Hershey, PA: IGI Global. doi:10.4018/978-1-5225-2452-6.ch002

Hucks, D., Sturtz, T., & Tirabassi, K. (2018). Insights, Next Steps, and Future Research. In *Fostering Positive Civic Engagement Among Millennials: Emerging Research and Opportunities* (pp. 65–72). Hershey, PA: IGI Global. doi:10.4018/978-1-5225-2452-6.ch005

Iguisi, O. V. (2018). Comparative Analysis of Hofstede's Culture Dimensions for West African Regions (WAF) and Nigeria. In S. Sarma (Ed.), *Global Observations of the Influence of Culture on Consumer Buying Behavior* (pp. 190–205). Hershey, PA: IGI Global. doi:10.4018/978-1-5225-2727-5.ch012

Islam, M. R. (2018). Abuse Among Child Domestic Workers in Bangladesh. In I. Tshabangu (Ed.), *Global Ideologies Surrounding Children's Rights and Social Justice* (pp. 1–21). Hershey, PA: IGI Global. doi:10.4018/978-1-5225-2578-3.ch001

Ito, K., & Hilliker, S. M. (2018). Supporting University International Students Through Supportive ESL Instruction and Corrective Feedback. In B. Blummer, J. Kenton, & M. Wiatrowski (Eds.), *Promoting Ethnic Diversity and Multiculturalism in Higher Education* (pp. 40–58). Hershey, PA: IGI Global. doi:10.4018/978-1-5225-4097-7.ch003

Iurato, G. (2018). A Brief Account of Ignacio Matte Blanco Theory and Other Related Psychoanalytic Themes. In *Computational Psychoanalysis and Formal Bi-Logic Frameworks* (pp. 114–135). Hershey, PA: IGI Global. doi:10.4018/978-1-5225-4128-8.ch003

Iurato, G. (2018). First Attempts to Formalize Some Main Aspects of Psychoanalysis: Towards a Computational Psychoanalysis. In *Computational Psychoanalysis and Formal Bi-Logic Frameworks* (pp. 136–205). Hershey, PA: IGI Global. doi:10.4018/978-1-5225-4128-8.ch004

Jacobsen, M., Friesen, S., & Brown, B. (2018). Teachers' Professional Learning Focused on Designs for Early Learners and Technology. In D. Polly, M. Putman, T. Petty, & A. Good (Eds.), *Innovative Practices in Teacher Preparation and Graduate-Level Teacher Education Programs* (pp. 417–438). Hershey, PA: IGI Global. doi:10.4018/978-1-5225-3068-8.ch022

Jensen, A. A., & Thomassen, A. O. (2018). Teachers' Reflective Practice in Lifelong Learning Programs. In Z. Djoub (Ed.), *Fostering Reflective Teaching Practice in Pre-Service Education* (pp. 25–45). Hershey, PA: IGI Global. doi:10.4018/978-1-5225-2963-7.ch002

Jiang, K., Barnett, G. A., Taylor, L. D., & Feng, B. (2018). Dynamic Co-Evolutions of Peace Frames in the United States, Mainland China, and Hong Kong: A Semantic Network Analysis. In B. Cook (Ed.), *Handbook of Research on Examining Global Peacemaking in the Digital Age* (pp. 145–168). Hershey, PA: IGI Global. doi:10.4018/978-1-5225-3032-9.ch010

Jiménez-González, S. G., Mendoza-González, R., & Luna-García, H. (2018). Guidelines Based on Need-Findings Study and Communication Types to Design Interactions for MOOCs. In F. Cipolla-Ficarra (Ed.), *Optimizing Human-Computer Interaction With Emerging Technologies* (pp. 210–231). Hershey, PA: IGI Global. doi:10.4018/978-1-5225-2616-2.ch008

Johnson, N. N. (2018). Effectively Managing Bias in Teacher Preparation. In U. Thomas (Ed.), *Advocacy in Academia and the Role of Teacher Preparation Programs* (pp. 146–160). Hershey, PA: IGI Global. doi:10.4018/978-1-5225-2906-4.ch008

Joseph, C. (2018). The Role of Government in a Liberal Market Economy: A Double-Edge Sword. In H. Levine & K. Moreno (Eds.), *Positioning Markets and Governments in Public Management* (pp. 53–61). Hershey, PA: IGI Global. doi:10.4018/978-1-5225-4177-6.ch005

Kade, D., Lindell, R., Ürey, H., & Özcan, O. (2018). Supporting Motion Capture Acting Through a Mixed Reality Application. In F. Cipolla-Ficarra (Ed.), *Optimizing Human-Computer Interaction With Emerging Technologies* (pp. 248–273). Hershey, PA: IGI Global. doi:10.4018/978-1-5225-2616-2.ch010

Karataş, S., Kukul, V., & Özcan, S. (2018). How Powerful Is Digital Storytelling for Teaching?: Perspective of Pre-Service Teachers. In D. Polly, M. Putman, T. Petty, & A. Good (Eds.), *Innovative Practices in Teacher Preparation and Graduate-Level Teacher Education Programs* (pp. 511–529). Hershey, PA: IGI Global. doi:10.4018/978-1-5225-3068-8.ch027

Kavaklı, N. (2018). Hate Speech Towards Syrian Refugees in Turkish Online Reader Comments. In C. Akrivopoulou (Ed.), *Global Perspectives on Human Migration, Asylum, and Security* (pp. 127–142). Hershey, PA: IGI Global. doi:10.4018/978-1-5225-2817-3.ch007

Kaynak, S. (2018). Pakistan. In S. Ozdemir, S. Erdogan, & A. Gedikli (Eds.), *Handbook of Research on Sociopolitical Factors Impacting Economic Growth in Islamic Nations* (pp. 293–313). Hershey, PA: IGI Global. doi:10.4018/978-1-5225-2939-2.ch015

Korstanje, M. E. (2018). Thana-Capitalism and the Sense of Reality: Lessons Unlearned. In C. Akrivopoulou (Ed.), *Global Perspectives on Human Migration, Asylum, and Security* (pp. 1–20). Hershey, PA: IGI Global. doi:10.4018/978-1-5225-2817-3.ch001

Korstanje, M. E. (2018). The Lost Paradise: The Religious Nature of Tourism. In H. El-Gohary, D. Edwards, & R. Eid (Eds.), *Global Perspectives on Religious Tourism and Pilgrimage* (pp. 129–141). Hershey, PA: IGI Global. doi:10.4018/978-1-5225-2796-1.ch008

Korstanje, M. E., & George, B. P. (2018). Emotionality, Reason, and Dark Tourism: Discussions Around the Sense of Death. In M. Korstanje & B. George (Eds.), *Virtual Traumascapes and Exploring the Roots of Dark Tourism* (pp. 1–25). Hershey, PA: IGI Global. doi:10.4018/978-1-5225-2750-3.ch001

Kougioumtzis, G. A., & Louka, D. (2018). Advocacy and Teacher Mentoring. In U. Thomas (Ed.), *Advocacy in Academia and the Role of Teacher Preparation Programs* (pp. 65–87). Hershey, PA: IGI Global. doi:10.4018/978-1-5225-2906-4.ch004

Kousar, H. (2018). Gender Violence in Academia. In N. Mahtab, T. Haque, I. Khan, M. Islam, & I. Wahid (Eds.), *Handbook of Research on Women's Issues and Rights in the Developing World* (pp. 144–155). Hershey, PA: IGI Global. doi:10.4018/978-1-5225-3018-3.ch009

Koutsafti, M., & Politi, N. (2018). Career Counseling: The "Model of Personal Career Management". In K. Koutsopoulos, K. Doukas, & Y. Kotsanis (Eds.), *Handbook of Research on Educational Design and Cloud Computing in Modern Classroom Settings* (pp. 410–429). Hershey, PA: IGI Global. doi:10.4018/978-1-5225-3053-4.ch020

Koutsopoulos, K. (2018). From Ground to Cloud: The School on the Cloud. In K. Koutsopoulos, K. Doukas, & Y. Kotsanis (Eds.), *Handbook of Research on Educational Design and Cloud Computing in Modern Classroom Settings* (pp. 1–21). Hershey, PA: IGI Global. doi:10.4018/978-1-5225-3053-4.ch001

Kovacevic, Z., Klimek, B., & Drower, I. S. (2018). Refugee Children and Parental Involvement in School Education: A Field Model. In K. Norris & S. Collier (Eds.), *Social Justice and Parent Partnerships in Multicultural Education Contexts* (pp. 139–161). Hershey, PA: IGI Global. doi:10.4018/978-1-5225-3943-8.ch008

Kratky, A. (2018). Personal Touch: A Viewing-Angle-Compensated Multi-Layer Touch Display. In F. Cipolla-Ficarra (Ed.), *Optimizing Human-Computer Interaction With Emerging Technologies* (pp. 232–247). Hershey, PA: IGI Global. doi:10.4018/978-1-5225-2616-2.ch009

Kuang, Y. (2018). Application of the "Teaching Innovation Practice Platform" in English Reading Instruction: A Case Study of a Public Middle School in Shanghai. In H. Spires (Ed.), *Digital Transformation and Innovation in Chinese Education* (pp. 249–271). Hershey, PA: IGI Global. doi:10.4018/978-1-5225-2924-8.ch014

Kubilay, S., & Yardibi, N. (2018). Refugee Parents' Preferential Values in Education. In Ş. Erçetin (Ed.), *Educational Development and Infrastructure for Immigrants and Refugees* (pp. 72–84). Hershey, PA: IGI Global. doi:10.4018/978-1-5225-3325-2.ch004

Kumar, T. P. (2018). Impact of Corporate Social Responsibility on Service Performance in Mediating Effect of Brand Equity With Reference To Banks in India. In Rajagopal, & R. Behl (Eds.), Start-Up Enterprises and Contemporary Innovation Strategies in the Global Marketplace (pp. 88-99). Hershey, PA: IGI Global. doi:10.4018/978-1-5225-4831-7.ch007

LaPlante, J. M. (2018). Unequal Opportunities and Inequitable Outcomes: Rethinking Education Finance Policy Design for a Global Society. In H. Levine & K. Moreno (Eds.), *Positioning Markets and Governments in Public Management* (pp. 209–239). Hershey, PA: IGI Global. doi:10.4018/978-1-5225-4177-6.ch016

Lau, B. T., & Win, K. M. (2018). Differentiated Animated Social Stories to Enhance Social Skills Acquisition of Children With Autism Spectrum Disorder. In V. Bryan, A. Musgrove, & J. Powers (Eds.), *Handbook of Research on Human Development in the Digital Age* (pp. 300–329). Hershey, PA: IGI Global. doi:10.4018/978-1-5225-2838-8.ch014

Lee, J. K., & Chirino-Klevans, I. (2018). Cosmopolitanism in a World of Teachers: American Student Teachers in a Chinese School. In H. Spires (Ed.), *Digital Transformation and Innovation in Chinese Education* (pp. 232–248). Hershey, PA: IGI Global. doi:10.4018/978-1-5225-2924-8.ch013

Lee, S. (2018). Expatriate Cantonese Learners in Hong Kong: Adult L2 Learning, Identity Negotiation, and Social Pressure. In D. Velliaris (Ed.), *Study Abroad Contexts for Enhanced Foreign Language Learning* (pp. 151–168). Hershey, PA: IGI Global. doi:10.4018/978-1-5225-3814-1.ch007

Lee, S. C. (2018). Mother America: Cold War Maternalism and the Origins of Korean Adoption. In F. Topor (Ed.), *Ethical Standards and Practice in International Relations* (pp. 157–186). Hershey, PA: IGI Global. doi:10.4018/978-1-5225-2650-6.ch007

Li, Y., & Wang, X. (2018). Seeking Health Information on Social Media: A Perspective of Trust, Self-Determination, and Social Support. *Journal of Organizational and End User Computing*, *30*(1), 1–22. doi:10.4018/JOEUC.2018010101

Livers, S. D., & Lin, L. (2018). Elementary Teacher Candidates' Perspectives on the Teaching and Learning of English Learners. In U. Thomas (Ed.), *Advocacy in Academia and the Role of Teacher Preparation Programs* (pp. 23–41). Hershey, PA: IGI Global. doi:10.4018/978-1-5225-2906-4.ch002

López-Cózar-Navarro, C., & Priede-Bergamini, T. (2018). Nascent Social Entrepreneurship: Economic, Legal, and Financial Framework. In A. Carrizo Moreira, J. Guilherme Leitão Dantas, & F. Manuel Valente (Eds.), *Nascent Entrepreneurship and Successful New Venture Creation* (pp. 132–152). Hershey, PA: IGI Global. doi:10.4018/978-1-5225-2936-1.ch006

Lu, S. (2018). Financial Literacy Education Program Post Financial Housing Crisis: Community Based Financial Literacy Education Program. In S. Burton (Ed.), *Engaged Scholarship and Civic Responsibility in Higher Education* (pp. 49–66). Hershey, PA: IGI Global. doi:10.4018/978-1-5225-3649-9.ch003

Luyombya, D. (2018). Management of Records and Archives in Uganda's Public Sector. In P. Ngulube (Ed.), *Handbook of Research on Heritage Management and Preservation* (pp. 275–297). Hershey, PA: IGI Global. doi:10.4018/978-1-5225-3137-1.ch014

Luyombya, D., Kiyingi, G. W., & Naluwooza, M. (2018). The Nature and Utilisation of Archival Records Deposited in Makerere University Library, Uganda. In P. Ngulube (Ed.), *Handbook of Research on Heritage Management and Preservation* (pp. 96–113). Hershey, PA: IGI Global. doi:10.4018/978-1-5225-3137-1.ch005

Lytras, M. D., Papadopoulou, P., Marouli, C., & Misseyanni, A. (2018). Higher Education Out-of-the-Box: Technology-Driven Learning Innovation in Higher Education. In S. Burton (Ed.), *Engaged Scholarship and Civic Responsibility in Higher Education* (pp. 67–100). Hershey, PA: IGI Global. doi:10.4018/978-1-5225-3649-9.ch004

Mafumbate, R. (2018). Child Resilience, Survival, and Development: Voices of Orphans in Zimbabwe. In I. Tshabangu (Ed.), *Global Ideologies Surrounding Children's Rights and Social Justice* (pp. 239–252). Hershey, PA: IGI Global. doi:10.4018/978-1-5225-2578-3.ch015

Malmierca, M. J. (2018). Cloud Computing for Rural and Isolated Schools. In K. Koutsopoulos, K. Doukas, & Y. Kotsanis (Eds.), *Handbook of Research on Educational Design and Cloud Computing in Modern Classroom Settings* (pp. 376–394). Hershey, PA: IGI Global. doi:10.4018/978-1-5225-3053-4.ch018

Maroofi, F. (2018). Knowledge Management and Organizational Performance in Service Industry: Transformational Leadership Versus Transactional Leadership. In N. Baporikar (Ed.), *Global Practices in Knowledge Management for Societal and Organizational Development* (pp. 194–212). Hershey, PA: IGI Global. doi:10.4018/978-1-5225-3009-1.ch009

Mattson, T., & Aurigemma, S. (2018). Running with the Pack: The Impact of Middle-Status Conformity on the Post-Adoption Organizational Use of Twitter. *Journal of Organizational and End User Computing, 30*(1), 23–43. doi:10.4018/JOEUC.2018010102

Medhekar, A., & Haq, F. (2018). Urbanization and New Jobs Creation in Healthcare Services in India: Challenges and Opportunities. In U. Benna & I. Benna (Eds.), *Urbanization and Its Impact on Socio-Economic Growth in Developing Regions* (pp. 198–218). Hershey, PA: IGI Global. doi:10.4018/978-1-5225-2659-9.ch010

Meletiou-Mavrotheris, M., & Koutsopoulos, K. (2018). Projecting the Future of Cloud Computing in Education: A Foresight Study Using the Delphi Method. In K. Koutsopoulos, K. Doukas, & Y. Kotsanis (Eds.), *Handbook of Research on Educational Design and Cloud Computing in Modern Classroom Settings* (pp. 262–290). Hershey, PA: IGI Global. doi:10.4018/978-1-5225-3053-4.ch012

Miller, J. (2018). Causes and Ramifications of Public Pension Fund Underfunding: A Case Study of the New Jersey Pension Funds. In H. Levine & K. Moreno (Eds.), *Positioning Markets and Governments in Public Management* (pp. 114–146). Hershey, PA: IGI Global. doi:10.4018/978-1-5225-4177-6.ch010

Milović, B. (2018). Developing Marketing Strategy on Social Networks. In S. Sarma (Ed.), *Global Observations of the Influence of Culture on Consumer Buying Behavior* (pp. 66–82). Hershey, PA: IGI Global. doi:10.4018/978-1-5225-2727-5.ch004

Mosweu, O., & Kenosi, L. S. (2018). Theories of Appraisal in Archives: From Hillary Jenkinson to Terry Cook's Times. In P. Ngulube (Ed.), *Handbook of Research on Heritage Management and Preservation* (pp. 24–46). Hershey, PA: IGI Global. doi:10.4018/978-1-5225-3137-1.ch002

Mukherjee, S., & Pradeep, K. (2018). Does Internationalization of Business-Group-Affiliated Firms Depend on Their Performance? In Rajagopal, & R. Behl (Eds.), Start-Up Enterprises and Contemporary Innovation Strategies in the Global Marketplace (pp. 153-165). Hershey, PA: IGI Global. https://doi.org/ doi:10.4018/978-1-5225-4831-7.ch011

Mutisya, P. M., & Conway, C. S. (2018). Quality Mentoring: A Prerequisite for Faculty at HBCUs. In C. Conway (Ed.), *Faculty Mentorship at Historically Black Colleges and Universities* (pp. 15–34). Hershey, PA: IGI Global. doi:10.4018/978-1-5225-4071-7.ch002

Nagabhushan, P. (2018). Mean Level Changes in College Students' Academic Motivation and Engagement. In *Engaging Adolescent Students in Contemporary Classrooms: Emerging Research and Opportunities* (pp. 142–174). Hershey, PA: IGI Global. doi:10.4018/978-1-5225-5155-3.ch006

Naranjo, J. (2018). Meeting the Need for Inclusive Educators Online: Teacher Education in Inclusive Special Education and Dual-Certification. In D. Polly, M. Putman, T. Petty, & A. Good (Eds.), *Innovative Practices in Teacher Preparation and Graduate-Level Teacher Education Programs* (pp. 106–122). Hershey, PA: IGI Global. doi:10.4018/978-1-5225-3068-8.ch007

Nirmala, T., & Aram, I. A. (2018). Newspaper Framing of Climate Change and Sustainability Issues in India. *International Journal of E-Politics*, *9*(1), 15–28. doi:10.4018/IJEP.2018010102

Novak, J. I., & Loy, J. (2018). Digital Technologies and 4D Customized Design: Challenging Conventions With Responsive Design. In V. Bryan, A. Musgrove, & J. Powers (Eds.), *Handbook of Research on Human Development in the Digital Age* (pp. 403–426). Hershey, PA: IGI Global. doi:10.4018/978-1-5225-2838-8.ch018

Ögeyik, M. C. (2018). Measuring Phonological and Orthographic Similarity: The Case of Loanwords in Turkish and English. In D. Buğa & M. Coşgun Ögeyik (Eds.), *Psycholinguistics and Cognition in Language Processing* (pp. 49–67). Hershey, PA: IGI Global. doi:10.4018/978-1-5225-4009-0.ch003

Oling-Sisay, M. (2018). Don't Touch My Hair: Culturally Responsive Engagement in Service-Learning. In O. Delano-Oriaran, M. Penick-Parks, & S. Fondrie (Eds.), *Culturally Engaging Service-Learning With Diverse Communities* (pp. 43–55). Hershey, PA: IGI Global. doi:10.4018/978-1-5225-2900-2.ch003

Ololube, N. P., Ingiabuna, E. T., & Dudafa, U. J. (2018). Effective Decision Making for Knowledge Development in Higher Education: A Case Study of Nigeria. In N. Baporikar (Ed.), *Global Practices in Knowledge Management for Societal and Organizational Development* (pp. 382–399). Hershey, PA: IGI Global. doi:10.4018/978-1-5225-3009-1.ch018

Oritsejafor, E. O. (2018). Enhancing Competitiveness of Public Utilities in Nigeria: The Case of the Power Holding Company of Nigeria (PHCN). In H. Levine & K. Moreno (Eds.), *Positioning Markets and Governments in Public Management* (pp. 240–252). Hershey, PA: IGI Global. doi:10.4018/978-1-5225-4177-6.ch017

Otunla, A. O., & Olatunji, O. T. (2018). Clients' Perception, Extent of Adoption, and Level of Satisfaction With Multi-Platform Advertising Media Strategies (MuPAMS): Among Business Organisations in Ibadan, South-Western Nigeria. In K. Yang (Ed.), *Multi-Platform Advertising Strategies in the Global Marketplace* (pp. 54–80). Hershey, PA: IGI Global. doi:10.4018/978-1-5225-3114-2.ch003

Owuor, N. A. (2018). Oil and Gas Discoveries in Kenya: Important Global Exploration and Production Value Chain Lessons for the Society. In M. Risso & S. Testarmata (Eds.), *Value Sharing for Sustainable and Inclusive Development* (pp. 322–337). Hershey, PA: IGI Global. doi:10.4018/978-1-5225-3147-0.ch015

Özdemir, E., & Yılmaz, M. (2018). Omni-Channel Retailing: The Risks, Challenges, and Opportunities. In A. Kumar & S. Saurav (Eds.), *Supply Chain Management Strategies and Risk Assessment in Retail Environments* (pp. 97–118). Hershey, PA: IGI Global. doi:10.4018/978-1-5225-3056-5.ch006

Panko, T. R., & George, B. P. (2018). Animal Sexual Abuse and the Darkness of Touristic Immorality. In M. Korstanje & B. George (Eds.), *Virtual Traumascapes and Exploring the Roots of Dark Tourism* (pp. 175–189). Hershey, PA: IGI Global. doi:10.4018/978-1-5225-2750-3.ch009

Paraschiv, M. M. (2018). Elif Shafak's Works: A Means of Preventing Honor Based Violence. In M. Badea & M. Suditu (Eds.), *Violence Prevention and Safety Promotion in Higher Education Settings* (pp. 36–49). Hershey, PA: IGI Global. doi:10.4018/978-1-5225-2960-6.ch003

Paravastu, N., Simmers, C. A., & Anandarajan, M. (2018). Non-Compliant Mobile Device Usage and Information Systems Security: A Bystander Theory Perspective. *International Journal of Information Systems and Social Change*, *9*(1), 1–25. doi:10.4018/IJISSC.2018010101

Pathak, B. (2018). Process Documentation of Interfaith Peacebuilding Cycle: A Case Study From Nepal. In B. Cook (Ed.), *Handbook of Research on Examining Global Peacemaking in the Digital Age* (pp. 70–93). Hershey, PA: IGI Global. doi:10.4018/978-1-5225-3032-9.ch006

Pathak, S. J. (2018). Women Painters of Mithila: A Quest for Identity. In N. Mahtab, T. Haque, I. Khan, M. Islam, & I. Wahid (Eds.), *Handbook of Research on Women's Issues and Rights in the Developing World* (pp. 370–381). Hershey, PA: IGI Global. doi:10.4018/978-1-5225-3018-3.ch023

Patro, C. S., & Raghunath, K. M. (2018). Corporate Social Responsibility: A Conscientious Take. In M. Risso & S. Testarmata (Eds.), *Value Sharing for Sustainable and Inclusive Development* (pp. 75–99). Hershey, PA: IGI Global. doi:10.4018/978-1-5225-3147-0.ch004

Pérez-Uribe, R. I., Torres, D. A., Jurado, S. P., & Prada, D. M. (2018). Cloud Tools for the Development of Project Management in SMEs. In R. Perez-Uribe, C. Salcedo-Perez, & D. Ocampo-Guzman (Eds.), *Handbook of Research on Intrapreneurship and Organizational Sustainability in SMEs* (pp. 95–120). Hershey, PA: IGI Global. doi:10.4018/978-1-5225-3543-0.ch005

Perrotta, K. A., & Mattson, M. F. (2018). Using Counterstories and Reflective Writing Assignments to Promote Critical Race Consciousness in an Undergraduate Teacher Preparation Course. In U. Thomas (Ed.), *Advocacy in Academia and the Role of Teacher Preparation Programs* (pp. 42–64). Hershey, PA: IGI Global. doi:10.4018/978-1-5225-2906-4.ch003

Poli, A., Gambini, A., Pezzotti, A., Broglia, A., Mazzola, A., Muschiato, S., ... Costa, F. (2018). Digital Diorama: An Interactive Multimedia Resource for Learning the Life Sciences. In F. Cipolla-Ficarra (Ed.), *Optimizing Human-Computer Interaction With Emerging Technologies* (pp. 52–82). Hershey, PA: IGI Global. doi:10.4018/978-1-5225-2616-2.ch003

Presadă, D. (2018). Literature and Aesthetic Reading as Means of Promoting Nonviolence. In M. Badea & M. Suditu (Eds.), *Violence Prevention and Safety Promotion in Higher Education Settings* (pp. 94–109). Hershey, PA: IGI Global. doi:10.4018/978-1-5225-2960-6.ch006

Punetha, H., Kumar, S., Mudila, H., & Prakash, O. (2018). Brassica Meal as Source of Health Protecting Neuraceutical and Its Antioxidative Properties. In A. Verma, K. Srivastava, S. Singh, & H. Singh (Eds.), *Nutraceuticals and Innovative Food Products for Healthy Living and Preventive Care* (pp. 108–131). Hershey, PA: IGI Global. doi:10.4018/978-1-5225-2970-5.ch005

Puri, R., & Sengupta, P. (2018). Application of Statistics in Human Resource Management. In D. Bhattacharyya (Ed.), *Statistical Tools and Analysis in Human Resources Management* (pp. 15–37). Hershey, PA: IGI Global. doi:10.4018/978-1-5225-4947-5.ch002

Putnik, N., & Milošević, M. (2018). Trends in Peace Research: Can Cyber Détente Lead to Lasting Peace? In B. Cook (Ed.), *Handbook of Research on Examining Global Peacemaking in the Digital Age* (pp. 1–18). Hershey, PA: IGI Global. doi:10.4018/978-1-5225-3032-9.ch001

Rana, S., & Sharma, R. (2018). An Overview of Employer Branding With Special Reference to Indian Organizations. In N. Sharma, V. Singh, & S. Pathak (Eds.), *Management Techniques for a Diverse and Cross-Cultural Workforce* (pp. 116–131). Hershey, PA: IGI Global. doi:10.4018/978-1-5225-4933-8.ch007

Randa, I. O. (2018). Leveraging Knowledge Management for Value Creation in Service-Oriented Organisations of Namibia. In N. Baporikar (Ed.), *Global Practices in Knowledge Management for Societal and Organizational Development* (pp. 145–167). Hershey, PA: IGI Global. doi:10.4018/978-1-5225-3009-1.ch007

Rekun, M. S. (2018). A Swift Kick: Russian Diplomatic Practice in Bulgaria, 1879-1883. In F. Topor (Ed.), *Ethical Standards and Practice in International Relations* (pp. 49–72). Hershey, PA: IGI Global. doi:10.4018/978-1-5225-2650-6.ch003

Rodil, K., Nielsen, E. B., & Nielsen, J. B. (2018). Sharing Memories: Co-Designing Assistive Technology with Aphasic Adults and Support Staff. *International Journal of Sociotechnology and Knowledge Development, 10*(1), 21–36. doi:10.4018/IJSKD.2018010102

Samli, R. (2018). A Review of Internet Addiction on the Basis of Different Countries (2007–2017). In B. Bozoglan (Ed.), *Psychological, Social, and Cultural Aspects of Internet Addiction* (pp. 200–220). Hershey, PA: IGI Global. doi:10.4018/978-1-5225-3477-8.ch011

Sánchez-García, J. C., & Hernández-Sánchez, B. R. (2018). Nascent Entrepreneurs, Psychological Characteristics, and Sociocultural Background: Psycho-Sociocultural Background of Nascent Entrepreneurs. In A. Carrizo Moreira, J. Guilherme Leitão Dantas, & F. Manuel Valente (Eds.), *Nascent Entrepreneurship and Successful New Venture Creation* (pp. 111–131). Hershey, PA: IGI Global. doi:10.4018/978-1-5225-2936-1.ch005

Santana-Mansilla, P., Costaguta, R., & Schiaffino, S. (2018). A Multi-Agent Model for Personalizing Learning Material for Collaborative Groups. In F. Cipolla-Ficarra (Ed.), *Optimizing Human-Computer Interaction With Emerging Technologies* (pp. 343–375). Hershey, PA: IGI Global. doi:10.4018/978-1-5225-2616-2.ch015

Santos, C. E., Lima de Oliveira, D., & Freitas, M. D. (2018). The Role of Pibid in Graduation Courses: Discussing Teachers' Education. In Z. Djoub (Ed.), *Fostering Reflective Teaching Practice in Pre-Service Education* (pp. 218–234). Hershey, PA: IGI Global. doi:10.4018/978-1-5225-2963-7.ch012

Sarkar, J. (2018). Methodological Considerations for Research in Compensation Management. In D. Bhattacharyya (Ed.), *Statistical Tools and Analysis in Human Resources Management* (pp. 142–168). Hershey, PA: IGI Global. doi:10.4018/978-1-5225-4947-5.ch007

Sarofim, S., & Tolba, A. (2018). When Age, Religion, and Culture Matter: The Impact of Aging, Religiosity, and Cultural Differences on Consumers' Emotions and Behavior. In S. Sarma (Ed.), *Global Observations of the Influence of Culture on Consumer Buying Behavior* (pp. 261–278). Hershey, PA: IGI Global. doi:10.4018/978-1-5225-2727-5.ch015

Schroth, S. T., & Helfer, J. A. (2018). Differentiated Fieldwork and Practicum Experiences: Matching Teacher Candidate Assignments to Their Skills and Needs. In D. Polly, M. Putman, T. Petty, & A. Good (Eds.), *Innovative Practices in Teacher Preparation and Graduate-Level Teacher Education Programs* (pp. 306–326). Hershey, PA: IGI Global. doi:10.4018/978-1-5225-3068-8.ch017

Schwartz, H. M. (2018). States via Markets and Markets via States: Symbiosis and Change, Not Conflict. In H. Levine & K. Moreno (Eds.), *Positioning Markets and Governments in Public Management* (pp. 1–10). Hershey, PA: IGI Global. doi:10.4018/978-1-5225-4177-6.ch001

Semali, L. M. (2018). Indigenous Knowledge as Resource to Sustain Self-Employment in Rural Development. In S. Chhabra (Ed.), *Handbook of Research on Civic Engagement and Social Change in Contemporary Society* (pp. 142–158). Hershey, PA: IGI Global. doi:10.4018/978-1-5225-4197-4.ch008

Seraphin, H., & Gowreesunkar, V. (2018). On the Use of Qualitative Comparative Analysis to Identify the Bright Spots in Dark Tourism. In M. Korstanje & B. George (Eds.), *Virtual Traumascapes and Exploring the Roots of Dark Tourism* (pp. 67–83). Hershey, PA: IGI Global. doi:10.4018/978-1-5225-2750-3.ch004

Shahidi, N., Tossan, V., & Cacho-Elizondo, S. (2018). Assessment of A Mobile Educational Coaching App: Exploring Adoption Patterns and Barriers in France. *International Journal of Technology and Human Interaction, 14*(1), 22–43. doi:10.4018/IJTHI.2018010102

Sikira, A. N., Matekere, T., & Urassa, J. K. (2018). Engaging Men in Women's Economic Empowerment in Butiama District, Mara Region, Tanzania. In N. Mahtab, T. Haque, I. Khan, M. Islam, & I. Wahid (Eds.), *Handbook of Research on Women's Issues and Rights in the Developing World* (pp. 252–268). Hershey, PA: IGI Global. doi:10.4018/978-1-5225-3018-3.ch015

Silveira, D. G. (2018). Diffusion of Innovation and Role of Opinion Leaders. In S. Sarma (Ed.), *Global Observations of the Influence of Culture on Consumer Buying Behavior* (pp. 83–93). Hershey, PA: IGI Global. doi:10.4018/978-1-5225-2727-5.ch005

Simard, D. A., Martin, M., Mockry, J., Puliatte, A., & Squires, M. E. (2018). Introduction: Mental Health and Well-Being of College Students. In M. Martin, J. Mockry, A. Puliatte, D. Simard, & M. Squires (Eds.), *Raising Mental Health Awareness in Higher Education: Emerging Research and Opportunities* (pp. 1–20). Hershey, PA: IGI Global. doi:10.4018/978-1-5225-3793-9.ch001

Sosnin, P. (2018). Experimental Actions With Conceptual Objects. In *Experience-Based Human-Computer Interactions: Emerging Research and Opportunities* (pp. 47–97). Hershey, PA: IGI Global. doi:10.4018/978-1-5225-2987-3.ch003

Sosnin, P. (2018). Lack of Naturalness in Human-Computer Interactions. In *Experience-Based Human-Computer Interactions: Emerging Research and Opportunities* (pp. 9–46). Hershey, PA: IGI Global. doi:10.4018/978-1-5225-2987-3.ch002

Spaseski, N. (2018). Fractal and Wavelet Market Analysis in Pattern Recognition. In *Alternative Decision-Making Models for Financial Portfolio Management: Emerging Research and Opportunities* (pp. 254–309). Hershey, PA: IGI Global. doi:10.4018/978-1-5225-3259-0.ch007

Spaseski, N. (2018). Theory and Modelling. In *Alternative Decision-Making Models for Financial Portfolio Management: Emerging Research and Opportunities* (pp. 1–19). Hershey, PA: IGI Global. doi:10.4018/978-1-5225-3259-0.ch001

Spires, H. A., Green, K. E., & Liang, P. (2018). Chinese Parents' Perspectives on International Higher Education and Innovation. In H. Spires (Ed.), *Digital Transformation and Innovation in Chinese Education* (pp. 272–287). Hershey, PA: IGI Global. doi:10.4018/978-1-5225-2924-8.ch015

Spires, H. A., Himes, M., & Wang, L. (2018). Designing a State-of-the-Art High School in Suzhou, China: Connecting to the Future. In H. Spires (Ed.), *Digital Transformation and Innovation in Chinese Education* (pp. 191–210). Hershey, PA: IGI Global. doi:10.4018/978-1-5225-2924-8.ch011

Squires, M. E., Martin, M., Mockry, J., Puliatte, A., & Simard, D. A. (2018). Campus-Wide Initiatives. In M. Martin, J. Mockry, A. Puliatte, D. Simard, & M. Squires (Eds.), *Raising Mental Health Awareness in Higher Education: Emerging Research and Opportunities* (pp. 77–104). Hershey, PA: IGI Global. doi:10.4018/978-1-5225-3793-9.ch005

Standing, K., & Parker, S. L. (2018). Girls' and Women's Rights to Menstrual Health in Nepal. In N. Mahtab, T. Haque, I. Khan, M. Islam, & I. Wahid (Eds.), *Handbook of Research on Women's Issues and Rights in the Developing World* (pp. 156–168). Hershey, PA: IGI Global. doi:10.4018/978-1-5225-3018-3.ch010

Stępień, B., & Hinner, M. (2018). From Love to Rebuff: How Culture Shapes the Perception of Luxury Goods Among Consumers. In S. Sarma (Ed.), *Global Observations of the Influence of Culture on Consumer Buying Behavior* (pp. 24–47). Hershey, PA: IGI Global. doi:10.4018/978-1-5225-2727-5.ch002

Tantau, A. D., & Frăţilă, L. C. (2018). Trends and Conclusions for Business Development in the Renewable Energy Industry. In *Entrepreneurship and Business Development in the Renewable Energy Sector* (pp. 351–376). Hershey, PA: IGI Global. doi:10.4018/978-1-5225-3625-3.ch010

Terry, D. L., & Amudalat, E. A. (2018). Data Documentation and Informed Consent in Research. In C. Sibinga (Ed.), *Ensuring Research Integrity and the Ethical Management of Data* (pp. 127–154). Hershey, PA: IGI Global. doi:10.4018/978-1-5225-2730-5.ch008

Toma, S. I., Marinescu, P., & Grădinaru, C. (2018). Creating Shared Value in the 21st Century: The Case of Toyota Motor Company. In M. Risso & S. Testarmata (Eds.), *Value Sharing for Sustainable and Inclusive Development* (pp. 155–184). Hershey, PA: IGI Global. doi:10.4018/978-1-5225-3147-0.ch007

Travis, F. T. (2018). Long-Term Changes in Experienced Yoga Practitioners: Growth of Higher States of Consciousness. In S. Telles & N. Singh (Eds.), *Research-Based Perspectives on the Psychophysiology of Yoga* (pp. 35–51). Hershey, PA: IGI Global. doi:10.4018/978-1-5225-2788-6.ch003

Tripp, L. O., Love, A., Thomas, C. M., & Russell, J. (2018). Teacher Education Advocacy for Multiple Perspectives and Culturally Sensitive Teaching. In U. Thomas (Ed.), *Advocacy in Academia and the Role of Teacher Preparation Programs* (pp. 161–181). Hershey, PA: IGI Global. doi:10.4018/978-1-5225-2906-4.ch009

Tshabangu, I. (2018). Child Poverty and Social Inequalities in Africa: A Social Justice Perspective. In I. Tshabangu (Ed.), *Global Ideologies Surrounding Children's Rights and Social Justice* (pp. 74–87). Hershey, PA: IGI Global. doi:10.4018/978-1-5225-2578-3.ch005

Tugjamba, N., Yembuu, B., Gantumur, A., & Gezel, U. (2018). Research Study on Climate Change Education for Sustainable Development in Mongolia. In P. Ordóñez de Pablos (Ed.), *Management Strategies and Technology Fluidity in the Asian Business Sector* (pp. 192–214). Hershey, PA: IGI Global. doi:10.4018/978-1-5225-4056-4.ch012

Upadhye, B. D., & Bandopadhyay, N. (2018). The Taxonomy of Methodological Approaches in Marketing Research: Retrospect and Prospect. In Rajagopal, & R. Behl (Eds.), Start-Up Enterprises and Contemporary Innovation Strategies in the Global Marketplace (pp. 276-293). Hershey, PA: IGI Global. https://doi.org/doi:10.4018/978-1-5225-4831-7.ch021

Uvanesh, K., Nayak, S. K., Sagiri, S. S., Banerjee, I., Ray, S. S., & Pal, K. (2018). Effect of Non-Ionic Hydrophilic and Hydrophobic Surfactants on the Properties on the Stearate Oleogels: A Comparative Study. In A. Verma, K. Srivastava, S. Singh, & H. Singh (Eds.), *Nutraceuticals and Innovative Food Products for Healthy Living and Preventive Care* (pp. 260–279). Hershey, PA: IGI Global. doi:10.4018/978-1-5225-2970-5.ch012

Vallverdú, J., Nishida, T., Ohmoto, Y., Moran, S., & Lázare, S. (2018). Fake Empathy and Human-Robot Interaction (HRI): A Preliminary Study. *International Journal of Technology and Human Interaction, 14*(1), 44–59. doi:10.4018/IJTHI.2018010103

Van Deur, P. (2018). Assessing Self-Directed Learning at School Level. In *Managing Self-Directed Learning in Primary School Education: Emerging Research and Opportunities* (pp. 61–77). Hershey, PA: IGI Global. doi:10.4018/978-1-5225-2613-1.ch003

Van Deur, P. (2018). Case Study: The Relationship Between Curriculum Focus on Inquiry and Self-Directed Learning. In *Managing Self-Directed Learning in Primary School Education: Emerging Research and Opportunities* (pp. 95–111). Hershey, PA: IGI Global. doi:10.4018/978-1-5225-2613-1.ch005

Van Deur, P. (2018). Describing Self-Directed Learning in Primary Students. In *Managing Self-Directed Learning in Primary School Education: Emerging Research and Opportunities* (pp. 33–59). Hershey, PA: IGI Global. doi:10.4018/978-1-5225-2613-1.ch002

Vargas-Hernández, J. G., Almanza-Jiménez, R., Calderón, P. C., & Casas-Cardenaz, R. (2018). Organizational Learning and Performance Under the Approach of Organizational Theories. In N. Baporikar (Ed.), *Global Practices in Knowledge Management for Societal and Organizational Development* (pp. 106–125). Hershey, PA: IGI Global. doi:10.4018/978-1-5225-3009-1.ch005

Vega, J. A., Arquette, C. M., Lee, H., Crowe, H. A., Hunzicker, J. L., & Cushing, J. (2018). Ensuring Social Justice for English Language Learners: An Innovative English as a Second Language (ESL) Endorsement Program. In D. Polly, M. Putman, T. Petty, & A. Good (Eds.), *Innovative Practices in Teacher Preparation and Graduate-Level Teacher Education Programs* (pp. 48–66). Hershey, PA: IGI Global. doi:10.4018/978-1-5225-3068-8.ch004

Verma, A. K., Singh, A., & Negi, M. S. (2018). Nutriproteomics: An Advance Methodology of Nutrichemical Analysis. In A. Verma, K. Srivastava, S. Singh, & H. Singh (Eds.), *Nutraceuticals and Innovative Food Products for Healthy Living and Preventive Care* (pp. 1–23). Hershey, PA: IGI Global. doi:10.4018/978-1-5225-2970-5.ch001

Verma, J., & Verma, R. (2018). Innovation in the Provision of Medical Services in India. In Rajagopal, & R. Behl (Eds.), Start-Up Enterprises and Contemporary Innovation Strategies in the Global Marketplace (pp. 16-27). Hershey, PA: IGI Global. doi:10.4018/978-1-5225-4831-7.ch002

Verrini, A. (2018). Strategists From the Past, as Encrypted Cognitive Maps, Whose Access Code Is the Will of Learning Solutions. In L. dall'Acqua, & D. Lukose (Eds.), Improving Business Performance Through Effective Managerial Training Initiatives (pp. 196-209). Hershey, PA: IGI Global. https://doi.org/ doi:10.4018/978-1-5225-3906-3.ch009

Veselinova, E., & Samonikov, M. G. (2018). Driving Brand Equity With Radical Transparency. In *Building Brand Equity and Consumer Trust Through Radical Transparency Practices* (pp. 18–62). Hershey, PA: IGI Global. doi:10.4018/978-1-5225-2417-5.ch002

Veselinova, E., & Samonikov, M. G. (2018). Henkel: Radical Transparency and Sustainability. In *Building Brand Equity and Consumer Trust Through Radical Transparency Practices* (pp. 337–389). Hershey, PA: IGI Global. doi:10.4018/978-1-5225-2417-5.ch009

Veselinova, E., & Samonikov, M. G. (2018). The 3M Company: How to Use Radical Transparency to Generate Value for the Company. In *Building Brand Equity and Consumer Trust Through Radical Transparency Practices* (pp. 185–318). Hershey, PA: IGI Global. doi:10.4018/978-1-5225-2417-5.ch007

Vila, A. R. (2018). Latin American and Caribbean Literature Transposed Into Digital: Corpus, Ecosystem, Canon, and Cartonera Publishing. In F. García-Peñalvo (Ed.), *Global Implications of Emerging Technology Trends* (pp. 34–58). Hershey, PA: IGI Global. doi:10.4018/978-1-5225-4944-4.ch003

Vorkapic, C. F. (2018). Yoga for Children. In S. Telles & N. Singh (Eds.), *Research-Based Perspectives on the Psychophysiology of Yoga* (pp. 104–120). Hershey, PA: IGI Global. doi:10.4018/978-1-5225-2788-6.ch007

Vu, N. T. (2018). Pros and Cons of Integrating Non-Financial Services in Microfinance. In S. Hipsher (Ed.), *Examining the Private Sector's Role in Wealth Creation and Poverty Reduction* (pp. 171–199). Hershey, PA: IGI Global. doi:10.4018/978-1-5225-3117-3.ch008

Wani, K. A., Manzoor, J., Anjum, J., Bashir, M., & Mamta. (2018). Pesticides in Vegetables: Their Impact on Nutritional Quality and Human Health. In A. Verma, K. Srivastava, S. Singh, & H. Singh (Eds.), *Nutraceuticals and Innovative Food Products for Healthy Living and Preventive Care* (pp. 132-157). Hershey, PA: IGI Global. https://doi.org/ doi:10.4018/978-1-5225-2970-5.ch006

Weiss-Randall, D. (2018). DOI Theoretical Framework: Adopting Innovative Technologies. In *Utilizing Innovative Technologies to Address the Public Health Impact of Climate Change: Emerging Research and Opportunities* (pp. 144–166). Hershey, PA: IGI Global. doi:10.4018/978-1-5225-3414-3.ch005

Weiss-Randall, D. (2018). Sustainable Development. In *Utilizing Innovative Technologies to Address the Public Health Impact of Climate Change: Emerging Research and Opportunities* (pp. 167–203). Hershey, PA: IGI Global. doi:10.4018/978-1-5225-3414-3.ch006

Whitelaw, L., & Taddei, L. M. (2018). Using Reflection to Explore Cultural Responsiveness of Preservice Teachers. In Z. Djoub (Ed.), *Fostering Reflective Teaching Practice in Pre-Service Education* (pp. 166–188). Hershey, PA: IGI Global. doi:10.4018/978-1-5225-2963-7.ch009

Wongsurawat, W., & Shrestha, V. (2018). Information Technology, Globalization, and Local Conditions: Implications for Entrepreneurs in Southeast Asia. In P. Ordóñez de Pablos (Ed.), *Management Strategies and Technology Fluidity in the Asian Business Sector* (pp. 163–176). Hershey, PA: IGI Global. doi:10.4018/978-1-5225-4056-4.ch010

Woodman, K., & Kourtis-Kazoullis, V. (2018). Facebook, Tele-Collaboration, and International Access to Technology in the Classroom. In F. Cipolla-Ficarra (Ed.), *Optimizing Human-Computer Interaction With Emerging Technologies* (pp. 274–286). Hershey, PA: IGI Global. doi:10.4018/978-1-5225-2616-2.ch011

Woods, R. J., Johnson, S., & Pope, M. L. (2018). Teaching in an Anti-Deficit Pedagogical Mindset. In U. Thomas (Ed.), *Advocacy in Academia and the Role of Teacher Preparation Programs* (pp. 190–205). Hershey, PA: IGI Global. doi:10.4018/978-1-5225-2906-4.ch011

Wright, M. (2018). Cyberbullying: Description, Definition, Characteristics, and Outcomes. In F. Cipolla-Ficarra (Ed.), *Optimizing Human-Computer Interaction With Emerging Technologies* (pp. 161–182). Hershey, PA: IGI Global. doi:10.4018/978-1-5225-2616-2.ch006

Xu, D. (2018). Multimodal Semiotics in China. In H. Spires (Ed.), *Digital Transformation and Innovation in Chinese Education* (pp. 60–79). Hershey, PA: IGI Global. doi:10.4018/978-1-5225-2924-8.ch004

Yaokumah, W., & Kumah, P. (2018). Exploring the Impact of Security Policy on Compliance. In F. García-Peñalvo (Ed.), *Global Implications of Emerging Technology Trends* (pp. 256–274). Hershey, PA: IGI Global. doi:10.4018/978-1-5225-4944-4.ch014

Yaokumah, W., & Okai, E. S. (2018). Inter-Organizational Study of Access Control Security Measures. *International Journal of Technology and Human Interaction, 14*(1), 60–79. doi:10.4018/IJTHI.2018010104

Zheng, X., Liu, H., Lin, D., & Li, J. (2018). Achieving Rural Teachers' Development Through a WeChat Professional Learning Community: Two Cases From Guangdong Province. In H. Spires (Ed.), *Digital Transformation and Innovation in Chinese Education* (pp. 307–318). Hershey, PA: IGI Global. doi:10.4018/978-1-5225-2924-8.ch017

About the Contributors

Remya Lathabhavan is an Assistant Professor of Indian Institute of Management Bodh Gaya, India. Her research interests include Glass Ceiling, Corporate Social Responsibility, Human Resource Management, Data Analytics, Artificial Intelligence, Career Progression, mental health and psychology. She authored many articles and book chapters in peer reviewed journals and books.

Prabir Padhy is working as an Assistant Professor (Sr.) in VIT Business School, Vellore Institute of Technology, Vellore, Tamil Nadu. Padhy has more than 14 years of experience in academics, research, corporate consultancy and have more than 32 publications in the journals of national and international repute. Padhy has a special interest for working in the areas of Human Resource Management and Organisational Behaviour.

***

Aarthi Chandrasantha Singh is a Research Scholar doing her Ph.D. in Industrial and Organizational Psychology from Vellore Institute of Technology. She has completed her Bachelors in Psychology from Ehtiraj College and Masters in HRD Psychology from University of Madras Campus, Chennai. She has worked as HR for Rane NSK Steering Systems Ltd. and served as Regional Manager for Chennai Reliable Pest Solutions Pvt. Ltd. before starting her Ph.D. for 8 years. Her specialization skills are employee engagement, counselling, Organizational Development and Change Management, Training, Learning and Development in Organizations.

Tanvi Daulatabadkar has a BA(Double majors psychology sociology) undergrad, Sophia college Mumbai.

Fatma Guneri was granted with Emerging Scholar Award on 2022 by Common Ground Research Networks. PhD in Marketing (2014, Institut of Business Admistrations, University of Lille, France), Executive Certificate in Designing for Social

Innovation and Leadership (2016), Higher Research Degree in the Creativity and Innovation Management (2018). Research engineer at HEMiSF4iRE, Lille Catholic University since 2017. Lecturer and thesis tutor in marketing and management at the faculties of Lille Catholic University, JUNIA, IESEG and Skema. Guest lecturer at the University of Toyo, Japan (2019-2020). Her current research topics concern the third places (fablabs, coworking spaces etc.), remote working and visualisation of work space data. Recently, she is interested in students online learning experiences. Recently associate member of European Association of Work and Organizational Psychology. Member of REMO (Researcher Mental Health Observatory) Cost Action CA19117 and Making Young Researchers' Voices Head For Gender Equality Cost Action CA20137.

Ayush Gupta was born in 2002 in Kanpur, Uttar Pradesh. Ayush Gupta is an undergrad student in the 3rd year of IPM (Integrated Programme in Management) at IIM Bodhgaya. His research interests lie in hrm, ob, well-being, mental health, and mindfulness.

Abdul Halim Hasanzada holds a master's degree in Marketing and Management from JUNIA, Lille Catholic University and a bachelor's degree in Agricultural Sciences from Kabul University. He's also holding an associate degree in Computer Science from ATVI Afghanistan. Abdul Halim is coming from a diverse background having 3 years of professional experience in Customer Service, Marketing and Project Management.

Gülrenk Hayırcıl holds a Ph.D. in American Literature and Media Studies from the University of Duisburg- Essen in Germany. Her focus was on the construction of cultural memory through mothering in African American and Black British women's neo-slave narratives. She was able to gain relevant professional experience in her previous work as a lecturer at departments such as English Language Teaching at Istanbul Bilgi University, Translation Studies at Beykent University, American Literature at Haliç University, and English Literature at Ayvansaray University in Istanbul. She is interested in memory and gender studies and has published several articles on cultural memory and black women's literature. She still continues to work as a volunteer spokesperson for the Afro-Turkish Association in Anatolia and is actively involved in projects regarding cultural memory.

Sanchit Khedkar is Pre-final year Information technology student.

Bhuvaneswari M. holds a Doctoral degree in Psychology and is currently working as an associate professor grade-1 at Vellore Institute of Technology, Vellore.

Bhuvaneswari M. hold a Doctoral degree in Psychology and is currently working as associate professor grade-1 at Vellore Institute of Technology, Vellore.

Akhil M P. is currently working as Assistant Professor at Faculty of Management studies & Commerce Alliance School of Business, Alliance University, Bangalore. He completed his doctoral degree under UGC Junior Research Fellowship (JRF) scheme from the department of commerce, University of Kerala. Prior to his research, he was a guest faculty at department of Commerce, Mahatma Gandhi College, Trivandrum. He has published a number of papers in refereed, indexed national and international journals. He also presented various academic as well as research based papers at several national and international conferences. His areas of interest include Income tax, Goods and Services Tax (GST), Sustainable development, Sustainable finance, Green finance, Climate finance etc

Aditya Mantri is a Pre-Final year Electronics & Communications student.

Annanya Negi is a Pre-Final year Biotechnology student.

Smita Panda has more than five years of experience in corporate and academics put together. She has presented several papers at national and international conferences. She has a particular interest in entrepreneurship culture, startup ecosystems, and talent management. She is currently pursuing a Ph.D. from VIT University, Vellore, Tamil Nadu.

Dharti Parikh has more than 8 years of academic career exposure with different universities. Parikh is currently pursuing PhD in the area of Organizational Behavior with special focus on Emotional Intelligence from the Department of Management Studies, Dharmsinh Desai University.

Niyati Patel is working as assistant professor at Navrachana University. Patel has more than 12 years of academic and corporate. Patel is more interested in research.

Syed Perwez is a M.A, MBA, Ph.D. & FDPM – (IIM-A). presently designated as Professor in OB & HR area, teaching since more than twelve years to under graduate, post graduate and doctoral management students in VIT Business School, VIT, Vellore, Tamil Nadu, India. He has more than 5 years of industry experience in reputed pharmaceutical company like Cipla Ltd, and Nicholas Piramal India Ltd. Dr.Syed has produced four doctorates under his guidance and also supervising 6 more Ph.D. research scholars. He has completed one funded research project grant aid of Rs- 5.64 lakhs sponsored by Indian Council for Social Science Research (ICSSR),

New Delhi. He has published 34 research journal publications in the reputed peered reviewed international and national journals indexed in Scopus as well as ABDC listed journal. He wrote two case study with teaching notes and published two book chapters. Dr. Syed has performed key administrative roles such as Divisional Chair for OB & HR Division, Program Chair - BBA, Time Table Coordinator, Exam Coordinator, NAAC Coordinator, RAAC Coordinator, Proctor Coordinator, MBA Capstone and Internship Project Coordinator, Entrepreneur-Cell Coordinator, and Sports Coordinator. He has conducted many training programs, MDPs, FDPs and also facilitated the training sessions. He has received many prestigious awards such as Best Research Award, Research Award for the contribution to research through Sponsored Research Project by VIT, Star Performer Award, I- Man Award by Nicholas Piramal India Ltd in Bangkok, Thailand, 2006, Received first prize in the faculty debate competition in Teachers Day, Received Best Management Student Talent Award in Utkal University, Bhubaneswar, Orissa by Shri. Sharat Kar (Education Minister of Orissa) in 2000, Passed the 34th Annual All India UN Information Test conducted all over India by Council for UN Information, a wing of USO and get a Pre-Senior UN Information Certificate by UNO, on 31st August, 1991. .

Krishna Priya B. holds a Bachelor's in Psychology and a Master's in Counselling Psychology. She's currently pursuing her Ph.D. in Psychology. Her passion for research has led her to conduct various research on diverse topics. She is a university rank hold at masters and bachelors level and a recipient of the best outgoing student award and Madras University merit fellowship in her bachelors and masters program respectively for consistently maintaining high academic performance and actively engaging with the curriculum. She has also received the best paper award from the Indian Academy of Applied Psychology and M.G.R Janaki College for Women. She is passionate about contributing her part to the community through evidence-based research.

Gaddam Rahul Paul - Contributing Author| **Gaddam Rahul Paul** is a research scholar in VIT Business School, Vellore Institute of Technology, Vellore. He is a postgraduate in MBA (Human Resource and Marketing) from Karunya University and MSc (Psychology) from Acharya Nagarjuna University. He has been conferred with the "National Teacher Innovation Award" for the year 2019 at the Indian Institute of Technology (IIT), Delhi, by Honourable Union Minister, Ministry of Human Resource Development (MHRD), Government of India. His research focuses on Organisational Psychology and Positive Psychology.

Rakshan S. is a student in second year B.Tech in the School of Mechanical Engineering, Vellore Institute of Technology, Vellore, Tamil Nadu, India. He is a dedicated Mechanical Engineer with the experience and technical expertise to provide the highest quality mechanical component and system support. He is skilled at formulating and implementing equipment designs, testing and producing specifications, and researching product applications.

Harman Singh is a Pre-Final year Biotechnology student.

Saubhagya Sooradas is a Final-year Mechanical Engineering student.

Rishwin Thayat is a fourth-year engineering student in the School of Mechanical Engineering of Vellore Institute of Technology Vellore, Tamil Nadu, India. He is a dedicated mechanical engineer with strong knowledge of technologies, tools, and best practices in mechanical design using AutoCAD and engineering drawings. He is a passionate Toastmaster, a member of VITAC, a senior mentor in various projects, and a football coach.

Rohan Varshney is a lPre-Final year Electrical Engineering student at VIT Vellore,2X Founder, Nationals Football and Karate winner.

Amisha Vatsa is a Pre-Final year Biotechnology student.

Index

N

O

P

R

S

T

U

W

www.ingramcontent.com/pod-product-compliance
Lightning Source LLC
LaVergne TN
LVHW081329300926
849161LV00008B/1918